Manipal

Practical
Orthopedics

- Orthopedic Clinical Cases
- X-ray, Implants, Prosthesis, Orthosis, Tractions and Plasters

Manipal
Practical
Orthopedics

- Orthopedic Clinical Cases
- X-ray, Implants, Prosthesis, Orthosis, Tractions and Plasters

Vivek Pandey MS
Associate Professor
Department of Orthopedics
Kasturba Medical College
Manipal, Karnataka
India

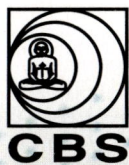

CBS

CBS Publishers & Distributors Pvt Ltd

New Delhi • Bengaluru • Chennai • Kochi • Kolkata • Mumbai

Bhopal • Bhubaneswar • Hyderabad • Jharkhand • Nagpur • Patna
• Pune • Uttarakhand • Dhaka (Bangladesh) • Kathmandu (Nepal)

Manipal

Practical Orthopedics

ISBN: 978-93-90046-15-7

First Edition: 2020

Published by Satish Kumar Jain and Produced by Varun Jain for

CBS Publishers & Distributors Pvt Ltd
4819/XI Prahlad Street, 24 Ansari Road, Daryaganj, New Delhi 110 002, India.

Ph: 011-23289259, 23266861, 23266867 Fax: 011-23243014   Website: www.cbspd.com
e-mail: delhi@cbspd.com;
cbspubs@airtelmail.in.

Corporate Office: 204 FIE, Industrial Area, Patparganj, Delhi 110 092, India
Ph: 011-4934 4934   Fax: 011-4934 4935   e-mail: publishing@cbspd.com;
publicity@cbspd.com

Branches

- **Bengaluru:** Seema House 2975, 17th Cross, KR Road,
  Banasankari 2nd Stage, Bengaluru 560 070, Karnataka, India
  Ph: +91-80-26771678/79   Fax: +91-80-26771680   e-mail: bangalore@cbspd.com
- **Chennai:** 7, Subbaraya Street, Shenoy Nagar, Chennai 600 030, Tamil Nadu, India
  Ph: +91-44-26260666, 26208620   Fax: +91-44-42032115   e-mail: chennai@cbspd.com
- **Kochi:** 42/1325, 1326, Power House Road, Opp KSEB, Kochi 682 018, Kerala, India
  Ph: +91-484-4059061-67   Fax: +91-484-4059065   e-mail: kochi@cbspd.com
- **Kolkata:** 6/B, Ground Floor, Rameswar Shaw Road, Kolkata-700014 (West Bengal), India
  Ph: +91-33-2289-1126, 2289-1127, 2289-1128   e-mail: kolkata@cbspd.com
- **Mumbai:** 83-C, Dr E Moses Road, Worli, Mumbai-400018, Maharashtra, India
  Ph: +91-22-24902340/41   Fax: +91-22-24902342   e-mail: mumbai@cbspd.com

Representatives

• Bhopal	0-8319310552	• Bhubaneswar	0-9911037372	• Hyderabad	0-9885175004
• Jharkhand	0-9811541605	• Nagpur	0-9421945513	• Patna	0-9334159340
• Pune	0-9623451994	• Uttarakhand	0-9716462459	• Dhaka	01912-003485
• Kathmandu (Nepal)	977-9818742655			(Bangladesh)	

Printed at Magic International Pvt. Ltd., Greater Noida, UP, India

to

my parents
Dr Kuldip Narain Pandey (MS, Surgical gastroenterology) and Manju Pandey

my wife, Deeksha Pandey (MS, ObG) and son, Krish

my brother and his family
Dr Abhishek (MS, Urology), Dr Susanne (MD, Radiology), Demira and Maya

my teachers, students and patients

Foreword

"The mediocre teacher tells.
The good teacher explains.
The superior teacher demonstrates.
The great teacher inspires" — William Arthur Ward.

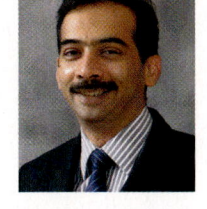

I have known Vivek Pandey ever since I started lecturing at conferences. Vivek caught my eye as we both seem to agree on most fundamentals but at the same time he does not allow me the comfort moment in agreement, as his scientific probity is always testing me. Vivek's zeal for teaching students at every level of medicine, right from UGs to clinicians is remarkable. So when Vivek requested me to review his latest book (and there are many) *Manipal Practical Orthopedics*, I promptly jumped at the opportunity to read a clinical book.

Am not one to be pessimistic but writing books can be counterintuitive as the goal posts change, knowledge is updated by the day and books can quickly become irrelevant. Vivek, who I have always insisted, is ahead of his time, has ensured the book, covers the subject comprehensively with recent advances too.

Knowledge ought to flow bidirectionally but that is rare. Along with the chapters that are replete with theory, Vivek also has sections on *viva voce* closing the loop from theory to the practical. The onus now lies upon the reader to soak in this detail and apply it real life.

As a seasoned examiner, Vivek has recreated scenarios of every possible condition and captured the milieu of possible questions arising from such a case. This is a rich harvest of cases and no doubt has been eloquently and painstakingly captured by Vivek in his inimitable style. This book is not only recommended for the exam appearing PG but also the ravenous clinician. Vivek has captured common clinical cases but also supplemented this with a chapter on orthosis. What I adore most is Vivek has covered all the recent advances (usually found lacking) on each condition, with easy to understand illustrations.

Without any hesitation I strongly recommend *Manipal Practical Orthopedics* as a must buy. My best wishes for another milestone by Vivek and may he continue to produce such books of utility; a laborious but desirable exercise.

Ashish Babhulkar
Shoulder Specialist and Joint replacement Surgeon
Founder Director, PSRP and Shoulder Conclave
Founder President of SESI
Pune, India

Preface

My passion for sharing clinical knowledge and experience continues with this edition of *Manipal Practical Orthopedics* which is a fusion of two of my old books; *Manipal Orthopedics: Short Case Viva Voce* and *Manipal Orthopedics: X-rays and Tools*. This academic material has been redesigned and upgraded with several new scenarios to enable a student who knows the subject but finds it difficult to articulate a precise answer especially during clinical viva and exams. Though it is a question–answer type of a series, I have never believed in rote learning and I firmly believe that this book will help a student only if they have grasped the basics of the subject in the form of sound theoretical knowledge and reasonable examination skills. This book is not a replacement for standard textbooks. Yet, I am sure that this manual will help them tremendously in their preparation for exams when time is short and stakes are high.

Vivek Pandey

Contents

Section II: Radiological Diagnosis

Section III: Orthopedic Implants

17. Implants

Section IV: Orthopedic Instruments

18. Instruments

Section V: Prosthesis and Orthosis

19. Prosthesis

20. Orthosis

Section VI: Ward Round

I

Short Cases and Viva Voce

1. **Trauma and its Complications:** Cubitus varus, cubitus valgus, malunion, myositis ossificans, nerve injury module—basics of nerve injury, wrist drop (radial and posterior interosseous nerve injury), clawhand (median nerve injury, ulnar nerve injury), footdrop non-union, reflex sympathetic dystrophy, complex regional pain syndrome, stiff joint, Volkmann's ischemic contracture

2. **Congenital Musculoskeletal Conditions:** Congenital talipes equinus (CTEV), developmental dysplasia of the hip (DDH), spina bifida

3. **Bone and Joint Infections:** Chronic osteomyelitis, TB of the knee

4. **Arthritis:** OA knee, rheumatoid arthritis

5. **Painful Hip:** Transient synovitis, tuberculosis of the hip, Perthes' disease

6. **Metabolic Disease:** Rickets, osteomalacia

7. **Bone Tumours:** Ewing's sarcoma, osteosarcoma, solitary exostosis (osteochondroma), giant cell tumor

8. **Low Back Pain:** Intervertebral disc prolapse, spondylolysis/spondylolisthesis, lumbar canal stenosis, ankylosing spondylitis

9. **Pott's Spine**

10. **Painful Shoulder:** Frozen shoulder, rotator cuff tendinitis, rotator cuff tear, glenohumeral arthritis

11. **Spine Injury its Complications and Rehabilitation**

12. **Unstable Knee (ligament injury of the knee):** ACL tear, PCL tear, meniscal injury, patella dislocation

13. **Miscellaneous Conditions:** Carpal tunnel syndrome, tendo Achillis rupture, lateral epicondylitis, medial epicondylitis, De Quervain's tenosynovitis

14. **Case Taking Format**

Trauma and its Complications

ELBOW DEFORMITY (CUBITUS VARUS, CUBITUS VALGUS)

Common Presentation of Patient with Cubitus Varus of Elbow

Case summary: An 8-year-old boy presented with a deformity of his left elbow since two years. Two years back, there was history of fall on outstretched hand followed by a fracture around the elbow. He was taken to a local hospital where an above elbow cast was applied. Three week later, cast was removed. He underwent regular physiotherapy which led to restoration of movement and function of his left elbow. He regained complete movements only later to observe that his elbow was progressively showing a deformity with forearm moving closer to the body. Local examination revealed cubitus varus deformity of left elbow. There was bony irregularity felt over the distal humerus. Three bony point relationship was intact. Flexion range of motion was 0–160° with no limb length discrepancy. Neurovascular examination, and the examination of shoulder and wrist-hand was normal.

Q. What is the clinical diagnosis?

The clinical diagnosis is malunited supracondylar fracture with cubitus varus deformity of left elbow (Fig. 1.1).

Q. Why do you say so?

It is because of following reasons.
1. History of trauma with **fall on outstretched hand**
2. Presence of cubitus varus deformity
3. Intact three bony point (medial and lateral epicondyle, olecranon) relationship
4. Bony irregularity over the distal humerus (indicates a healed fracture in that region)

Note: Carrying angle is the inner angle formed between the axis of humerus and forearm (Fig. 1.1). Carrying angle/Cubitus varus/Cubitus valgus is assessed with elbow in complete extension. If elbow cannot be completely extended due to flexion deformity, the exact assessment of carrying angle is not possible, and its assessment should be avoided.

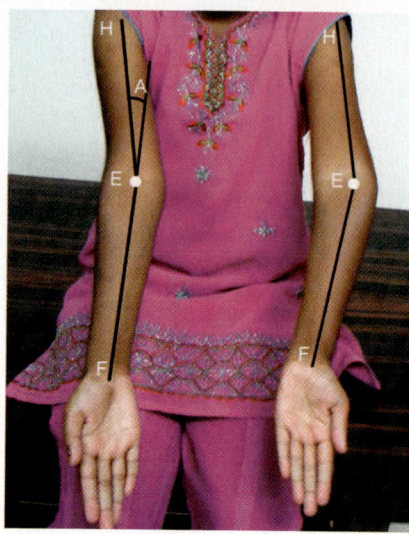

Fig. 1.1: Clinical picture of a child with cubitus varus deformity of left elbow. On the right upper limb, line HE represents humerus-elbow longitudinal axis and line EF represents elbow-forearm longitudinal axis. Normal carrying angle is represented by A which is an inner angle between line HE and EF

Q. What is the normal alignment of the elbow?

Normal alignment of the elbow is "cubitus valgus", i.e. the forearm is drifted outwards with respect to the midline (or arm). This is also known as carrying angle (normal carrying angle in males is 7° and females is 15°).

Q. Why carrying angle is greater in females?

It is greater because of broader pelvis in females.

Q. How will you comment upon the cubitus varus, if there is flexion deformity of elbow?

Cubitus varus or valgus **should not be commented** upon, **if there is flexion deformity** of elbow as varus or valgus tends to become less obvious with increasing flexion of the elbow joint.

Q. What is the methodology to palpate three bony points (lateral epicondyle, medial epicondyle and tip of olecranon)?

For lateral and medial epicondyles, first supracondylar ridge is palpated which is situated in the supracondylar region over medial and lateral side of the elbow above the two epicondyles. As the ridge is traced downwards, the most prominent point palpated over these ridges is medial and lateral epicondyle respectively.

For palpation of tip of the olecranon, first posterior ulnar border is palpated and then traced upwards. The most prominent point situated over the olecranon is the tip.

Q. What is the normal relation between these points?

In a normal elbow, these three bony points form a straight line in an extended elbow and form a triangle in 90° flexed elbow. Pronated/supinated forearm does not make

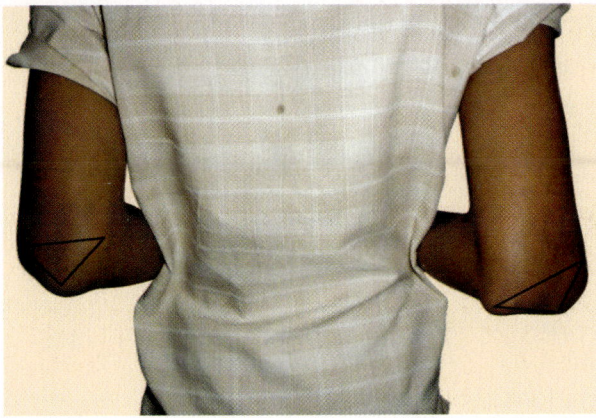

Fig. 1.2: Clinical photograph showing altered three bony point relation over the right elbow as compared to left elbow

any difference. Figure 1.2 shows altered relationship between the two triangles formed on right and left elbow in flexion.

Note: Remember; the type of triangle, i.e. scalene/isosceles is not important. What is important is that is it comparable with normal side or not!

Q. Which conditions around the elbow could result in disturbed three bony point relation?

a. Posterior dislocation of elbow
b. Intercondylar fracture of humerus
c. Lateral or medial condyle fracture of elbow
d. Fractures of medial or lateral epicondyle.

Q. Which condition other than malunited supracondylar fracture humerus could result in cubitus varus deformity of the elbow?

Trochlear avascular necrosis.

Q. Which nerve is more prone for injury in supracondylar fracture?

Anterior interosseous nerve is most commonly affected in extension type of supracondylar fracture followed by radial and ulnar nerve whereas **ulnar nerve** is most commonly **affected in flexion** type of supracondylar fracture (#).

Q. What is the difference between anterior interosseous nerve (AIN) and median nerve?

AIN is a branch of median nerve on volar aspect which supplies deeper muscles of forearm, viz. flexor pollicis longus (FPL), pronator quadratus (PQ), and the radial two tendons of flexor digitorum profundus (FDP).

Commonest fracture around the elbow joint in children is supracondylar fracture

Q. What are the complications of supracondylar fracture?

Acute

1. Compartment syndrome or Volkmann's ischemia
2. Anterior interosseous nerve or radial nerve injury (extension type) and ulnar nerve (flexion type)
3. Brachial artery injury

Chronic

1. Volkmann's ischemic contracture
2. Myositis ossificans
3. Malunion leading to cubitus varus deformity

Q. How will you treat this patient?

I will ask for X-ray of the elbow, AP and lateral view

Q. What will be the X-ray finding?

X-ray will reveal
a. Healed supracondylar fracture
b. Cubitus varus deformity

Q. What is the treatment of the cubitus varus deformity?

Since this deformity is **non-progressive** for last 6 months, corrective osteotomy should be performed.

Q. What if the deformity would have been progressive?

If the deformity is progressive; it is important to wait till the deformity ceases to progress as if osteotomy is performed in progressive stage, deformity can later recur or correction would be lost.

Q. Which osteotomy you will perform?

Modified French osteotomy. It is a lateral closing wedge osteotomy performed in the supracondylar region of elbow (Fig. 1.3).

Q. Is there a possibility that the three bony point relation can get disturbed in a malunited supracondylar fracture too?

Yes, it is possible. Sometimes during fall over elbow, there can be

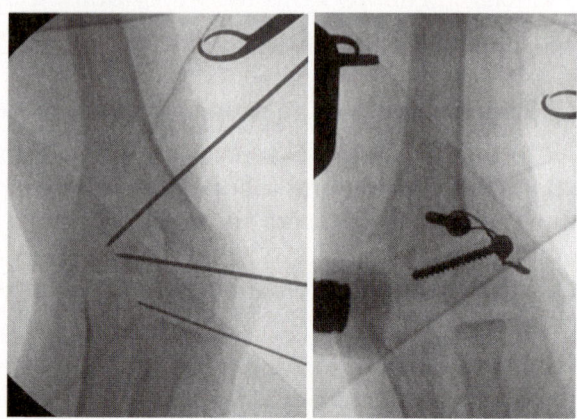

Fig. 1.3: X-ray of a varus elbow (left image) undergoes corrective osteotomy and fixation by screws and tension band wiring (right image)

injury to distal humerus physis/growth plate which could result in disturbed relation between three points.

Q. Mention a common condition in which cubitus valgus deformity is observed?

Cubitus valgus is observed in **non-union of lateral condyle fracture** of humerus.

Q. What is lateral condyle?

Lateral condyle is comprised of:
a. Lateral epicondyle
b. Capitellum
c. Lateral half of trochlea

Q. Why fracture lateral condyle of humerus results in non-union?

The lateral condyle fragment gets displaced and rotated due to pull from common extensor muscles which are attached over it.

Q. Which other complication can happen with non-union of lateral condyle associated with cubitus valgus?

Tardy ulnar nerve palsy.

Q. Why does tardy ulnar nerve palsy happen?

Tardy ulnar palsy is a result of **friction neuritis of ulnar nerve** behind medial epicondyle due to constant friction because of **progressively increasing valgus of elbow.**

Q. What is the treatment of tardy ulnar nerve palsy?

Anterior transposition of ulnar nerve should be done (ulnar nerve is surgically transposed anterior to medial epicondyle. This prevents further damage to the ulnar nerve due to friction and results in gradual recovery of the ulnar nerve due to friction neuritis).

Q. What is the treatment of non-union of lateral condyle?

In children, **non-union should be treated with internal fixation and bone grafting.** However, in adults it can be left alone.

Q. What should be done with cubitus valgus deformity?

If asymptomatic and minimal deformity: It should be left alone.

In adults: It can be left alone without any consequence after ulnar nerve transposition. However, if patient demands, it should be corrected.

In children: It can be corrected by corrective osteotomy along with internal fixation of non-union.

MALUNITED COLLES' FRACTURE

Common presentation of patient with malunion of fracture around wrist:

Case summary: A 55-year-old female patient case of mild pain and deformity in her right wrist for 6 months. 6 months back, she had a fall on outstretched hand and sustained a fracture around the wrist. She underwent closed reduction and below elbow cast was application. The cast was removed after 6 weeks. After cast removal, she noticed a deformity which has been non-progressive. She also complains of mild pain during daily routine activities. There was no history of fever, loss of weight or appetite. General and systemic examination was normal. Local examination revealed manus valgus deformity with bony irregularity over the distal radius. There was tenderness over distal radioulnar joint. The radial styloid process was at the level of ulnar styloid process. Palmar and dorsiflexion were limited but not painful while pronation and supination were limited and painful. Neurovascular examination was normal.

Q. What is the clinical diagnosis?

The clinical diagnosis is malunited distal radius fracture with stiffness of wrist joint.

Q. Why do you say so?

It is because of the following reasons:
1. History of fall on outstretched hand (common mechanism to cause distal radius fracture)
2. History of cast application for 6 weeks (indicates a fracture)
3. Presence of manus valgus deformity (Fig. 1.4) (common after malunited Colles' fracture)
4. Irregularity at lower end of radius (healed fracture site)
5. Radial and ulnar styloid process at same level (indicates malunion of distal radius)
6. Limited movements at the wrist joint (indicates stiffness)

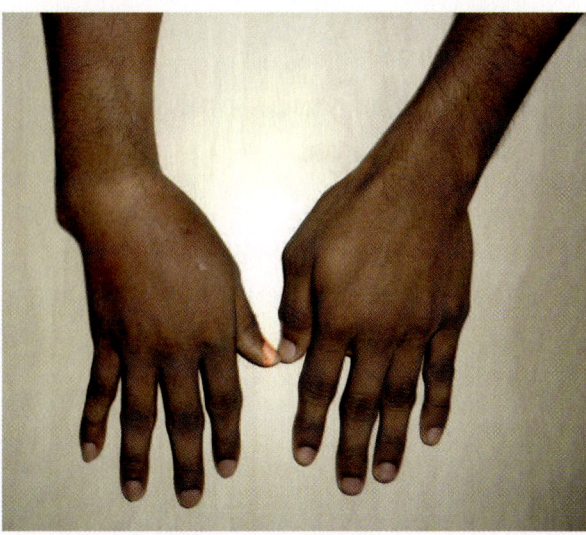

Fig. 1.4: Clinical photograph of both hands showing manus valgus deformity of right wrist

Q. What is the relationship between age and sex with distal radius fracture?

In elderly females, osteoporosis ensues faster especially after the menopause resulting in a weak bone. After fall on the outstretched hand; this is the commonest fracture around the wrist.

> Bones which are prone for osteoporotic fractures are mostly cancellous bones, e.g. dorsal and lumbar vertebrae, neck of the femur, distal radius, proximal humerus and pelvis.

Q. What are the common injuries due to fall on the outstretched hand?

1. Colles' fracture
2. Scaphoid fracture
3. Radial head fracture
4. Supracondylar fracture
5. Humeral neck fracture
6. Clavicle fracture

Q. What is principal clinical finding to suggest that it is a malunited Colles' fracture?

1. Manus valgus deformity
2. Radial and ulnar styloid process are at same level

> Note: Sometimes, the radial styloid process can be at a higher level than ulnar styloid process. Also, the relationship between the two styloid process should always be compared with the normal side.)

> **Normal relation between radial and ulnar styloid process**
> Radial styloid process is 8–14 mm lower than ulnar styloid process

Q. Define malunion.

When fracture does not unite in original anatomical alignment, it is called malunion.

Q. What is the clinical presentation of malunion?

Clinically, malunion presents as deformity and/or functional deficit.

Q. Do you think that his distal radioulnar joint is also involved and why do you say so?

Yes. Because patient has limited and painful pronation and supination indicating involvement of the distal radioulnar joint.

> Note: Pronation and supination occurs at radioulnar joint and not at the wrist joint).

Q. Is Colles' fracture is synonymous with distal radius fracture?

No. Colles' fracture is a type of distal radius fracture.

Q. Define Colles' fracture?

Colles' fracture is defined as fracture at the distal end of radius 2 cm proximal to the distal radius articular margin at cortico-cancellous junction characterized by six displacements.

1. Lateral tilt
2. Lateral displacement
3. Dorsal tilt
4. Dorsal displacement
5. Supination, and
6. Impaction.

Q. What is the classical deformity seen in acute Colles' fracture?

Dinner fork deformity.

Q. How will you confirm the diagnosis of malunited Colle's fracture?

X-ray of the wrist (posteroanterior and lateral view).

> In the wrist, posteroanterior view is asked for rather than anteroposterior.

Q. Which other investigation would delineate the fracture lines and comminution in better way?

CT scan with 3D reconstruction of distal radius is a great tool to assess the complex distal radius fracture.

Q. What are the common findings in a X-ray of malunited distal radius fracture?

1. Radial and ulnar styloid process relation is disturbed, i.e. the radial styloid process is often at the same level or above the ulnar styloid process.
2. Healed fracture in a malunited position.

> **Normal distal radius radiological parameters**
> 1. The radial styloid process is 8–18 mm distal to the ulnar styloid process
> 2. The average radial inclination is 22°
> 3. The average volar inclination is 11°
> It should be compared with normal side.

Q. What is the common method to treat Colles' fracture?

Closed reduction and below elbow cast application.

Q. How long cast is kept on Colles' fracture?

6 weeks.

Q. What are the other methods to treat Colles' fracture?

1. ORIF with plate and screws
2. Closed reduction and external fixator application.

Q. If there is patchy osteoporosis over various bones of wrist and hand, what else must be clinically ruled out?

If there is **patchy osteoporosis,** one must suspect **reflex sympathetic dystrophy** (complex regional pain syndrome/sudeck's osteodystrophy).

Q. How will you treat this patient?

Since patient is still having pain and stiffness, I would do the following measures.

1. *General Measures*
   a. Activity modification (avoiding lifting heavy weight and excess pronation–supination movements)

2. *Medications*
   a. Analgesics sos (as and when required)

3. *Physiotherapy*
   a. Moist heat
   b. Short wave diathermy/local ultrasound therapy
   c. Wrist and finger mobilization exercises
   d. Intrinsic muscle of hand strengthening exercises

Q. Should the deformity of distal radius be corrected at this stage?

Not now. Because
1. First; goal is to achieve "functional, painless range of movement"
2. Then, reassess the function of hand and wrist

If the deformity still hampers in restoration of adequate function (poor movements and strength, residual pain) despite appropriate physiotherapy, deformity correction should be considered. However, most malunited lower end radius fractures especially Colles' fracture may not need corrective osteotomy as after few months, patients do not have any major functional deficit hampering the activities of daily living.

Remember that **not all malunion need surgical correction**. As long as deformity does not cause any major functional deficit, it may not require surgical correction except when it is cosmetically not acceptable like cubitus varus or it may be causing any functional deficit.

Three basic function of hand
1. Pinch
2. Grasp
3. Hook

Q. If required, which surgery is performed for the malunited distal radius fracture?

Corrective osteotomy, internal/external fixation with or without bone graft is performed to correct the deformity.

Corrective osteotomy is the general term used to indicate **surgical correction of bony deformity**.

Q. What are the other common fractures around wrist?

1. Colles' fracture
2. Smith's fracture
3. Chauffeur's fracture (radial styloid fracture)
4. Scaphoid fracture
5. Volar and dorsal Barton #

Q. What are the common complications of Colles' fracture?

1. Malunion
2. Stiffness of wrist and hand
3. Carpal tunnel syndrome
4. Reflex sympathetic dystrophy (also known as Sudeck's dystrophy/complex regional pain syndrome)
5. Rupture of extensor pollicis longus tendon
6. Osteoarthritis of the radiocarpal and distal radioulnar joint

Note: Rupture of extensor pollicis longus tendon is more commonly observed in undisplaced fractures of distal radius. It happens due to fracture callus resulting in attritional rupture of tendon.

Q. What is the clinical presentation of malunited fracture of forearm bones?

1. Deformity of forearm
2. Restricted pronation-supination

Q. Name some fractures which are classically prone for malunion?

Upper Limb

1. Clavicle #
2. Supracondylar humerus fracture in children
3. Colles' fracture

Lower Limb

1. Intertrochanteric fracture
2. Calcaneum #

Colles' # was described by Abraham Colles in 1814 even before X-rays were discovered.

MYOSITIS OSSIFICANS

Common Presentation of Patient with Myositis Ossificans

Case summary: A 15-year-old boy complained of pain and stiffness in his left elbow since one year. The problem started after trauma to his left elbow due to fall following which he sustained olecranon fracture. The fracture was managed by open reduction and plate fixation followed by cast application. Mobilisation of the elbow was started after 3 weeks of surgery. Patient initially gained some movements but later, he gradually started losing movements till the elbow became very stiff. His father gave history of massage around elbow and forcible passive mobilization during the phase of mobilization. There was no history of fever or swelling.

General and systemic examination was normal. There was bony irregularity over the Olecranon. The three bony point relationship was normal. A hard bony mass was palpable in front of the cubital fossa which was non-tender. The range of movement was 40°–90° with normal neurovascular examination.

Q. What is the clinical diagnosis?

The clinical diagnosis is operated olecaranon fracture with post-traumatic myositis ossificans of left elbow.

Q. Why do you say so?

It is because of the following reasons.

1. History of trauma
2. **History of massage and vigorous passive mobilisation** (massage and vigorous passive mobilisation could initiate myositis ossificans)
3. Healed scar over the olecranon along with bony irregularity over the olecranon (indicates operated fracture)
4. Palpable bony mass in front of the elbow (indicates myositis ossificans)
5. Regaining some movement while physiotherapy and then again loss of movement may indicate myositis ossificans.

Q. Which history is relevant for myositis ossificans?

a. Massage around the elbow, and
b. Passive forcible mobilization.

Massage and **forcible passive mobilization** of a stiff joint during the phase of early mobilisation could increase the chance of myositis ossificans. (Both factors can result in bleeding in the muscles adjacent to the joint which in turn leads to myositis ossificans.)

Q. How does myositis ossificans occurs?

Myositis ossificans around elbow occurs due to bleeding in the brachialis muscle. Later, the hematoma gets converted into a bony mass (myositis ossificans) due to osteoblastic proliferation. The reasons behind osteoblastic proliferation remains idiopathic.

Q. Is there any inflammation in the muscle as name suggests (myositis)?

No. There is **no** inflammation in the muscle. It is a **misnomer**. There is an ossified (not calcified) hematoma in the substance of the brachialis muscle.

Q. How will you confirm the diagnosis?

I would like to take X-ray. X-ray shows a myositis mass in front of the humerus and a *in situ* plate over olecranon indicating an operated olecranon # (Fig. 1.5).

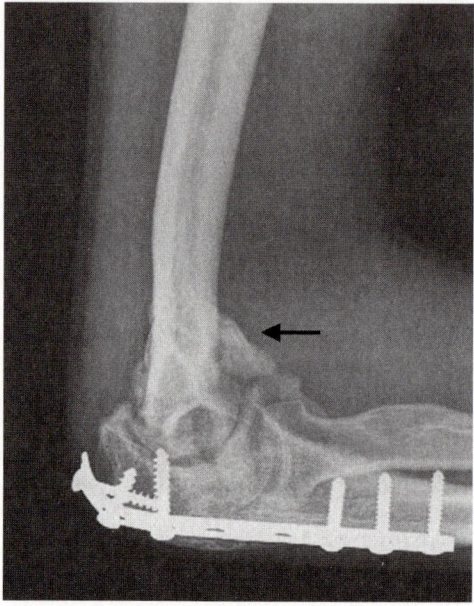

Fig. 1.5: Lateral view of elbow reveals myositis mass (black arrow) in front of the humerus

Q. Is there any clinical-radiological staging of myositis ossificans?

Yes. There are **two clinical-radiological** stages of myositis ossificans

1. *Early stage:* It starts after few days of mobilization. There is local rise in temperature and tenderness around the joint. **The movements suddenly become more painful and much less than what patient gained in the period of mobilization.**

   Radiographs of the region reveals a **"cotton wool appearance"** as early myositis.

2. *Late stage:* After a few weeks, pain and inflammation subsides and a bony mass is gradually formed due to ossification of hematoma. The bony mass is clinically palpable. The range of movement is restricted but is painless.

   Radiologically, a **"bony mass"** is seen in front of the bone with **usually a clear line of demarcation between the mass and bone.**

Q. Is there any other investigation which can reveal the bone mass in a more accurate way?

CT scan can be done to confirm the bone mass and its extent.

Q. What could be the radiological differential diagnosis of myositis ossificans?

Parosteal osteosarcoma

Features Similar

1. Acute history
2. Young age
3. Pain and swelling at the lower end of humerus (near metaphysis which is site for osteosarcoma)
4. Localized tenderness and swelling
5. Radiologically, cotton-wool appearance and bony mass can confuse the picture with periosteal reaction.

Features Against

1. History of trauma (though, it can be present in case of tumor and infection too!!)
2. Both cotton-wool appearance and bony mass of myositis are slightly away from bone (gap between them) whereas in case of osteosarcoma, the bony mass or periosteal reaction is in continuity with bone.
3. Serum ALP (alkaline phosphatase) is very high in case of osteosarcoma.

Q. How will you manage a case of myositis ossificans?

The management depends upon the **clinical and radiological stage.**

A fact need to be remembered that once the process of myositis ossificans starts, it is inevitable. It will form a mature bony mass in future. So, the treatment is aimed at reducing the further extent of bony mass and not to prevent the formation!

Early Stage

Goal is to reduce pain, inflammation and edema and prevent extent of myositis mass formation

a. **Re-immobilization** in the POP cast for two to three weeks
b. **NSAIDs** (indomethacin is the drug of choice unless there is a contraindication)
c. **Anti-edema measures** (limb elevation)
d. **Cold pack** to the elbow

After two to three weeks, the limb is taken out of POP and re-mobilized. Only **gentle active mobilization is permitted**.

Late Stage

Once mature bony mass is formed, it can be **surgically excised if it hampers the function.**

Q. What is the complication of myositis ossificans excision surgery?

Re-formation of the myositis mass is the commonest complication after the surgery as the post-surgical hematoma in the muscle can re-form the mass and it can lead to re-stiffness of the joint. (This has to be explained to the patient before the surgery.)

Q. How much is the flexion deformity in this patient?

It is 40°.

Q. What is the meaning of flexion deformity?

Flexion deformity means that the joint cannot be fully extended, actively or passively.

Q. Do you think that is it a stiff joint or ankylosed joint?

It is a stiff joint as joint with any degree of loss of movement is known as stiff joint. However, in an ankylosed joint, there is just a jog of movement or no movement at all. So, an ankylosed joint is a stiff joint but not all stiff joints are ankylosed.

This patient has ROM of 40° to 90° which indicates that it is stiff joint but not ankylosed.

Q. What do you mean by ankylosis?

Ankylosis means pathological fusion of a joint which hardly exhibits any movements.

Note: Arthrodesis means surgical fusion of a joint)

Q. What are the types of ankylosis?

There are two types of ankyloses.
a. True ankylosis: Fusion in the joint
b. False ankylosis: Stiffness in the joint due to extra-articular causes.

Q. What are the types of true ankylosis?

There are two types of true ankyloses: Fibrous and bony.

a. *Fibrous Ankylosis Occurs due to*

1. Tuberculous arthritis of peripheral joints
2. Gonococcal arthritis
3. Rheumatoid arthritis

- Fibrous ankylosis occurs due to dense fibrous adhesions running across the joint surfaces, and tight capsule-synovium-ligament complexes.
- Fibrous ankylosis is characterized by **painful, but slight jog of movement.**
- Any attempted movements are painful as highly innervated dense adhesions and contracted capsule-synovium-ligament are stretched during attempted movements.
- Jog of movements are present due to slightly flexible and pliable nature of fibrous adhesions.
- X-ray reveals relatively preserved joint space as there might not be complete damage to the articular cartilage.

b. *Bony Ankylosis Occurs due to*

1. Septic arthritis
2. Occasionally when tuberculous arthritis becomes infected
3. Tuberculosis of the vertebrae ends with bony fusion of the two vertebrae.

- Bony ankylosis occurs when subchondral bone from **both the articular surfaces** is denuded of the articular cartilage and subchondral bone is exposed resulting in bony fusion of the two articular surface.
- Bony ankylosis is characterized by **painless joint, with no movements.** It is painless as the two articulating surfaces are fused due to bony trabeculae formation across the joint due to severe or complete destruction of cartilage.
- X-ray of the joint reveals obliteration of joint space with bony trabeculae crossing the joint (Fig. 1.6).

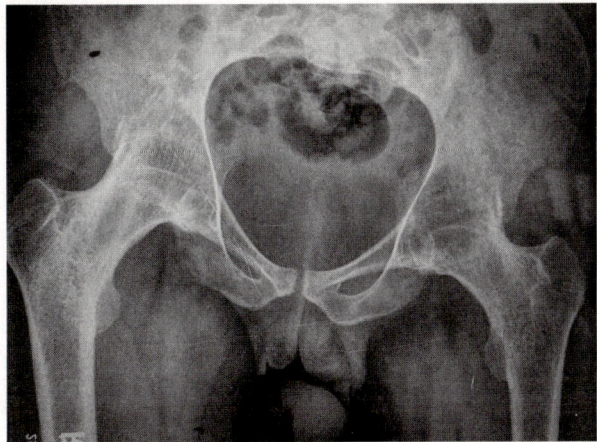

Fig. 1.6: Ankylosed hip with total obliteration of hip joint space copy

Q. What are the causes of false ankylosis?

The causes of false ankylosis vary from skin to the joint.

a. *Skin contracture:* Burn scar, surgical or open wound scars
b. *Underlying soft tissue contracture:* Subcutaneous tissue/fascia scars, Dupuytren's contracture.
c. *Muscles tendon units contracture* which fails to slide while joint is attempting to move.
d. *Joint capsule contracture* after prolonged immobilisation, trauma, inflammation or surgical procedure . It fails to relax while joint is attempting to move.
e. *Intra- and extra-articular ligaments contracture*
f. *Bone:* New bone formation (myositis) or excess callous formation after fracture healing or malunited displaced bone fragment.

Q. How will you manage true ankylosis?

a. *Bony Ankylosis*

1. **Arthrodesis in sound position** if bony ankylosis is in unsound position of the joint.
2. **Joint replacement if there is no evidence of infection.** At least few (5–10) years after the episode of septic arthritis and 1–2 years after complete treatment of tuberculosis, if ESR and CRP are normal.

b. *Fibrous Ankylosis*

Initial attempt of physiotherapy can be tried to overcome the tight intra-articular adhesions and other reasons for a stiff joint.

However, if it fails to improve open or arthroscopic adhesiolysis should be performed.

Q. How will you manage false ankylosis?

False ankylosis is managed according to the structure affected.

a. *Skin:* Lengthening of scar by Z or V-Y plasty. Scar excision and reconstruction by flap
b. Tight fascia or subcutaneous tissue-excision
c. *Tight muscle tendon unit:* Lengthening of tendon by Z plasty or V-Y plasty
d. *Tight capsule:* Capsulectomy and/or capsulotomy.
e. *Tight ligaments:* Lengthened if possible otherwise should be left alone lest it would lead to instability.

Q. What should be done after release of ankylosed or stiff joint?

Patient needs to undergo extensive supervised physiotherapy to retain the movements; otherwise joint is prone for stiffness.

Q. What is the complication of surgery done for release of stiff joint?

It can lead to re-stiffness, however may not be same degree. Hence, guarded prognosis about movement should be given.

NERVE INJURY MODULE

To understand the clinical symptoms, signs, management and prognosis of nerve injury; it is important to understand the anatomy of the nerve (Fig. 1.7), causes of nerve injury and pathophysiology (wallerian degeneration and regeneration) of nerve injury (Table 1.1).

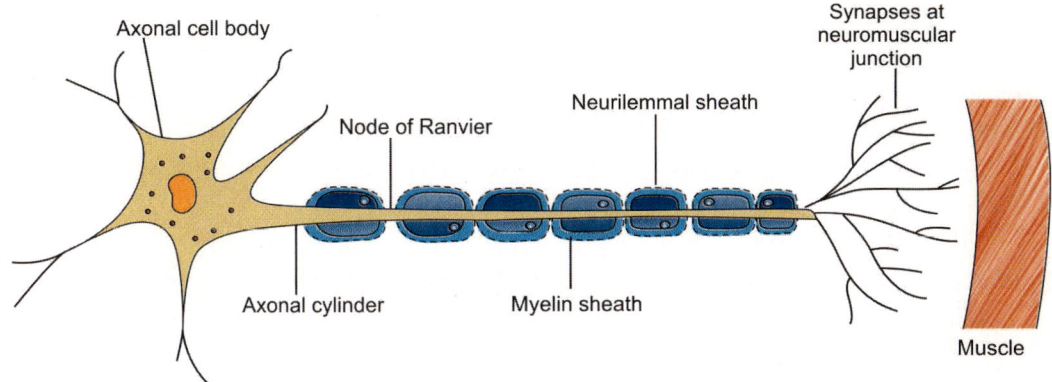

Fig. 1.7: Illustrated diagram of a single nerve axon

Table 1.1: Summary of wallerian degeneration and regeneration

Any structural injury to axonal cylinder and/or neurilemmal sheath leads to **wallerian degeneration (WD)**. WD is characterized by:

1. Complete breakdown of axonal cylinder and myelin sheath in both proximal and distal segments, proximally up to the node of Ranvier just proximal to the level of injury and distally up to the motor end plate.
2. The broken down material of axonal cylinder and myelin is engulfed and, area is further cleared of debris by macrophages. However, **neurilemmal sheath is not broken down**. This phenomenon is wallerian degeneration.

Wallerian regeneration (WR) is characterized by:

1. Growth of new axonal sprouts (50–100) from the end of the proximal axon terminal. Only one of them makes connection with neurilemmal sheath and continues to grow as axonal cylinder at the rate of **1 mm/day**.
2. New axon is further myelinated by Schwann cells. Finally, it meets with motor end plate.

Nerve regeneration (WR) is characterized by two phenomena.

A. **Tinel's sign:** Hence, Tinel's sign is **NOT seen in neuropraxia where there is neither WD and WR**.
B. **Motor march:** Nerve re-innervates in the order of its innervation pattern to the muscles, i.e. proximal to distal which known as motor march. Hence, **motor march too is not seen in neuropraxia** as there is no injury/regeneration.

Q. What are the causes of nerve injury/affection?

Peripheral nerve involvement is seen in:

1. **Infective:**
   a. Poliomyelitis—history polio in childhood
   b. Hansen's disease—history of patchy loss of sensation over body, thickened and tender nerves like CPN, greater auricular, ulnar, superficial radial nerve
2. **Traumatic:** Traumatic injury to spinal cord or peripheral nerves
3. **Acute or chronic pressure over the nerves:** Intervertebral disc prolapse, carpal or tarsal tunnel syndromes
4. **Charcot-Marie-tooth** disease
5. **Neoplastic:** Tumors compressing the nerves; neurofibroma, neurofibromasarcoma
6. **Metabolic:** Vitamin B_1, B_{12} deficiency, diabetes mellitus, chronic alcoholism, porphyria
7. **Chemical:** Lead poisoning

Note: Students must take pertinent history in cases of nerve affection.

Q. Classify nerve injuries?

Seddon's Classification of Nerve Injury

1. *Neuropraxia:* **Focal conduction block** at axonal cylinder but no demonstrable anatomical disruption.
2. *Axonotmesis:* **Injury to the axonal cylinder** but the **neurilemmal sheath is intact.**
3. *Neurotmesis:* Complete injury to the nerve including neurilemmal sheath.

Description of Type of Nerve injury

1. *Neuropraxia:* Since there is only focal conduction block and no anatomical damage to the nerve in neuropraxia, there is no wallerian degeneration of the nerve. As there is no demonstrable structural damage to nerve, nerve function is restored within a few weeks (3–6 weeks). It carries **excellent prognosis**.

   Neuropraxia is comparable to a vehicle overturn on a highway and a resultant traffic blockade. However, there is no damage to road. Hence, complete restoration of traffic is expected once blockade is over. Likewise, neuropraxia resolves once axonal blockade resolves.

2. *Axonotmesis:* It is observed after traction or compression injury of the nerve. The axonotmesis is characterized by **damage to the axonal cylinder but intact neurilemmal sheath.** It undergoes WD and WR. Further, recovery period of axontmesis is characterized by presence of **Tinel's sign and motor march phenomena.** Recovery is **usually complete** because neurilemmal sheath is intact

Once in exam, there was a question on "classify nerve injury". A student wrote correct classification. However, he/she fumbled on the name! Rather than Seddon's, it was mentioned as Saddam's classification!!

Choice is yours, Seddon or Saddam!

but may take a few months according to the length of the nerve damaged. It carries **good prognosis**.

3. *Neurotmesis:* The nerve is **completely severed including axonal cylinder and neurilemmal sheath** and is characterized by:
   a. Wallerian degeneration.
   b. Since the **neurilemmal sheath is also severed,** the **two ends of the nerve along with sheath retract.** When the nerve starts regenerating from proximal end; axonal sprout **fails to connect** with the distal end of the nerve since both ends are retracted, and gap is filled with scar tissue.
   c. Also, it may lead to **neuroma formation** at the regenerating end of axon as it fails to makes a connection with sheath.
   d. Unless surgical intervention is done, neurotmesis may not recover and carries **poor prognosis**.
   e. Motor march and Tinel's sign could be observed if nerve starts regenerating after the two severed ends are surgically repaired.

Any of the three types of nerve injury would result in various clinical feature.

1. **Sensory loss:** Anaesthesia/hypoaesthesia/paresthesia
2. **Motor dysfunction:** Paresis/palsy
3. **Loss of reflexes**
4. **Autonomic dysfunction:** Trophic changes in skin and nails

Clinical facts
1. By and large, **all closed fractures and dislocations commonly result in neuropraxia or axonotmesis.** Since neuropraxia/axonotmesis usually recover, the line of treatment is usually expectant.
2. **Open fractures or open injuries** result in **neurotmesis** unless proved otherwise. Hence, nerve should always be explored in open injuries to ascertain its anatomical status. If the nerve is completely severed, it should be approximated to ensure recovery.

Diagnosis of nerve injury is established by
1. *Nerve conduction velocity (NCV) test: **Usually performed at the end of three weeks.*** It is useful in ascertaining
   a. Location of the lesion
   b. Type of lesion
   c. Prognostic
2. *Electromyography (EMG):* **Not useful till 3 weeks of acute injury.** After 3 weeks, EMG is performed. It shows fibrillations and positive sharp waves in axonotmesis and neurotmesis.
3. *Specific investigation* as per the etiology, e.g. Hansen's and carpal tunnel.

   With this background information of nerve injuries and understanding of pathology, we will proceed with case history and questions.

Points to remember
1. ***Best prognosis:*** Neuropraxia (since no nerve damage)
2. ***Worst prognosis:*** Neurotmesis (since the nerve is completely severed)

3. ***Tinel's sign and motor march never observed in:*** Neuropraxia (as there is no WD)
4. ***Tinel's sign and motor march always observed in:*** Axonotmesis (as WD is followed by WR)
5. ***Tinel's sign and motor march may be observed in:*** Neurotmesis (if surgical repair is done)
6. ***Since neuropraxia always recovers:*** Line of treatment is expectant!
7. ***Since neurotmesis will not recover:*** Surgical intervention is must
8. ***Since axonotmesis mostly recovers:*** Line of treatment is expectant initially and surgical intervention only if incomplete or no recovery.

WRIST DROP

Case summary: A 25-year-old man met with RTA, 2 months back following which he sustained fracture shaft of the humerus. At the time of injury, he had weakness at the wrist and finger with inability to extent wrist, thumb and fingers. He underwent open reduction and internal fixation of fracture shaft humerus with plate. Current clinical examination reveals mild tenderness at the fracture site. Elbow and shoulder examination is normal. Distal neurological examination revealed wrist and finger drop with decreased sensation in 1st web space.

Q. What is the clinical diagnosis?

The clinical diagnosis is healing operated fracture shaft humerus with radial nerve palsy.

Q. What is the impression you get about the wrist and finger drop?

Wrist and finger drop means that there is radial nerve palsy.

Q. Why patient is having wrist and finger drop?

Wrist and finger drop is due to:
a. *Paralysis of wrist extensor:* Extensor carpi radialis longus (ECRL) and brevis (ECRB)
b. *Paralysis of finger extensor:* Extensor digitorum (ED), extensor indicis (EI)
c. *Paralysis of thumb extensor:* Extensor pollicis

Q. Which nerve injury results in only finger drop?

Posterior interosseous nerve injury.

Q. Which condition results in posterior interosseous nerve (PIN) injury?

PIN palsy is observed in Monteggia fracture dislocation.

Q. Why there is only finger drop in PIN palsy?

PIN palsy results in thumb and finger drop because of paralysis of finger extensors (EDC, EI) and extensor polllicis whereas wrist extensor ECRL and ECRB escape paralysis as latter are supplied by the radial nerve.

Q. What do you mean by high and low radial nerve palsy?

In **high radial nerve palsy,** the radial nerve is paralyzed in the radial groove affecting the function of brachioradialis, ECRL, ECRB and other common extensors originating from lateral epicondyle. Hence, patient has wrist, thumb and finger drop. Since triceps is supplied before the radial nerve enters the radial groove, hence elbow extension is not affected (Fig. 1.8).

In **low radial nerve palsy,** the nerve is injured after it has supplied brachioradialis, ECRL and ECRB. It is known as PIN after it enters substance of supinator. So, only common extensors are affected causing palsy of finger-thumb (Fig. 1.8).

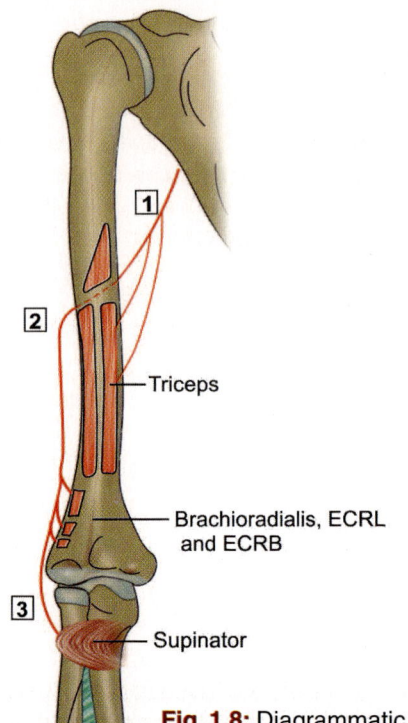

Radial nerve, after crossing the elbow joint enters the supinator muscle which is around the radial head and neck. From this point, radial nerve is known as posterior interosseous nerve (PIN).

In Monteggia fracture dislocation; there is proximal ulna fracture with dislocation of proximal radioulnar joint. The PIN which winds around neck of radius, sustains traction injury due to dislocated head radius (Fig. 1.8).

— Triceps

— Brachioradialis, ECRL and ECRB

— Supinator

Fig. 1.8: Diagrammatic representation of course of radial nerve. Point 1 represents area of the radial nerve before it enters the radial groove. Point 2 represents radial nerve in the groove and point 3 represents radial nerve to be called posterior interosseous nerve (PIN) just after it crosses the elbow joint and enters supinator muscle

Points to examine in nerve injury
a. Wasting of muscle
b. Deformity at joints
c. Scar and tenderness over nerve course
d. Trophic change in hand and nails
e. Joint movement
f. Tinel's sign, motor march
g. Sensori-motor examination, reflexes

Q. What are the clinical factors indicating a recovering nerve?

1. Improving sensory perception and motor power
2. Motor march phenomena
3. Progressive Tinel's sign
4. Return of reflexes

Q. How did you elicit Tinel's sign and what is its relevance?

Tinel's sign is elicited by gently tapping along the nerve its course from **distal to proximal**. In case of "**positive Tinel's sign**", patient will experience current/shock-like sensation along the course of the nerve.

If the Tinel's sign is progressive (means, it is progressing distally with every follow up of patient), it suggests a recovering nerve. If the Tinel's sign is static (not progressive at every follow up), it indicates a neuroma formation and is a bad sign.

Q. What is motor march?

In recovering phase of nerve injury, there is proximal to distal recovery of muscle power.

Q. How will you confirm the diagnosis of nerve injury?

Diagnosis is confirmed by NCV and EMG.

Q. What is the role of X-ray?

X-ray is done to look for any associated
a. Fracture
b. Foreign body/lesion which can affect nerve.

Q. What type of nerve injury is suspected in this patient?

It is most likely either neuropraxia or axonotmesis.

Q. Why do you think that this is neuropraxia or axonotmesis?

Generally, all closed fractures and dislocation result in neuropraxia or axonotmesis type of nerve injury.

Q. When do you suspect neurotmesis?

In case of open fracture/dislocation/any other open injury with nerve palsy.

Q. Why it is important to differentiate between these type of nerve injuries?

It is important to differentiate between these nerve injuries because neuropraxia is always managed on expectant lines whereas axonotmesis initially is managed on the expectant line of treatment. However, neurotmesis always needs a surgical intervention.

Q. How will you treat radial nerve injury in this patient?

Since the nerve injury in this patient is associated with closed fracture, hence it will be either neuropraxia or axonotmesis type of nerve injury. These type of nerve injury usually recover in due course of time with expectant line of treatment. Hence, one must follow expectant/conservative line of treatment.

Q. What is expectant or conservative treatment of nerve injury?

The meaning of expectant line is:
a. **Passive mobilization of wrist and fingers** several times a day (passive mobilization of affected joint to prevent stiffness of affected joints)
b. **Active mobilization of unaffected joints**

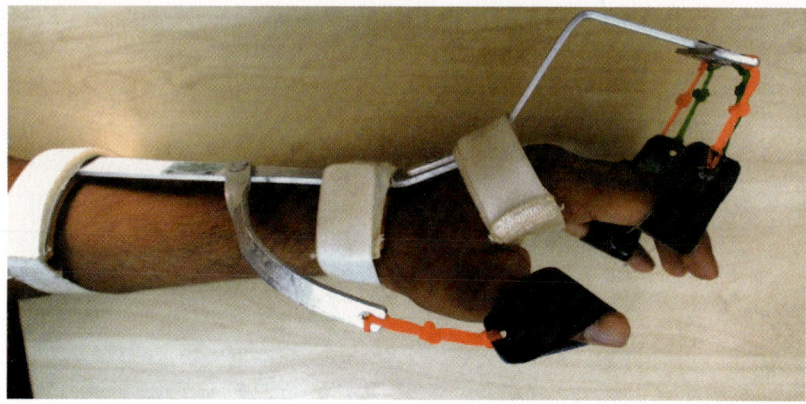

Fig. 1.9: Dynamic cock up splint applied on forearm, wrist and hand. It keeps finger in extended position

c. **Application of dynamic cock-up splint:** Encourages mobilization and keeps wrist and finger in functional position at the time of rest (Fig. 1.9)
d. **Electrical stimulation to the affected muscle:** Prevents disuse atrophy
e. Oral and/injectable vitamins B_1, B_6, B_{12} can be used but are of questionable value.

Q. How will you follow this patient?

Since nerve recovery is a slow process (1 mm/day), patient should be followed every 6–8 weeks. At every follow-up, clinico-electrophysiological examination must be performed which includes:

a. **Sensory examination** and recovery
b. **Motor examination** and its recovery **(motor march)**
c. **Tinel's sign** which must be progressive: It means that the point over skin where Tinel's sign was last elicited, should migrate at least 30–40 mm as nerve grows at the rate of 1 mm/day from the last follow up. So, after 6–8 weeks (42–56 days) a regenerating nerve should move 30–40 mm distally, if it is regenerating at the rate of 1 mm/day.

Note: A **static Tinel's sign** indicates a **neuroma** formation which is a bad sign and indicates that nerve is not recovering)

d. **NCV**
e. **EMG** (shows fibrillation and positive sharp waves)

Q. What is the next step if there is no nerve recovery?

a. **Explore** the nerve
b. **Neurolysis** if nerve is adhered within fibrous tissue or fracture callus
c. **Neurorrhaphy** (nerve repair) with or without nerve grafting **if nerve is found to be completely severed**

Q. What will you do after neurolysis/neurorrhaphy?

I would again follow the expectant line of treatment

Q. What is the next step if nerve still does not recover even after neurolysis/neurorrhaphy?

Tendon transfer should be performed to restore wrist, thumb, and finger extension.

Remember, before you answer tendon transfer!! Ensure that
- Joint is NOT stiff, i.e. it is mobile
  - Stiff joint need to be mobilized before tendon transfer
  - At least grade 4 powered tendon to be transferred

Q. Which tendon transfer is performed for radial nerve palsy?

Modified Jones transfer:

To restore wrist extension: Transfer pronator teres to ECRL and ECRB

To restore finger extension at MCP joint: Transfer FCU/FDS to EDC

To restore thumb extension and abduction: Transfer palmaris longus to EPL

FCU, flexor carpi ulnaris; FDS, flexor digitorum superficialis; EDC, extensor digitorum communis; EPL, extensor pollicis longus.

Q. What could be done if there are no viable tendons to transfer?

Wrist arthrodesis in functional position

Note: Functional position for wrist and hand is **glass holding position**

Various surgical procedures performed for a paralysed nerve
1. Neurolysis
2. Neurorrhaphy (nerve repair) with or without nerve graft
3. Tendon transfer
4. Arthrodesis

Q. What are the prerequisite for tendon transfer?

1. **Age >5 years:** After tendon transfer, patient need to be re-educated to use the **new muscle tendon unit in new location and new function.** Children lesser than 5 years may not be able to cooperate with re-education and rehabilitation programme.
2. **Mobile joints:** If involved joint is/are stiff, then tendon transfer should not be performed till the joints become passively mobile and free.
3. **Muscle to be transferred should have minimum grade IV power**
4. Preferably muscle tendon unit from same action group also known as **synergistic/phasic** (i.e. flexor to flexor and extensor to extensor).

Note: Muscle-tendon unit tends to **lose one grade power** after transfer. Hence, muscle with grade IV power post-transfer will retain grade III power which is sufficient to act against the gravity and accomplish reasonable function. However, if we transfer muscle with grade III power, the resultant power post-transfer would be grade II which would be insufficient to act against gravity and perform the optimal function.

Q. How do you grade muscle power?

According to medical research council (MRC), muscle power is graded from 0 to 5.

0 = no power

1 = flicker of contraction

2 = contraction with gravity eliminated

3 = contraction against gravity but no resistance

4 = contraction against mild-moderate resistance

5 = normal power

Note: Refrain using + or − with power, e.g. patient has 3+ power in elbow flexion. There is no standardization of + or − and has not been suggested by MRC.

Q. What are the factors which affect the nerve recovery?

1. **Age: Younger** the person, better is recovery
2. **Distal** lesion: **Better** recovery
3. **Predominantly motor (radial) or sensory** nerve: **Better** recovery
4. Mixed nerves/nerve with fine function (median/ulnar)—poor recovery
5. **Type of nerve injury:** Neuropraxia → axonotmesis → neurotmesis in order of bad prognosis

Q. What you would have done if this nerve injury was associated with open wound in arm?

Then, this should be treated like an open fracture of humerus with radial nerve injury. It involves:

1. **Debridement** of the wound
2. **Fixation** of fracture by external fixator (usually, internal fixation is avoided in open fracture)
3. **Exploration of nerve**
4. If nerve is found to be intact, then expectant line of treatment should be followed
5. If nerve is found to be severed (neurotmesis); primary repair of nerve is performed if the wound is clean. However, if the wound is quite contaminated, then secondary repair is performed after a few weeks once the wound is clean after repeated debridements.

Principle of nerve repair

1. **Repair in clean, vascular field** (that is why no primary repair is attempted if wound is contaminated)
2. **Tensionless repair** (it means that if there is defect in nerve length, then either nerve graft is used or joint is flexed to perform and protect repair from tension at repair site).

Q. What is the reason of persistent pain after the nerve injury in the area of nerve distribution?

It is known as causalgia. It is another type of reflex sympathetic dystrophy associated with nerve injury (also known as Type 2 complex regional pain syndrome).

Q. What is the root value of radial nerve?

The root value of radial nerve is C5, 6, 7, 8 and T1.

Q. What do you mean by autonomous zone?

Autonomous zone is the sensory area which is exclusively supplied by a single nerve without overlap by other nerve.

Q. What is the location of the autonomous zones of radial, median, ulnar and axillary nerve in upper limb?

a. *Radial nerve:* Dorsal 1st web space
b. *Median nerve:* Volar aspect of index finger
c. *Ulnar nerve:* Ulnar border of little finger
d. *Axillary nerve:* Upper lateral aspect of arm (known as regimental badge sign)

Q. Outline the treatment plan for all three types of peripheral nerve injury.

A brief outline of management of all three types of nerve injuries has been explained in Flowchart 1.1.

Flowchart 1.1: Management of three types of nerve injuries

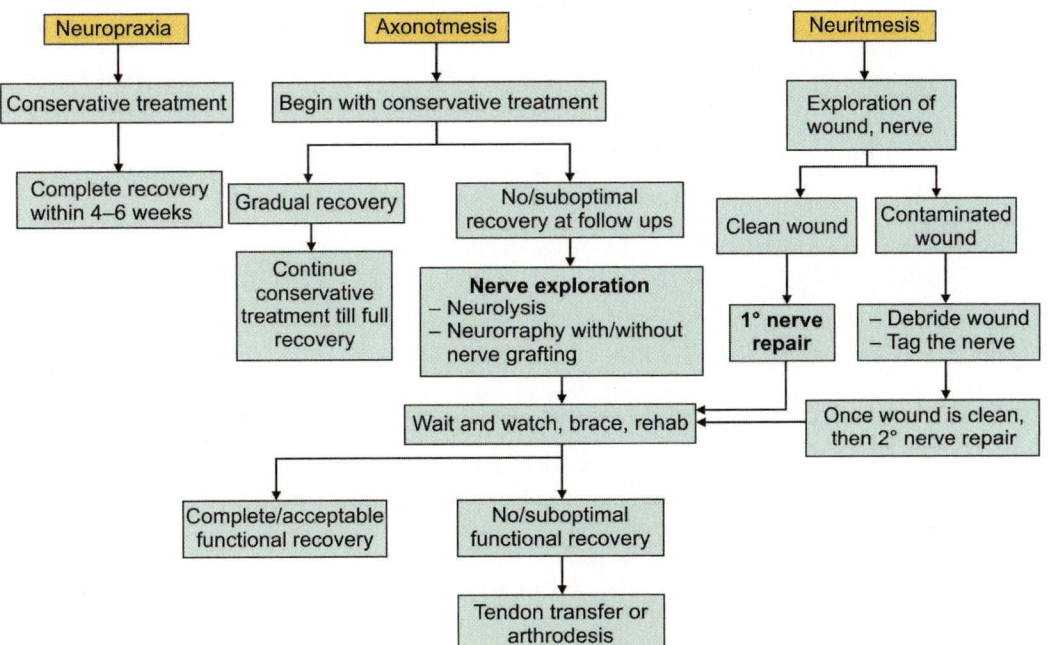

CLAWHAND

Q. Define clawhand?

Clawhand is characterized by hyperextension at the metacarpophalangeal (MCP) joint and hyperflexion at the interphalangeal (IP) joint (Figs 1.10a and b).

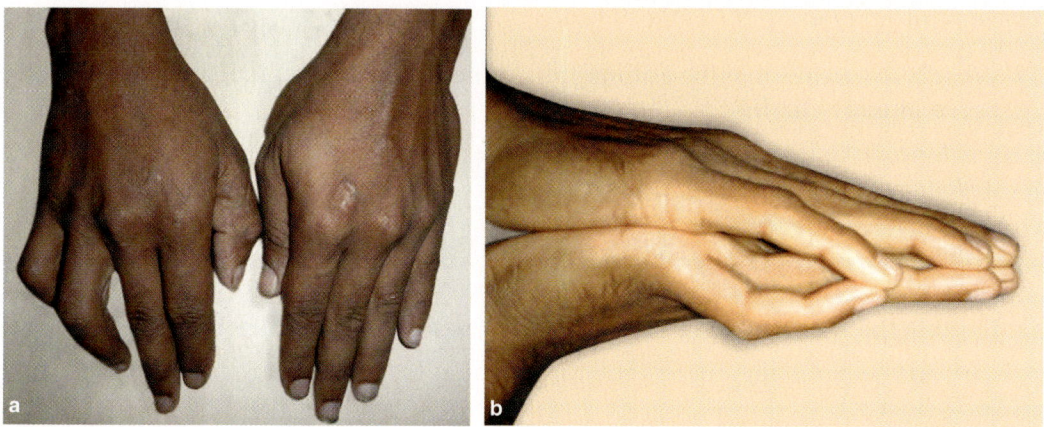

Figs 1.10a and b: Clinical picture of hand shows a classical clawhand which becomes clear in folded hand or *namaste* position

Q. Which nerve injury causes clawhand?

Clawhand deformity is seen after ulnar nerve injury or combined injury to both ulnar and median nerve.

Q. What is the difference between the clawhand pattern in 'ulnar' and 'ulnar with median' nerve injury?

In ulnar nerve injury: Partial clawhand affecting only little and ring fingers is observed.

In combined injuries of median and ulnar nerve: Complete clawhand deformity is observed affecting all four fingers.

Q. What is the reason behind clawhand after ulnar nerve injury?

Ulnar nerve supplies medial two lumbricals and all Interossei muscles. The combined action of interossei and lumbricals is to flex metacarpophalangeal (MCP) and extend interphalangeal (IP) joints. When these muscles are paralysed due to injury to the ulnar nerve, it results in MCP hyperextension and IP flexion due to unopposed action from finger extensors acting at MCP and flexors acting at the IP joints respectively.

Q. Why clawhand is not seen after isolated median nerve palsy?

Absence of clawhand deformity after the median nerve injury, even though the lateral two lumbricals are paralysed, is based upon a fact that the 'predominant MCP flexor and IP extensor of finger is interossei muscle and not lumbrical'. The lumbricals only assist interossei in above said action.

In case of ulnar nerve injury, both interossei and lumbricals are paralyzed resulting in clawhand.

In case of median nerve injury; even though there is paralysis of lateral two lumbricals but the interossei muscles are not involvement. Hence, there is no significant weakness in MCP flexion and IP extension and thereby, the clawhand is not observed.

Q. What is the nerve supply to the lumbricals and interossei?

Lateral two lumbricals: Median nerve
Medial two lumbricals: Ulnar nerve
Interossei (palmar and dorsal): Ulnar nerve

Q. What is the function of lumbricals and interossei?

1. *Lumbricals:* MCP joint flexion and IP joint extension
2. *Interossei: Palmar*—adduction of fingers; *dorsal*—abduction of fingers
   Furthermore *interossei assist lumbricals in MCP flexion and IP extension.*

Q. Which specific muscles are to be tested for median nerve?

1. Flexor pollicis longus
2. Flexor digitorum superficialis
3. Lateral two tendons of flexor digitorum profundus (FDP) **(Ochsner's clasping index sign)**
4. Abductor pollicis brevis **(pen test)**
5. Opponens pollicis **(test opposition of thumb to rest of fingers)**
6. Lateral two lumbricals
7. Pronators

Q. Which specific muscles are to be tested for ulnar nerve?

1. Flexor carpi ulnaris
2. Medial two tendons of flexor digitorum profundus
3. Adductor pollicis **(book test or Froment's sign)**
4. Palmar interossei **(finger adduction/card test)**
5. Dorsal interossei **(finger abduction)**
6. Abductor digiti minimi

Note: It is important that student must know the test for each muscle

Q. What is 'Hand of benediction' or 'Preacher's sign'?

In median nerve injury or compression at the elbow or forearm level, where it affects long flexors of fingers along with lateral two lumbricals of hand, patient finds difficult to flex his finger at the PIP and DIP joints in index and middle finger while attempting to make a fist.

This gives hand an appearance of 'benediction'.

Q. What is intrinsic plus hand?

It is a condition where extrinsic muscles of hand (long flexor group and extensor digitorum communis) are paralysed whereas intrinsics muscles are normal resulting in overpowered intrinsics causing MCP flexion and IP joint extension (Fig. 1.11).

Q. What do you mean by intrinsic minus hand?

Intrinsic minus means paralysis of intrinsic muscles of hand whereas extrinsic muscles of hand (long flexors and extensors) are normal.

It is observed after paralysis of ulnar nerve or ulnar and median nerve palsy at the level of wrist resulting in clawing of the hand.

Q. Which splint is used to prevent deformity in clawhand?

Knuckle bender splint is used in clawhand. It keeps MCP and IP in functional position (Fig. 1.12).

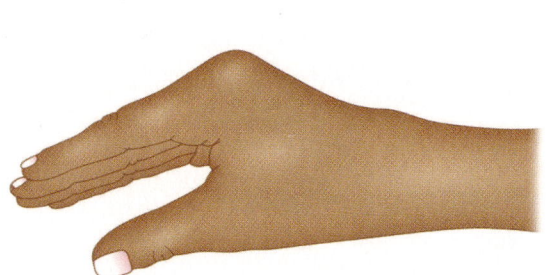

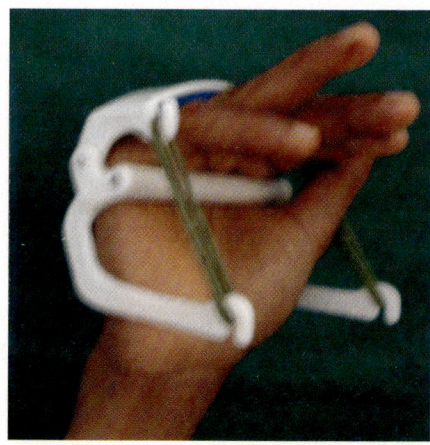

Fig. 1.11: Diagrammatic representation of intrinsic plus hand

Fig. 1.12: Clinical picture of hand with knuckle bender splint

Q. What are the various procedure(s) for ulnar nerve injury?

1. Exploration of the nerve followed by neurolysis
2. Neurorrhaphy (nerve repair) with or without nerve grafting
3. Tendon transfers

Q. What is ulnar paradox?

The ulnar nerve innervates medial two tendons of FDP proximally, and intrinsic muscles of hand (interossei and medial two lumbricals) distally. When ulnar nerve is paralysed near the elbow; two medial FDP, medial two lumbricals and interossei lose its power and hence, fingers lay flat due to no action from FDP.

However, when ulnar nerve is paralyzed below the elbow or near the wrist, medial two FDP retains its innervation but lumbricals and Interossei remain paralysed. Hence, normal FDP results in unopposed flexion at of PIP and DIP resulting in typical clawing of hand.

Thus distal palsy (lower lesion) results in "more deformed appearance (claw)" of the hand as compared to the proximal palsy (higher lesion) where less deformity is apparent in the hand.

So, this is the paradox! Higher the lesion, lesser is the apparent deformity in hand whereas lower the lesion, severe is the appearance! Normally one would expect more severe deformity with higher lesion and lesser deformity with lower lesion.

Q. What is tardy ulnar nerve palsy?

Tardy means "Late onset". Tardy ulnar nerve palsy is **most commonly observed in gradually progressive cubitus valgus deformity with non-union of lateral condyle fracture of humerus.** As the lateral condyle goes in for non-union, it results in progressive cubitus valgus deformity of the elbow. The progressive valgus deformity results in traction over the ulnar nerve. Further, every flexion-extension movement of the elbow results in frictional neuritis of the ulnar nerve followed by the fibrosis of ulnar nerve. So, this causes a slow onset of paralysis of ulnar nerve (tardy ulnar nerve palsy), usually a few months to years later after valgus deformity sets in.

Q. How do you treat tardy ulnar nerve palsy?

Tardy ulnar nerve palsy is treated by neurolysis and anterior transposition of ulnar nerve (anterior to medial epicondyle) to prevent further friction.

Q. What is the classical deformity after the median nerve injury?

Ape thumb deformity.

Note: The thumb abductor (abductor pollicis brevis) is paralysed with overacting adductor pollicis results in adducted thumb.

Q. Which splint is used after median nerve injury?

Thumb abductor splint.

Note: After abductor palsy, the thumb remains in adduction which could result in adduction contracture. Hence, an abduction splint keeps thumb in abduction avoiding adduction contracture.

Q. What is Klumpke's paralysis?

Klumpke's paralysis commonly occurs at birth during vaginal delivery. Occasionally, it happens due to catching a tree branch while fall from tree. It is due to **involvement of lower trunk of brachial plexus (C8, T1).** Mostly, **ulnar nerve is involved** resulting in paralysis involving intrinsic muscles of hand (interossei, medial two lumbrical, adductor pollicis and other hypothenar muscles) leading to clawhand and weakness of wrist and finger flexors (FCU, medial two FDP). Due to T1 involvement, there can be Horner's syndrome.

Q. What is Erb's paralysis?

Erb's paralysis is caused by injury to the upper trunk of the brachial plexus (C5, 6) in conditions wherein there is excess lateral flexion of the neck.

Most commonly, it happens during vaginal delivery in babies with shoulder dystocia when head and neck is excessively pulled sideways with respect to body axis to aid delivery of the trunk. Another common cause is fall on to the tip of shoulder during RTA.

Both conditions result in excess traction on upper trunk of Brachial plexus causing the palsy of upper trunk. The commonly involved nerves (with muscles) are:

- Suprascapular nerve (supra- and infraspinatus muscle),
- Musculocutaneous nerve (biceps and brachialis), and
- Axillary nerve (deltoid and teres minor)

The paralysis of shoulder abductors (deltoid, supraspinatus), external rotators (infraspinatus, teres minor), elbow flexors and forearm supinators (biceps, brachialis) result in:

- Arm hang by side in adduction
- Internal rotation at shoulder
- Extended elbow
- Pronation at forearm.

The classic deformity is known as **"policeman hand/waiter tip hand"**.

What is Erb's point?

Erb's point is a point at upper trunk of brachial plexus with confluence of six nerves (C5, C6 root, suprascapular nerve, nerve to subclavius, anterior and posterior divisions of C5 and C6).

It is located 2–3 cm above the clavicle and is named after Wilhelm Heinrich Erb.

FOOTDROP

Q. What do you mean by footdrop?

Footdrop means inability to actively dorsiflex the ankle.

Q. Which nerve paralysis can lead to footdrop?

1. Lateral popliteal/common peroneal nerve (CPN) injury
2. Sciatic nerve (SN) injury

Q. Are there any other causes for footdrop other than nerve injury?

Complete severance of extensor tendons especially tibialis anterior (TA) can also lead to footdrop even though the nerve is intact.

Q. How will you differentiate that footdrop is due to CPN or SN injury?

Understand the basic anatomy before you can answer this question. In the beginning of its course in gluteal and upper thigh region, sciatic nerve (SN) first supplies the knee flexors (hamstring). After descending the back of thigh, SN divides into common peroneal nerve (CPN) and the tibial nerve at the upper end of popliteal fossa.

The tibial nerve: It continues straight down to supply muscles on back of calf followed by the muscles in the plantar aspect of the foot. Important ones are plantar flexor at ankle (tendo Achillis), tibialis posterior, other toe long flexors and foot plantar intrinsic muscles.

CPN: It winds around the fibular neck and then divides into superficial and deep peroneal nerve. It supplies the various muscles of anterior and lateral compartment of the leg (Table 1.2).

Table 1.2: Summary of important muscles of anterior, lateral, and posterior compartment of the leg	
Muscle	**Function**
Anterior compartment supplied by deep peroneal nerve	
Tibialis anterior	Dorsiflexion at ankle, inversion at subtalar joint
Extensor hallucis longus	Great toe dorsiflexion
Extensor digitorum longus	Small toe extension
Peroneus tertius	Dorsiflexion at ankle joint, eversion at subtalar joint
Lateral compartment supplied by superficial peroneal nerve	
Peroneus longus	Eversion, plantar flexion
Peroneus brevis	Eversion, plantar flexion
Posterior compartment and foot muscles supplied by tibial nerve	
Tendoachilles	Plantar flexion at ankle
Tibialis posterior	Plantar flexion at ankle, inversion at subtalar joint
Flexor hallucis longus	Flexion of great toe
Flexor digitorum longus	Flexion of small toes

So **in case of SN palsy**, patient will lose
1. Knee flexion
2. All movements at the ankle (dorsiflexion, plantar flexion, eversion and inversion) resulting in flail foot (no strength as all foot intrinsic and extrinsic muscles paralysed)

Note: Knee extension is normal as knee extensors (quadriceps) are supplied by femoral nerve.

In case of CPN palsy, patient will lose ability to:
1. Dorsiflex the ankle
2. Dorsiflex the great toe
3. Dorsiflex the small toes
4. Eversion of subtalar joint

Note: In **case of isolated tibial nerve palsy**, patient will lose his ability to plantarflex and invert whereas he will retain dorsiflexion of ankle, toes and eversion of subtalar joint.

So, by examining the various functions of knee and ankle-foot, we can differentiate between sciatic nerve, tibial nerve and common peroneal nerve palsy.

Q. Which splint is used for footdrop?

Ankle-foot orthosis (AFO) (Fig. 1.13).

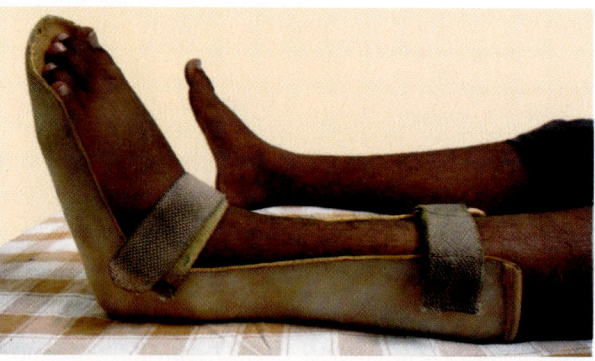

Fig. 1.13: Clinical picture of ankle-foot orthosis (AFO) applied on left foot-ankle

Q. What will happen if AFO is not used?

The foot will remain in plantar flexion position resulting in equinus deformity at the ankle.

Q. What could be done if SN/CPN fail to recover after a period of conservative treatment?

1. Explore the nerve
2. Neurolysis, neurorrhaphy with/without nerve graft
3. Tendon transfer

Q. Which tendon transfer is done for footdrop due to CPN palsy?

Tibialis posterior (TP) is transferred to correct footdrop. It is transferred onto the dorsum of foot. There are two classic tendon transfers for footdrop.

Ober's transfer: Circumtibial re-routing of TP and anchoring onto the 3rd metatarsal base.

Watkin's interosseous transfer: Re-routing through the interosseous membrane onto the 3rd metatarsal base.

Note: Do not forget to check the power of tibialis posterior as it could also be paralyzed or ineffective. If that is the case, then it cannot be transferred. Many at times, students are allotted case of sciatic nerve palsy or Volkmann's ischemic contracture of the leg and foot following a compartment syndrome of the leg where all/most muscles of leg and foot are ineffective. Answering TP transfer in such a case where no muscles are working a mistake!

Q. What is the role of examining ankle and foot movement in a case of foot-ankle paralysis?

If there is stiffness in the ankle-foot complex, the tendon transfer is not suitable till the ROM is restored to functional level.

Q. What should be done if ankle is stiff in equinus position?

1. First, patient should be advised physiotherapy of ankle and foot to restore the ROM of stiff joints.
2. If conservative measures (physiotherapy) fail, then surgical release of stiff joint can be performed.

Note: Commonly, tendo Achillis lengthening and posterior ankle joint capsule release is done to correct ankle equinus. It is important to have a good range of movements at the involved joint before tendon transfer. There is no point supplying electricity to a fan which is jammed and rusty!

Q. What will you do if there is no tendon remaining to be transferred?

Such patients can be managed in two possible ways:
a. AFO for the ankle-foot to keep ankle foot in functional position.
b. Arthrodesis of ankle and subtalar joint in neutral position.

Note: Avoid ankle-foot arthrodesis in patients with sensory loss over the foot especially over the plantar aspect as it may result in non-healing ulcers due to a rigid-foot result from arthrodesis.

Q. What are the other causes of footdrop?

Apart from other general causes of nerve palsy, there are some other causes of footdrop.

1. Infective:
   a. Poliomyelitis—history of polio in childhood

   b. Hansen's disease—history of patchy loss of sensation over body, thickened and tender nerves like CPN, greater auricular, ulnar, superficial radial nerve

2. **Traumatic**
   a. CPN, sciatic nerve injury
   b. Spinal cord injury
3. **Lumbar intervertebral disc prolapse:** History of lifting heavy weight, low back pain with radiation to the lower limb, Laségue and straight leg raising test positive
4. **Spastic cerebral palsy (since birth)**
5. **Cerebrovascular accidents:** History of CVA
6. **Charcot-Marie-Tooth** disease
7. Rupture of tibialis anterior and other ankle-foot extensor tendons
8. **Neoplastic:** Tumors compressing the nerves

Note: In non-traumatic nerve palsy, student must take history to rule out other causes of nerve injury.

NON-UNION

Common Presentation of Patient with Non-union

Case summary: A 32-year-old male case of inability to bear weight over his right lower limb. He had a RTA 6 months back following which he sustained fracture of tibia and fibula. He was taken to a local hospital where fracture was managed by a POP cast. Cast was changed twice in three months. Currently, patient cannot bear weight over right lower limb. There is no pain over the fracture site. General and systemic examinations are normal. Local examination of right tibia revealed painless abnormal mobility over lower fourth of shaft of the tibia. The right lower limb is short by 3 cm and shortening is in the tibia. Knee movements are normal but ankle joint is stiff having only 10° plantar and dorsiflexion each. Neurovascular examination is normal.

Q. What is the clinical diagnosis?

The clinical diagnosis is non-union of tibia with stiffness of ankle joint and shortening of tibia.

Q. Why do you say so?

It is because of the following reasons.
1. History of RTA
2. Presence of **painless abnormal mobility** over the fracture site (lower fourth of shaft tibia)
3. Stiffness of the ankle joint
4. Shortened tibia

Q. What is the main evidence to say that it is a non-union of the tibia?

Painless, abnormal mobility at the fracture site

Q. How will you confirm the diagnosis?

Plain X-ray of the leg (anteroposterior and lateral view).

Q. What are the common finding in a X-ray of non union?

Following are the common findings in the X-ray of non-union (Fig. 1.14)
1. Gap at the fracture site
2. Closed medullary canal
3. Sclerotic ends of fracture
4. Callus could be absent, minimal or in excess.

Q. What are the principles of treatment of non-union?

The treatment of non-union consists of the following principle:
a. Correct any systemic factor, if present: Stop smoking; correct anemia, control diabetes mellitus
b. Local principles involve
   1. **Open reduction** of the fracture site

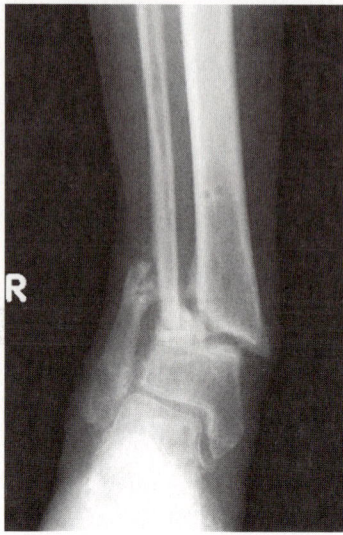

Fig. 1.14: Plain radiograph of tibia and fibula showing non-union at lower fourth shaft with gap at fracture site

2. **Excision of sclerotic ends** with **freshening of bone ends** till fresh bleeding is evident
3. **Open the medullary canal**
4. **Internal or external fixation:** If the patient has history of infection/currently having local infection, external fixation is a safer option. If there was no infection or infection is completely cured, then internal fixation can be safely performed)
5. **Bone grafting:** Essential for atrophic type whereas hypertrophic type may not require grafting.**

> **Bone grafting should not be done if there is slightest doubt of infection otherwise the graft will act like a dead piece of bone and will become a sequestrum and infection will flare up.

Q. What is atrophic and hypertrophic type of non-union?

Atrophic and hypertrophic type of non-union is a radiographic presentation/classification of callus in patients with non-union.

Q. What is the radiological classification of non-union?

This radiological classification (atrophic or hypertrophic type) is based upon presence/absence of callus
1. *Atrophic type:* Poor callus
2. *Hypertrophic type:* Excess callus

Q. What is the rationale behind this classification?

1. *Atrophic type:* It indicates "poor vascularity or deficient biological activity at the fracture site" resulting in nil or minimal callus.

2. *Hypertrophic type:* It indicates "poor mechanical stability at the fracture site" wherein the callus is present in reasonable or in abundance but two ends of callus could not stabilise due to persistent instability (or poor mechanical stability) at the # site.

Q. How can one use this classification in treating the patient?

1. Since atrophic type of non-union reflects poor vascularity or biological activity at the fracture site, *fresh autologous cancellous bone graft or vascularized bone graft* is applied at the fracture site along with fracture fixation to stimulate the fracture union after the fixation of fracture.

2. Since hypertrophic type of non-union reflects poor mechanical stability, the *stability at the fracture site is improved by using stronger/larger/different implant (nail/plate) to stimulate union.*

Q. Define non-union?

Non-union of fracture is defined as 'when there is no clinical or radiological evidence of union of fracture for three consecutive months, and there is no possibility of fracture union without further intervention'.

US FDA definition of non-union

The US Food and Drug Administration (FDA) defines a non-union as a fracture that is at least 9 months old and has not shown any signs of healing for 3 consecutive months.

Q. What are the local causes of non-union?

Common local causes are:
1. Infection
2. Inadequate vascularity
3. Intact fellow bone
4. Interposition of soft tissue
5. Inadequate reduction
6. Inadequate immobilization
   (Note: All causes start with "I")

Important systemic causes are:
1. Smoking
2. Diabetes
3. Osteoporosis
4. Malnutrition and vitamin deficiency

Q. Why lower end tibia is more prone for non-union?

Lower end tibia is prone for non-union because of precarious vascularity. There is minimal soft tissue envelope around the lower end of tibia reducing the vascularity of the lower end of tibia.

Q. Why does infection cause non-union?

Infection result in destruction to the callus, damage to the vascularity of the soft tissue envelope around the bone and fibrosis at the fracture site resulting in non-union.

Q. Why open fracture causes non-union?

Open fracture causes non-union because:
a. Soft tissue damage, periosteal stripping compromise the local vascularity
b. Infection
c. Loss of bone fragment

Q. What are the common sites of non-union?

Upper Limb

1. *Scaphoid waist fracture:* Disrupted vascularity which enters scaphoid from distal to proximal
2. *Lateral condyle # of humerus:* The fragment gets rotated and displaced due to pull from extensor muscles attached over the lateral condyle.

Lower Limb

1. *Fracture neck femur:* Disrupted retinacular blood supply, absent cambium layer in periosteum, no fracture hematoma formation as it gets lysed by synovial fluid
2. *Fracture lower end of tibia #:* Less vascularity at the lower end, poor soft tissue envelope over the lower end of tibia
3. *Fracture talus neck:* Disrupted blood supply

Q. How you would have treated a patient with a non-union and local infection (osteomyelitis) as well?

It can be treated as "two-staged procedure".

First, the local soft tissue and bony infection must be treated as per standard principles to treat chronic osteomyelitis.

Once infection heals completely, one should treat non-union on the standard principles.

Q. So, it means one has to undergo two-stage procedure for infective non-union. Is there a way to treat both simultaneously?

Yes. It can be treated in the same setting by Ilizarov's technique wherein, the infected bony segment is excised completely and the new bone is regenerated using Ilizarov's technique or limb reconstruction system.

Q. What is delayed union?

Delayed union refers to *a fracture in which union is not complete within the interval expected for that specific fracture.* Nevertheless, the clinical and radiographic evidence of healing is present and if given a proper milieu, has the potential to unite.

Q. What is the difference between delayed and non-union?

In non-union, the biological process of union is **completely halted** and there are no more biological attempts at union of fracture whereas in delayed union, the biological process of union is going on, albeit slow. The non-union will not unite without surgical intervention whereas in delayed union, fracture may unite with the current treatment plan without any intervention.

Q. What is the treatment of delayed union?

1. **Wait and watch:** Regular follow ups and continuing the present method of treatment
2. **Correct any local or systemic factor responsible for delayed union.**

   If above two does not work, then
3. **Bone marrow injections** at the fracture site to accelerate the healing process
4. **Bone grafting** at the fracture site
5. **Ultrasonic stimulation** at the fracture site

Q. How will you manage ankle stiffness?

Ankle stiffness can be managed by:
1. Physiotherapy
2. If physiotherapy fails to achieve any significant improvement in ROM, surgical release of stiff joint should be performed (*refer* to page 47: Stiff joint)

Q. How will you manage shortening of tibia?

Since shortening is only 3 cm, it can be managed by shoe raise or limb lengthening.

Q. What are the various ways in which shortening of a limb can be managed?

General principles of managing shortening of limb
1. *Shortening <4 cm:* Shoe raise
2. *Shortening >4 cm:* Limb lengthening by Ilizarov's technique.
   In paediatric patients with shortening, two more undermentioned methods can be utilized
3. Shortening of other limb
4. Epiphysiodesis

Q. How will you manage shortening of tibia?

Since shortening is only 3 cm, it can be managed by shoe raise or limb lengthening.

REFLEX SYMPATHETIC DYSTROPHY (RSD) OR SUDECK'S DYSTROPHY/CRPS

Common Presentation of Patient with Reflex Sympathetic Dystrophy (RSD)

Case summary: A 35-year-old male gave history of fall on outstretched left hand following which he sustained fracture of lower end radius. He underwent closed reduction and below elbow cast application for 6 weeks. After removal of cast, patient was advised physiotherapy of hand and fingers. However, patient noticed swelling of his fingers and hand. He experienced severe pain while moving the wrist and fingers and altered sensations over his hand. Now, after 12 weeks of injury, the swelling is still present over the hand and finger with quite painful movements of joints of wrist and finger. Examination revealed shiny skin with mottled bluish hue, spindle shape fingers with pulp atrophy with cold and sweaty feel over the skin of wrist-hand. Movements of wrist and finger are grossly restricted and painful. Mild paraesthesia was noted over the hand without any motor deficit. There was bony irregularity at distal end of radius but no abnormal mobility elicited.

Q. What is the clinical diagnosis?

The clinical diagnosis is united fracture lower end radius with reflex sympathetic dystrophy/RSD/complex regional pain syndrome (CRPS).

Q. Why do you say so?

I say so because of the following reason:

History
1. History of trauma with POP applied for fracture lower end radius
2. Swelling of hand and finger (Fig. 1.15)
3. Exaggerated pain while attempted movements
4. Painfully restricted movements of wrist and fingers even after a few weeks of active and passive mobilization/physiotherapy.

Examination
5. Bluish mottled hue of hand and finger.
6. Shiny skin with spindle shaped finger and finger pulp atrophy

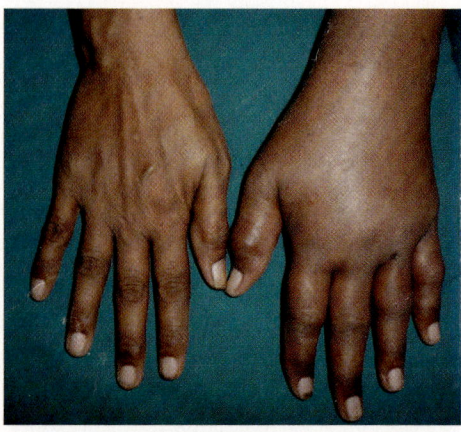

Fig. 1.15: Clinical photograph of left hand with RSD showing swelling and spindle shape fingers

7. Cold, sweaty hand
8. Grossly restricted and painful movement of fingers
9. Altered sensations (paraesthesia)

Q. How will you confirm the diagnosis?

Diagnosis is essentially clinical. However, some investigation may aid in diagnosis.
a. X-ray shows **patchy osteoporosis** in the bones of wrist and hand (Fig. 1.16).
b. **Phase III positive bone scan**

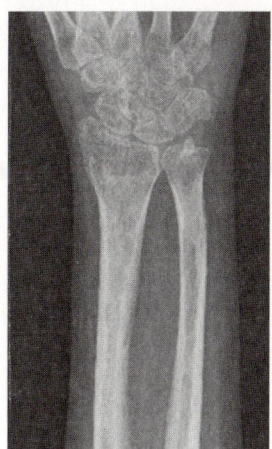

Fig. 1.16: Plain X-ray of left wrist and hand shows united fracture of distal radius with patchy osteoporosis in bones of forearm, wrist and hand

Q. What are the other synonyms for RSD?

1. Sudeck's osteodystrophy
2. Complex regional pain syndrome

Q. Which terminology is more appropriate?

Currently, CRPS is more appropriate and acceptable terminology.

Q. What it CRPS type 1 and type 2?

Type 1 CRPS: CRPS without any underlying cause
Type 2 CRPS: CRPS after a nerve injury

Q. What is causalgia?

Causalgia is a type 2 CRPS or RSD associated with nerve injury.

Q. What is the fundamental pathology in RSD?

The principal pathology in RSD is **idiopathic overactivity of sympathetic nervous system** (or exaggerated response to injury) in the affected limb **due to constant pain stimulus.**

Q. What are the predisposing factors which can lead to RSD?

a. Patient not mobilizing the affected limb effectively
b. Persistent edema
c. Pain, if not controlled well, could result in RSD

Note: By controlling these predisposing factors pre- and postoperatively, RSD could be mostly prevented.
a. Encourage active and passive mobilization of limb
b. Limb elevation and compression bandage to prevent edema
c. Adequate analgesics to control pain

Q. How will you treat patients with RSD/CRPS?

The aim of the treatment is

a. Break the pain-stiffness cycle by appropriate conservative measures such as
1. Appropriate **analgesia** (NSAIDs, opioids, etc.)
2. **Control limb edema** by limb elevation, compression bandage
3. Prolonged supervised physiotherapy to **mobilize the limb** is the key to success
4. Other medical measures:
   a. Calcium channel blockers: Nifedipine
   b. Pregabalin, Gabapentin
   c. Vitamin C

If above conservative measures for few weeks fail to provide relief, one could opt for

b. Blocking the sympathetic nerve supply to the limb

Block the sympathetic ganglion supplying the extremity by locally injecting lignocaine/phenol/alcohol. For example, stellate ganglion for the upper limb which is situated anterior to transverse process of C7 vertebra and coeliac ganglion for lower limb situated next to L1 vertebra.

The sympathetic ganglion block decreases pain in the affected part by blocking sympathetic response enabling the clinician to aggressively mobilize the limb and reduce stiffness.

Q. What you would have done if this patient presented with grossly malunited lower end of radius affecting his hand function with RSD?

First, RSD must be completely treated to reduce pain and swelling along with restore the movements.

Then **reassess the malunion** affecting the functional disability. If needed, then treat malunion.

Note: However, **no elective surgical intervention** should be done in presence of RSD. (Note: Also, all malunited fractures may not need surgical intervention)

Q. Why not to treat malunion in the setting of RSD?

RSD will aggravate if any surgical procedure is performed without treating RSD.

Note: Any surgical procedure around a joint with RSD is usually contraindicated as it can further aggravate the RSD by exacerbating pain stimulus.

STIFF JOINT

Common Presentation of Patient with Stiff Joint

Case summary: A 35-year-old man case of pain and difficulty in bending his right knee for 4 months. Four months back, following a RTA, he sustained distal femur intercondylar fracture. He underwent open reduction and internal fixation (ORIF)of fracture by a plate followed by knee immobilisation in a brace for three weeks. Three weeks later, active knee mobilisation was started. There was no history of infection or open fracture. Currently, he is full weight bearing but unable to squat or sit cross leg. General and systemic examination were normal. Local examination revealed a 16 cm long primarily healed scar over lateral aspect of thigh. The knee flexion range of movement was 0–90°. The limb lengths on both sides were equal and neurovascular examination was normal.

Q. What is the clinical diagnosis?

Healed fracture of lower end of femur with stiffness of the knee.

Q. Why do you say so?

I say so because of the following reasons:

History

1. History of trauma
2. ORIF of distal femur fracture and immobilisation (both could lead to stiffness)
3. Full weight bearing (indicates a healed fracture)

Examination

4. Decreased range of flexion movement (0–90°) (Fig. 1.17)
5. Irregular lower end femur (suggestive of a fracture)

Q. What is role of massage or forcible passive physiotherapy (often done by quacks) in the history of a stiff joint?

Massage and/or forcible passive physiotherapy could lead to myositis ossificans (read Myositis ossificans on page 13).

Q. How will you proceed?

I would like to take an X-ray.

Q. What would you see on X-ray?

X-ray can reveal
• United fracture with implant *in situ*.

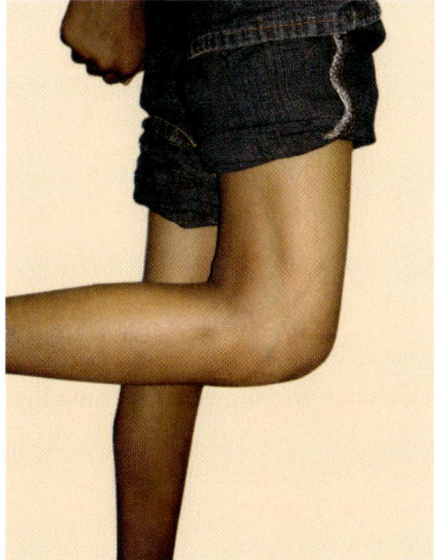

Fig. 1.17: Right knee showing decreased movements

Q. What is the treatment of a patient with stiff joint?

1. Physiotherapy
   a. Gentle active and assisted passive mobilization
   b. Moist heat, short wave diathermy (SWD)

Note: Moist heat and SWD help in relaxing the tight fibrous tissue and then active and gentle passive mobilisation of joint helps in regaining movements)

2. If physiotherapy for few weeks to months fails to result in significant improvement in range of movements, then surgical release could be considered to restore a functional or total range of movements.

Q. What surgery can be performed for a stiff joint?

In a stiff joint, one or more following structures can be tight. They can be released surgically.

1. **Skin** if scarred: Scar excision/lengthening (Z or V-Y plasty)
2. **Subcutaneous tissue** and **deep fascia:** Excise/divide them
3. **Muscles** are fibrotic and contracted: Concerned tendon should be lengthened using **Z or V-Y plasty.**
4. **Joint capsule is tight:** Capsulotomy/capsulectomy
5. **Intra-articular adhesions:** Release
6. **Finally a gentle manipulation:** It may also help in getting over some adhesions in and around joint.

Q. How can we prevent stiffness of joint after fracture or any injury?

Stiffness of a joint can be prevented or minimised by appropriate management of fracture or injury and early mobilization and physiotherapy of the joint.

Q. What do you mean by ankylosis?

Ankylosis is an abnormal stiffness of the joint means that the joint which exhibits hardly any movements.

Note: Ankylosis implies pathological fusion of the joint.

Q. What are the types of ankylosis?

There are two types of ankyloses: True and false

True ankylosis
1. Bony ankylosis
2. Fibrous ankylosis
   (Read false ankylosis on page 17)

Q. What is bony and fibrous ankylosis? How do you differentiate between them?

In **bony ankylosis**, after the denudation of cartilage due to trauma/infection/ inflammation; new bone forms across the two articular surfaces bridging two articular ends of bone resulting in complete fusion of the two articular surfaces. So there is no movement elicited across the joint and is painless **(painless, no movements)**.

In **fibrous ankylosis,** dense and tough fibrous bands run across the two articular surfaces and in the joint. Since there are fibrous bands running across, some movement can be elicited, and that is painful **(painful, jog of movement)**.

Q. What will be the X-ray finding in two types of ankyloses?

Bony Ankylosis

- Bony trabeculae cross the joint joining the two articular surface, and
- Joint space will be obliterated.

Fibrous Ankylosis

- Joint space is seen
- No bony trabeculae crossing the joint.

Q. What is the treatment of choice of bony ankylosis?

In case of bony ankylosis, physiotherapy is of no use as there is bony bridge between the two ends which would not allow any movements to be regained by physiotherapy, surgery is the preferred treatment option.

1. **If the joint is in sound functional position of bony ankylosis:** It could be left alone as long as it satisfies the functional demands of the patient.
2. **If the joint is in unsound position of bony ankylosis,** it should be converted into fusion (arthrodesis) in sound functional position.
3. However, above two options would not restore the movement at the fused joint. To restore ROM at the joint, total joint replacement can be performed.

Functional position means the position of joint in which several important functions can be performed. Functional position of various joints is mentioned below

Functional position of upper limb joints:
1. Shoulder: 30° forward flexion; 30° abduction and 30° internal rotation
2. Right elbow: 90° flexion; left elbow: 30° flexion
3. Forearm: Mid prone
4. Wrist and hand: Glass holding position

Lower limb joints
1. Hip: Neutral in extension and slight abduction
2. Knee: Full extension
3. Ankle and foot: Neutral

Q. If there is myositis ossificans, what will you do?

Management will depend upon the type of myositis ossificans (discussed in detail in chapter of myositis osssificans).

VOLKMANN'S ISCHEMIC CONTRACTURE (VIC)

Common Presentation of Patient with VIC of Forearm and Hand

Case summary: A 6-year-old boy case of pain and stiffness in his right forearm and hand. He had RTA one year back and fractured his both forearm bones. He was taken to a local hospital where an above elbow cast was applied after the fracture reduction, and was discharged. After reaching home, he developed severe pain in the forearm. He was rushed to the nearest hospital where the cast was removed. Examination revealed painful passive stretch of his fingers. His fracture was further managed on above elbow slab. Later, he developed gradually progressive flexion deformity in the hand and finger. Presently, he has difficulty in using his hand. Examination reveals wasting of forearm and hand muscles. On dorsiflexion of the wrist, the fingers become flexed at MCP and IP joint while palmar flexion of the wrist allows straightening of the fingers at the IP joint. There is sensory loss over forearm and hand over the median and ulnar nerve distribution areas with motor weakness in muscles supplied by the ulnar nerve.

Q. What is the clinical diagnosis?

Post-traumatic Volkmann's ischemic contracture (VIC) of right forearm and wrist.

Q. Why do you say so?

It is because of following reasons.

History

1. History of trauma with fracture forearm bone (susceptible for compartment syndrome)
2. History of above elbow cast application followed by severe pain in forearm (symptom of compartment syndrome)

Examination

3. Wasting of forearm muscles (Fig. 1.18)
4. Volkmann's sign present (this is the most important late clinical sign of VIC)
5. Median and ulnar nerve involvement

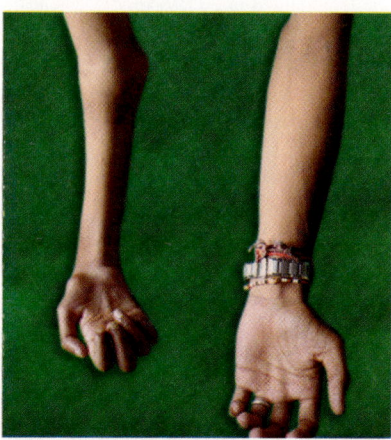

Fig. 1.18: Clinical photograph of VIC of right forearm reveals gross wasting of forearm muscles and flexion contracture of fingers

Q. What is Volkmann's sign?

In Volkmann's sign; when the wrist is dorsiflexed, the fingers become palmar flexed and cannot be extended passively or actively. However, when the wrist is brought to neutral or palmar flexion, the fingers can be extended passively or actively.

> VIC was first described in 1881 by Richard von Volkmann of Germany.

Q. What is the mechanics of Volkmann's sign?

It is due to **bow stringing effect** of fibrosed flexor muscle tendon unit over a fixed length of bone.

Q. What is Volkmann's ischemic contracture?

VIC is the **contracture and fibrosis of flexor muscles of forearm (deep and superficial)** after an episode of ischemia to the muscles due to the compartment syndrome.

Q. What is Volkmann's ischemia?

Volkmann's ischemia is also known as **compartment syndrome.**

Q. Which areas are prone for Volkmann's ischemia?

Although Volkmann's ischemia or compartment syndrome could occur in any area, it frequently occurs in following locations:
a. *Injury around the elbow:* Fracture supracondylar humerus, elbow dislocation
b. Fracture both bones forearm
c. Fracture both bones leg
d. Fracture of metacarpal or metatarsals
e. *Injuries around the knee:* Knee dislocation, fractures around the knee.

> Note: Compartment syndrome usually occurs where there are parallel bones (forearm, leg, hand or foot).

Q. What is compartment syndrome and its pathophysiology?

Normally the pressure in the osseofibrous compartment is less than 10 mm Hg. If the intracompartment pressure increases more than 30 mm of Hg, it indicates an established compartment syndrome.

The gradually increasing intracompartment pressure from 10 mm Hg and above results in decreased venous outflow while arterial inflow is maintained. This causes increased venous capillary pressure which results in increased transudation and exudation in extravascular space further increasing the compartment pressure.

The increasing compartment pressure causes ischemia to the smaller arteries supplying the muscle and the nerves resulting in painful gradual onset global ischemia of the muscles. If remains untreated within the stipulated time, nerves and muscles suffer irreversible damage.
a. *Muscles:* Ischaemic necrosis followed by fibrosis and contracture.
b. *Nerves:* Ischemia of arteria nervosa results in damage to nerves followed by partial or total sensorimotor dysfunction.

c. Complete arterial obstruction of the limb is very rare. Hence, gangrene is quite rare in compartment syndrome.

Q. What is the commonest cause of compartment syndrome?

Tight bandage/cast in the areas prone for compartment syndrome.

Q. What are other causes of compartment syndrome?

Burns, vascular injuries, reperfusion injuries, crush injuries, bleeding disorders, infections, intense athletic activity, and poor positioning during surgery.

Q. How do you clinically diagnose compartment syndrome?

The **most common clinical symptom is "pain out of proportion of the injury".**

Normally after the injury, pain decreases once patient receives medical aid in form of analgesics and splintage/cast application of the affected limb.

But in case of compartment syndrome, pain is quite severe and even after primary medical aid or splint/cast application, it remains very uncomforting or out of proportion of the injury and patient keeps demanding more analgesics.

Q. Why patients with compartment syndrome have pain out of proportion of injury?

It is due to the ischemia to the nerves (crying of the dying nerves!).

Treatment of compartment syndrome is
1. Remove all tight bandages, splint or cast
2. Urgent fasciotomy.
If untreated or treatment is delayed, it could result in VIC.

Q. What is the treatment of VIC of forearm and hand?

a. *Mild cases:* Splinting in functional position, stretching of tight structures.
b. *Moderate cases*
   1. Excision of fibronecrotic muscle mass in the compartment
   2. Flexor-pronator muscle sliding surgery *(Maxpage operation)*. The flexor groups of muscles are released (slided) from medial epicondyle.
   3. Lengthening (Z plasty) of muscle tendon unit.
   4. Neurolysis of the nerves as they are surrounded by thick fibrous tissue
   5. Bone shortening, proximal row carpectomy, wrist arthrodesis
c. *Severe cases*
   1. Free muscle transfer
   2. Nerve grafting and reconstructions
   3. Flap coverage of skin.

2

Congenital Musculoskeletal Conditions

CONGENITAL TALIPES EQUINUS VARUS (CTEV) OR CLUBFOOT

Common Presentation of Patient with CTEV

Case summary: A 6-month-old boy was brought to the hospital with deformity in his both feet since birth. The deformity was painless and non-progressive. There were no other associated congenital deformities in the body. He achieved all his milestones at regular interval. Prenatal and perinatal history was uneventful. General and systemic examinations are normal. On examination, both ankle–feet were in equinus, inversion and adduction. Both medial malleoli were hardly visible whereas lateral malleoli were more prominent. There were prominent medial and posterior creases. The neurovascular, spine and hip examinations were normal.

Q. What is the clinical diagnosis?

The clinical diagnosis is bilateral idiopathic congenital talipes equinus varus (it can also be called bilateral idiopathic congenital talipes equino cavo varus).

Q. Why do you say so?

It is because of the following reasons (Fig. 2.1):

History

1. Deformity present since birth

Examination

2. Ankle joint in plantar flexion: Equinus

Deformities in CTEV

A. Ankle-hindfoot:
   1. Equinus at ankle,
   2. Inversion at subtalar joint
B. Midfoot-forefoot:
   1. Adduction: Midtarsal
   2. Supination: Forefoot
   3. Midfoot cavus

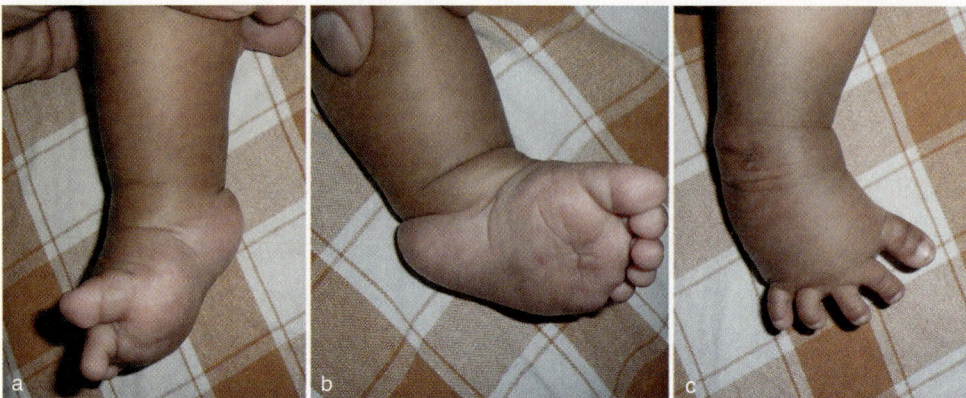

Figs 2.1a to c: Clinical photographs of idiopathic clubfoot showing hindfoot equinus, subtalar inversion and forefoot adduction

3. Subtalar joint inversion
4. Forefoot in adduction
5. Cavus

Q. What is the relevance of assessment of the flexibility of the deformed foot?

Flexibility of the foot implies whether the deformity present in the feet is passively over correctable/just correctable/partially correctable/not correctable.
a. If the deformity is passively correctable, it would respond very well to manipulation and plaster cast application.
b. If it is not passively correctable, then it implies it is a rigid deformity and
   1. Deformity may not respond easily to passive manipulation and cast application.
   2. The number of plaster required to correct the deformity would be more, and the chance of surgical interventions are higher.

Q. What are the other clinical findings in CTEV?

1. Tight tendo Achillis
2. Small heel in varus
3. Prominent lateral malleolus whereas medial malleolus is difficult to palpate
4. Splaying of toes
5. Small great toe
6. Prominent medial and posterior creases
7. Larger lateral border and smaller medial border of feet
8. Sole facing inward/medial wards
9. Older children who start walking, would have callosities over lateral border of foot and calf muscle wasting.

Q. What is the role of general, systemic and head to toe systematic examination?

Since this is a congenital abnormality, one must look for other congenital abnormalities in other systems.

Q. Why do you say that it is idiopathic CTEV?

Hip, spine and other joints of limbs are normal. There are no signs of spine anomalies and multiple congenital contractures.

Q. What is the need of examination of hip and spine?

In hip, there can be associated congenital dislocation of hip [developmental dysplasia of hip (DDH)].

In spine, there can be spina bifida (aperta or occulta)

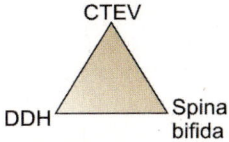

Always remember to look for TRIAD—feet, hip and spine.

Q. Why it is important to look for spina bifida?

Spina bifida (SB) can cause sensori-motor deficit in the lower limb resulting in weakness or paralysis of several muscle groups. Often, there is paralysis of ankle dorsiflexors and evertors of ankle-foot resulting in a foot which is **deformed in equinus and inversion** (TEV) as a result of muscle imbalance between dorsiflexor-evertor (weak/paralysed) and plantarflexor-invertor (normal and strong). A persistently strong muscle group initially causes a dynamic deformity. However, a persistent dynamic deformity ensues secondary static component due to local soft tissue contractures and deformed bones.

In case of CTEV with associated spine bifida, mere local soft tissue or bony correction of the deformity would correct the deformity temporarily. However, the deformity would soon recur as the primary etiology of the deformity (neurological deficit causing muscle imbalance) is not addressed. So in child with SB, **muscle imbalance due to neurological deficit must be addressed along with correction of local deformity.**

The muscle imbalance must be corrected either at the neurological level or by tendon transfers to **achieve a balanced normal foot**.

Further, same neurological deficit which causes foot deformity can also cause dislocation of hip due to powerful flexor and adductors of hip and weak extensor and abductors of the hip joint. Hence, examination of hip is must in cases of CTEV!

Q. What is the etiology/classification of a clubfoot?

a. *Idiopathic/primary:* No known causes
   1. *Uterine causes resulting in foot malposition:* Hydramnios
   2. *Muscular:* Local fibrosis of muscle
   3. Bony, tendon or ligamentous abnormalities
   4. Genetic
B. *Secondary*
   1. *Neurogenic or teratologic disorder:* Spina bifida, myelodysplasia
   2. *Syndromic:* AMC, tibial hemimelia, dystrophic dwarfism, amniotic band syndrome

Q. How to classify clubfoot/CTEV as per etiology?

1. *Idiopathic clubfoot*
   a. Postural (extrinsic): Deformity due to external pressure or faulty posture. It is easily correctable
   b. Rigid (intrinsic): Local internal contracture of muscle, tendon, capsule, muscle
2. *Neurogenic/Syndromic*

Q. What is the role of X-ray of ankle-foot in management of CTEV?

X-ray of the ankle-foot should be done to assess various angles which are helpful in assessing the severity of the deformity. The objective change in various angles during deformity correction also helps in monitoring the correction.

Q. Which clinical score is used to assess severity of the CTEV?

Pirani score is used to classify the severity of CTEV, and also helps in monitoring the progress of the correction. The scoring system allocates 0, 0.5 and 1.0 for each of following six clinical features.

Posterior crease, empty heel, ankle dorsiflexion, lateral border of foot, lateral head of talus, medial crease

Higher the score, severe is the deformity. A lowering score during manipulation indicates correction.

Q. How age of the patient determines the treatment of the CTEV?

The treatment of CTEV is according to age at presentation (Flowchart 2.1).
a. *From birth till one year:*
   • Most feet respond to serial manipulation followed by above knee case application. One can adopt Kite's or Ponseti method.
   • Rarely, the failed manipulation would require posteromedial soft tissue release (PMSTRs)
b. *Age; 1–3 years*
   Most patient require PMSTRs
c. *Age 3–13 years*
   All require PMSTRs along with bony osteotomy.
d. *Age >14 years*
   Triple arthrodesis

Q. How would you manage this patient (idiopathic bilateral CTEV)?

Since this child is 6 month old, I would like to do serial manipulation and above knee cast application.

Q. What is the order and technique of deformity correction by manipulation in CTEV??

Order of correction: Cavus, adduction, varus and then equinus with manipulation and serial cast application.

Technique: The manipulation and casting is done as an outpatient procedure with/without sedation.

Flowchart 2.1: Treatment of CTEV

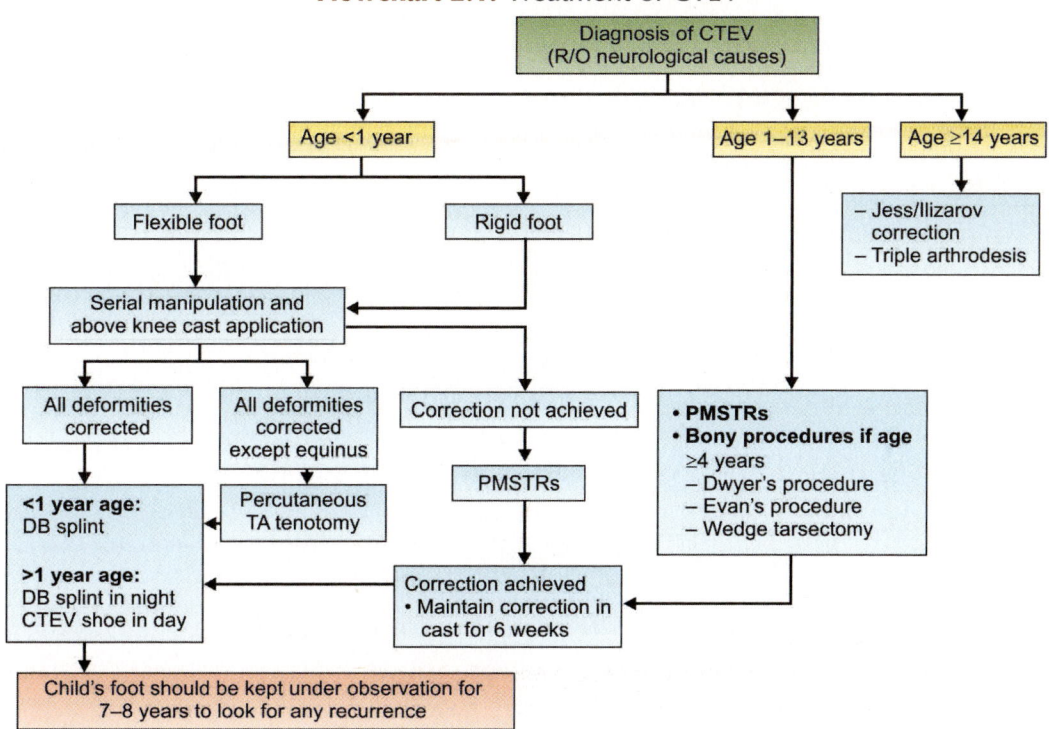

Diagnosis of CTEV
(R/O neurological causes)

Age <1 year | Age 1–13 years | Age ≥14 years

Age ≥14 years:
– Jess/Ilizarov correction
– Triple arthrodesis

Flexible foot | Rigid foot

Serial manipulation and above knee cast application

All deformities corrected | All deformities corrected except equinus | Correction not achieved

Age 1–13 years:
• PMSTRs
• Bony procedures if age ≥4 years
– Dwyer's procedure
– Evan's procedure
– Wedge tarsectomy

<1 year age: DB splint

Percutaneous TA tenotomy

PMSTRs

>1 year age: DB splint in night CTEV shoe in day

Correction achieved
• Maintain correction in cast for 6 weeks

Child's foot should be kept under observation for 7–8 years to look for any recurrence

- **After the manipulation and correction, above knee POP** cast is applied (Fig. 2.2)
- Cast is changed at **weekly or once in 15 days** interval. Response to serial casting is to be monitored on each visit after removal of the previous cast.
- All deformities are corrected by manipulation in Kite's technique whereas the equinus is corrected by TA tenotomy in Ponseti technique.

Once the correction is achieved, the correction is maintained in Denis-Browne (DB) splint/foot abduction brace (clubfoot brace) in a child <12 months. Once child starts walking, CTEV shoes are provided in the daytime and DB splint is continued in night the night.

> **Order of deformity correction (CAVE)**
> Cavus, adduction, varus and equinus

Q. Why above knee cast is applied in CTEV?

Above knee cast is applied due to several reasons.

a. Muscles causing equinus are gastrocsoleus complex which originate above the knee joint. So, by keeping the knee flexed, gastrocsoleus complex is relaxed and equinus correction becomes easy.

b. The plaster bandage to correct inversion is pulled over the femur (thigh) giving a support for correction of inversion.

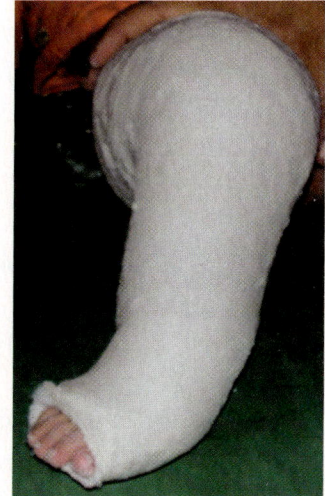

Fig. 2.2: Clubfoot correction with above knee cast

Q. What are the different methods of manipulation and cast techniques for treatment of clubfoot? Which one is more popular?

Ponseti and Kite methods are used to correct CTEV. Currently, Ponseti method is more popular. Table below outlines the difference between the two techniques.

Deformity correction	Ponseti's method	Kite's method
Cavus	Corrected first	Not mentioned
Fulcrum for correction: Correction achieved	Lateral part of talar head 1. Forefoot adduction, 2. Hindfoot varus	Calcaneocuboid joint 1. Forefoot varus Hindfoot varus corrected by direct calcaneum eversion
Hind foot equinus correction	Achieved by TA tenotomy	By cast wedging

Q. Why Ponseti technique is very popular nowadays?

Ponseti technique has shown to give more rapid and constant correction than any other technique of manipulation and casting.

Q. How early is treatment of CTEV is started?

It is advisable to start treatment as early as possible as initiation of early treatment is associated with good results.

Q. What will happen if 'CAVE' order of correction is not followed?

The foot will end up in rocker bottom foot deformity.

Note: Rocker bottom foot is a deformity wherein the sole of foot becomes convex like rocker bottom chair!

Q. Which other condition could result in "rocker bottom foot" deformity?

Congenital vertical talus.

In case rocker bottom deformity develops, the deformity of CTEV is re-created and then correct order of correction is followed.

Q. How to correct a deformity if soft tissue manipulation fails?

Soft tissue and or bony surgeries should be performed as per the age of the patient to achieve correction of the deformity.

Q. What is the name of soft tissue surgery for CTEV?

It is known as **posteromedial soft tissue release surgery** (PMSTRs).

No bony surgery (osteotomy) to be performed before 4 years of age.

Q. What is the minimum age of soft tissue surgery for CTEV and why?

Currently, minimum age for CTEV surgery is about one year because:

1. Most deformities are correctable with serial casting with/without TA tenotomy. So, the chance that a foot would require PMSTRs is quite rare.
2. Even if surgery is required, serial casting reduces the extent of deformity leading to lesser soft tissue release requirement during surgery.

The results of serial manipulation and cast application in CTEV are excellent. All attempts must be done to correct all deformities in CTEV by conservative treatment before embarking upon surgical correction as the results of conservative treatment are superior to operative treatment.

Q. Which structures are released in PMSTRs?

1. *Posterior*

   a. *Tendon:* Tendo Achillis—tenotomy/lengthening
   b. *Capsule:* Ankle and subtalar joint capsule—capsulotomy, capsulectomy
   c. *Ligaments:* Posterior talofibular, calcaneofibular—release ligaments

2. *Medial*

   a. *Tendon:* Lengthening of tibialis posterior, flexor digitorum, flexor hallucis longus
   b. *Capsule:* Subtalar, talonavicular
   c. *Ligament:* Talonavicular, deltoid and spring

3. *Plantar*

   a. *Muscle-tendon:* Flexor digitorum brevis and abductor hallucis is released from calcaneum
   b. *Fascia:* Plantar fascia released from calcaneum

Once the soft tissue release is over, the **correction must be maintained in above knee cast for 6 weeks.** After cast removal, foot is maintained in DB splint till one year followed by DB splint (nights) and CTEV shoes (day walking time) after one year.

Q. What is special about DB splint?

It appears to be a static splint. However, **it is a dynamic splint** as when infant kicks one side of DB splint, the other foot goes in eversion and dorsiflexion due to central connecting bar (Fig. 2.3).

Q. What are the characteristics of CTEV shoe?

Following are the characteristics of CTEV shoe (Fig. 2.4):

1. *No heel:* Prevents ankle equinus
2. *Lateral border shoe raise:* Prevents subtalar inversion
3. *Medial border straight and stiff:* Prevents forefoot adduction

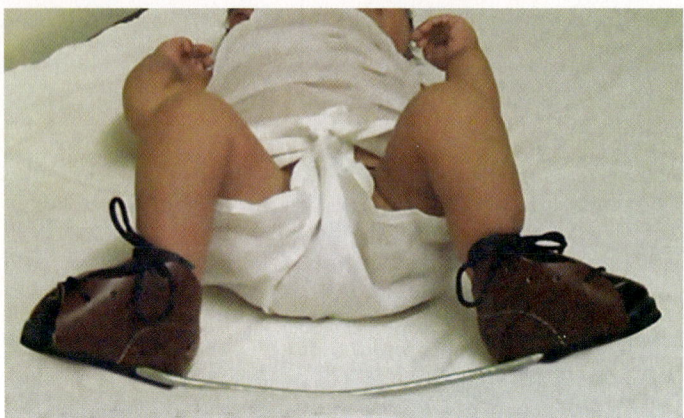

Fig. 2.3: Clinical photograph of clubfoot child treated with DB splint with its interconnecting bar after full correction of the clubfoot

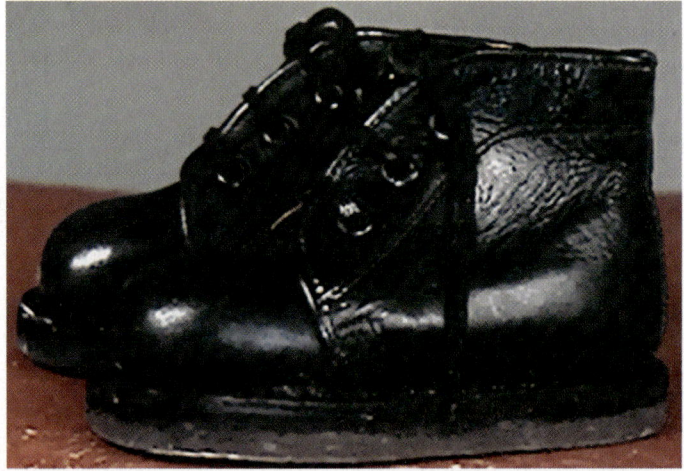

Fig. 2.4: CTEV shoe showing lateral sole raise, no heel and medial straight border

Q. What is the minimum age of bony surgery for CTEV and why?

The **minimum age for bony surgery is 4 years** because the bones are mostly cartilaginous before the age of four years.

1. If osteotomy is performed before 4 years, it would end up removing excess cartilage resulting in short foot.
2. The osteotomy performed in a cartilaginous bone would not heal, and the osteotomy fusion site might end up in non-union.

Q. What are the commonly performed osteotomies or bony surgeries in CTEV correction?

1. *Dwyer's osteotomy:* Lateral closing wedge calcaneal osteotomy to **correct heel varus**
2. *Dilwyn-Evans osteotomy:* Calcaneocuboid fusion to **correct forefoot adduction**

3. *Triple arthrodesis:* It is performed in children older than 14 years to achieve correction in a neglected CTEV foot. In triple arthrodesis, three joint are fused: Talocalcaneal, calcaneocuboid and talonavicular.

Q. In which condition, CTEV is associated with multiple contractures all over the body?

It is known as arthrogryposis multiplex congenita (AMC) which is associated with contracture over the shoulder, hip, knee, elbow, ankle, etc. It is also called multiple congenital contracture (MCC).

Q. Which is the most commonly recurring deformity?

Equinus at the ankle joint.

Q. Which component of CTEV deformity often remains uncorrected?

Forefoot adduction.

Q. What surgery can be performed in a neglected CTEV after 14 years?

Following surgeries can be performed:
1. Triple arthrodesis
2. Ilizarov's correction

Q. Which three joints are fused in triple arthrodesis operation?

Subtalar, talonavicular and calcaneocuboid joints are fused in triple arthrodesis.

DEVELOPMENTAL DYSPLASIA OF HIP (DDH)

Common Presentation of Child with DDH

Case summary: A one-year-old girl was brought to the hospital with painless limp after walking age. There were no other associated congenital deformities. All developmental milestones were normal. Prenatal and perinatal history was uneventful. General and systemic examination was normal. On examination, left lower limb was short with asymmetrical gluteal crease. Left side abduction of the hip joint was limited with exaggeration of both rotations. Left side Galeazzi test, telescopy and Trendelenburg were positive. There was 1 cm true supratrochanteric shortening on left side. Neurovascular examination of distal limbs and examination of spine were normal.

Q. What is the clinical diagnosis?

The clinical diagnosis is left side developmental dysplasia of the hip (DDH).

Q. Justify your clinical diagnosis.

History
1. Painless limp since child started walking
2. Female child

Examination
3. Asymmetrical gluteal fold
4. Limitation of passive abduction on left side
5. True shortening (supratrochanteric)
6. Positive Galeazzi, telescopic and Trendelenburg tests

Q. What is the meaning of dislocatable hip, relocatable hip and dislocated hip?

Dislocatable hip: When femoral head can be moved out of the acetabular socket by gentle force.

Relocatable hip: When femoral head can be moved inside the acetabular socket by gentle force.

Dislocated hip: When femoral head is already present outside of the acetabular socket.

Q. What is the meaning of dislocated hip?

When the **femoral head is present outside of the socket** of the acetabulum, it is called dislocated hip.

Q. What do you mean as dysplastic hip?

When the femoral head is present in the socket of the acetabulum with **flattening of the acetabulum,** it is called dysplastic hip.

Q. What are predisposing factors for occurrence of DDH?

Ligamentous laxity and acetabular dysplasia are main predisposing factors for occurrence of DDH.

Risk factors for DDH

- First born
- Female child
- Breech delivery
- Postmaturity
- Left side
- Ligamentous laxity
- Positive family history

Q. What are clinical screening tests for DDH at birth?

Barlow and Ortolani tests are useful to detect DDH at birth.

Q. How do you perform Barlow test?

Barlow test is a provocative test. It is performed with child lying supine with hip flexed to 90°. Examiner's thumb is placed on medial aspect of the thigh with index and middle fingers placed on lateral aspect of greater trochanter. Examiner adducts the thigh while applying lateral pressure with the thumb. If the hip dislocates, the Barlow test is considered to be positive.

Q. What is the inference of positive Barlow test?

A positive Barlow test indicates that the **hip is dislocatable.**

Q. How do you perform Ortolani test?

Ortolani test is performed with child lying supine and hip flexed to 90°. Examiner's thumb is placed on medial aspect of the thigh with index and middle fingers placed on lateral aspect of greater trochanter. Examiner abducts the thigh while applying pressure on the greater trochanter. If the femoral head relocates into the acetabulum with a palpable click, the Ortolani test is considered to be positive.

Q. What is the inference of positive Ortolani test?

A positive Ortolani test indicates that the **hip is relocatable** (reducible).

Q. Why Ortolani test is not possible to perform after the age of 6 months?

In children older than 6 months, the chronic contracture of soft tissues around the dislocated femoral head does not allow it to be relocatable by the examiner during Ortolani test. Therefore, the utility of Ortolani test is not established in patients older than 6 months.

Q. Which investigation is necessary to confirm your clinical diagnosis?

Plain radiograph-pelvis with both hips; AP and Von Rosen view.

Q. What are the parameters to be observed in the radiograph of pelvis with hips in a child with DDH?

AP view of the pelvis is quite important which reveals following signs (Fig. 2.5).

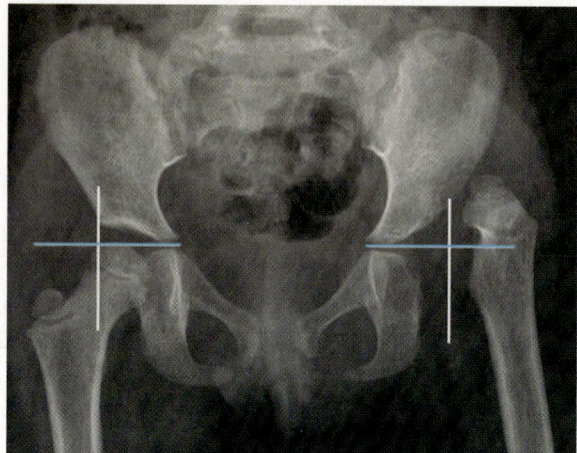

Fig. 2.5: Plain radiograph DDH child showing left side hip dislocation with marking of Perkin's (white) and Hilgenreiner's (blue) line

1. **Break in the Shenton's line** (line along the lower border of the superior pubic ramus should pass along lower border of neck of the femur)
2. **Abnormal position of the femoral epiphysis**; proximal to Hilgenreiner's line (horizontal line connecting the triradiate cartilages), lateral to Perkin's line (vertical line from outer margin of acetabulum)
3. **High acetabular angle** (angle between Hilgenreiner line and another line joining triradiate cartilage to superior outer margin of acetabular)
4. **USG of the hip:** In a child younger than 4 months or *in utero*.

Q. How do you diagnose DDH in neonatal period?

Clinically DDH is suspected with positive Ortolani and Barlow tests. It can be confirmed with ultrasound of the hip.

Q. Why do you use ultrasound to diagnose DDH rather than a plain radiograph in neonatal child?

The proximal capital femoral epiphysis is not ossified before 4–6 months, so the proximal femur is not visible in plain radiograph. Therefore, ultrasound is used to diagnose DDH in neonates.

Q. What is the goal of treatment in DDH?

The principle goal of treatment in DDH is to obtain **concentric reduction of the hip joint till the hip joint is stable and congruent, and follow up till skeletal maturity.**

Q. What is the plan of management of a patient with DDH?

The treatment plan is based upon the age of the patient and feasibility of reduction by closed or open method (Flowchart 2.2).

1. *Newborn to 6 months:* Closed reduction (CR) and maintain by Pavlik harness (Fig. 2.8)

2. *6–18 months:* Closed/open reduction and maintained in hip spica for 2–3 months. Once hip is stable, DDH splint (Denis Browne splint) is applied.
3. *18 months to 6 years:* "Closed reduction is not possible"

Open reduction and maintain in hip spica. Additional procedure like
   - Adductor tenotomy
   - Femoral shortening
   - Varus derotation osteotomy (VDO) on femur
   - Acetabular reconstruction by various osteotomies like Salter's, Dega's or Pemberton
4. *7–10 years:* Unilateral DDH: OR and VDO, femoral shortening, acetabuloplasty.
   Bilateral DDH: It can be left alone
5. *Age >10 years:* Uni- or bilateral DDH, it can be left alone.

Q. What is the plan to manage this patient who is one-year-old?

Since this patient is one-year-old, the DDH can be managed with CR/OR and spica application under general anesthesia (Fig. 2.6). Hip spica should be retained for 3 months.

Q. Which surgery is commonly performed on femoral side to achieve reduction?

On femoral side, two surgeries are performed.
1. Open reduction of dislocation
2. Varus derotation osteotomy (VDO) is performed to achieve concentric and stable reduction into the acetabular cavity (Fig. 2.7).

Q. What would a concentrically reduced hip would do on bony morphology of femoral head and acetabulum in children with DDH?

Once femoral head is concentrically reduced and maintained in the acetabulum, the remodeling of the femoral head and acetabulum will occur resulting in a stable hip joint.

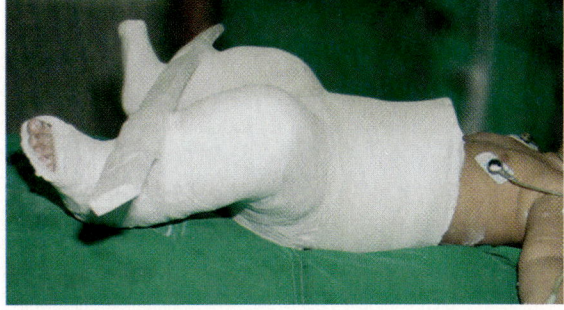

Fig. 2.6: Hip spica after closed reduction of DDH

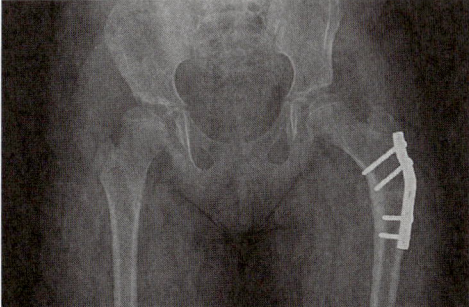

Fig. 2.7: Plain X-ray of child with left side DDH treated with varus derotation osteotomy showing reduced hip with union at osteotomy site

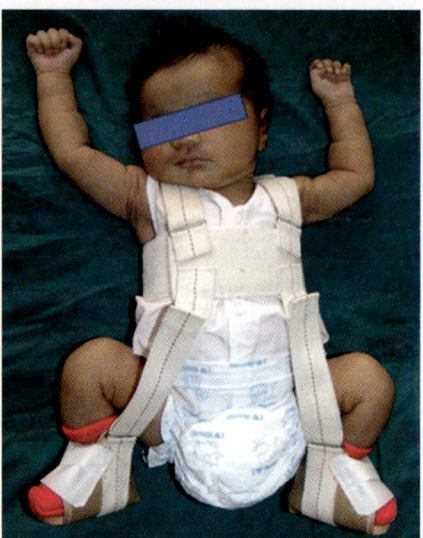

Fig. 2.8: Infant with DDH treated with Pavlik harness

Flowchart 2.2: Hip DDH management

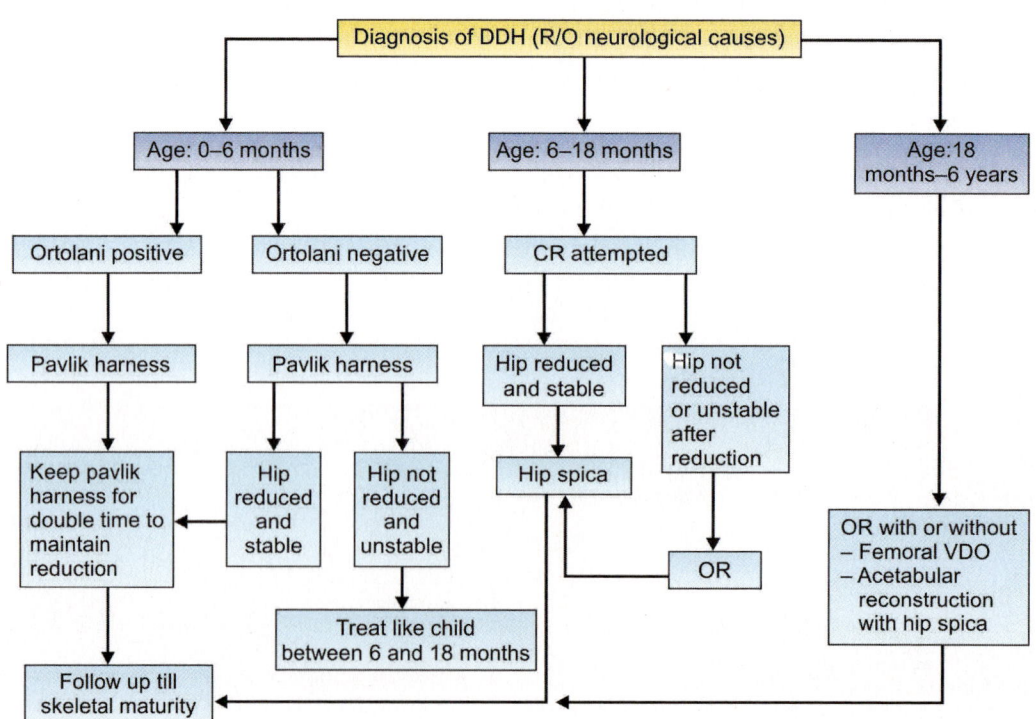

SPINA BIFIDA

Common Presentation of Patient with Spina Bifida

Case summary: A one-year-old boy was brought to the hospital with deformity in his left feet since birth which was gradually progressive. He achieved all his milestones at regular interval. Prenatal and perinatal history was uneventful. General and systemic examination was normal. Lumbar spine revealed tuft of hair with a palpatory underlying bony defect. O/E, left foot was in equinus, inversion and adduction. Child was not responding to deep touch on dorsum of the left foot. Active movements of toes and ankle were absent. Hips and upper limbs examination was normal.

Q. What is the clinical diagnosis?

The clinical diagnosis is left-sided **neurogenic congenital talipes equinus varus** due to spina bifida.

Q. Why do you say so?

It is so because of following reasons:

History
1. Deformity in foot present since birth,
2. Tuft of hair at the lower back (indicates spina bifida occulta) (Fig. 2.9)

Examination
3. Ankle joint in plantar flexion (equinus), hindfoot varus and forefoot in adduction
4. Child is not responding to deep touch on left foot dorsum (sensory loss)
5. Palpable interspinous step at lumbosacral area
6. Active movements of left foot and ankle are absent

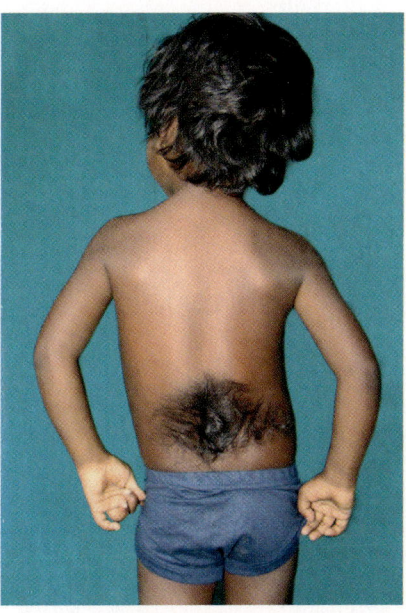

Fig. 2.9: Child with spina bifida occulta showing tuft of hair on lower lumbar spine

Q. What other clinical findings should be looked for?

1. Tight tendo Achillis
2. Small heel
3. Small great toe
4. Small foot **(asymmetrical size of the foot is always secondary to underlying neurological disorder)**
5. Older children may have callosities over lateral border of foot as they start walking (if sensory system is normal)
6. Older children may present with **neuropathic ulceration of lateral border of the foot** as they start walking (if sensory system is affected)

Q. How neurogenic clubfoot is different than idiopathic clubfoot clinically?

There are several neurologic features present along with deformity in neurogenic clubfoot.
1. Motor deficit can lead to paralysis and deformity.
2. Sensory deficit leads to neuropathic ulcer.
3. Autonomic dysfunction leads to bladder and bowel incontinence.

Q. Why management in clubfoot secondary to spina bifida is different than idiopathic clubfoot?

The foot deformity secondary to spina bifida is due to **muscle imbalance (paralysis of dorsiflexors and evertors of ankle)**. Hence, mere correction of the deformity may not address the underlying muscle imbalance; there are high chances of recurrence if only soft tissue release and/bony osteotomy is done. **Muscle imbalance must be addressed** in child with underlying neurological deficit.

Q. What is the meaning of spina bifida?

Spina bifida means "split spine". It is due to failure of closure of the neural tube.

Q. What are types of spina bifida?

A. **Spina bifida cystica** (or spina bifida aperta) (Fig. 2.10)
   • Meningocele
   • Myelomeningocele
   • Myeloschisis
B. **Spina bifida occulta** (hidden)

Q. Which other systems must be examined in patients with spina bifida?

I would like to examine from head to toe as **associated hydrocephalus, renal damage** due to ascending infection to neurogenic bladder and spinal deformities are common associated features in spina bifida.

Q. Which investigations are required before treatment?

1. *Radiographs of spine and pelvis:* To confirm spina bifida, sacral agenesis, DDH
2. *MRI of spine/brain:* To rule out intraspinal anomalies.

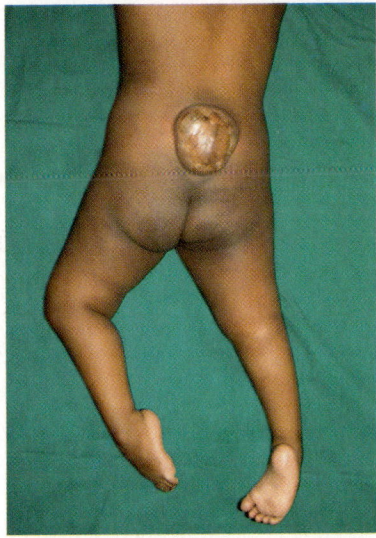

Fig. 2.10: Child with meningomyelocele (spina bifida aperta) showing swelling on lower lumbar spine with bilateral clubfeet

Q. What is the treatment of clubfoot due to spina bifida in infant?

The clubfoot can be treated by **serial manipulation and serial casting like idiopathic clubfoot**. Special care is needed while casting these feet as **neuropathic ulcers can develop** if the cast is not well moulded and padded.

1. So, **well-padded cast** is required.
2. **Tenotomy of Achilles tendon is mandatory** and **excision of a segment of tendon may be preferred** to a simple tenotomy as relapses are quite frequent in neurogenic clubfoot.

Q. How do you treat child above one year?

1. Posteromedial soft tissue releases (PMSTRs) with excision of contracted tendons is required in this child.
2. The gastroc-soleus and the tibialis posterior are functioning normal**, they may be transferred** to **restore muscle balance** and thus reduce the chance of recurrence.
3. The child must be protected with soft liner orthosis to prevent early recurrence of the deformity.

Q. How do you treat same deformity in older children?

1. PMSTR combined with tendon transfers and extra-articular osteotomies.
2. A**void fusing joints** of the foot especially **if sensation of the sole is lost** as fusion increases the risk of neuropathic ulceration.

Q. How do you treat sensory loss in child with spina bifida?

It is important to prevent complication of sensory loss (neuropathic ulceration). One must educate the parents and child for proper care of anesthetic feet and use of soft-lined footwear.

If there are deformities in the foot, it should be corrected to obtain plantigrade foot which minimizes the risk of neuropathic ulceration by increasing the area of contact of the sole, thereby decreasing the pressure.

Q. Which periconceptional vitamin deficiency in mother is associated with spina bifida?

Folic acid deficiency in periconceptional period.

Q. How to detect neural tube defects during the pregnancy?

It can be detected with the help of perinatal ultrasound scan and alpha fetoprotein levels in amniotic fluid.

Q. What is the treatment of spina bifida aperta?

Open spina bifida (cystica/aperta) must be closed by neurosurgeons.

Q. Will that change the prognosis of neurological deficit?

It may not. It will help in reducing the chance of meningitis but the neurological deficit may or may not recover.

3

Bone and Joint Infections

CHRONIC OSTEOMYELITIS

Common Presentation of Patient with Osteomyelitis

Case summary: A 16-year-old boy case of pain, swelling and discharging sinus from right arm for last six months. Six month back, he met with a RTA and sustained open fracture of humerus. He underwent debridement and above elbow cast application. 2 weeks later, he developed multiple sinuses around the fracture site with purulent discharge. There was minimal pain at rest and occasional history of fever. There was no loss of weight or appetite. General and systemic examination was normal. Local examination revealed single discharging sinus with a bead of pus at the tip of sinus at the upper end of arm with several other healed sinuses. Adjacent skin was hyperpigmented and scarred. On palpation, humerus shaft was thickened, tender and irregular. Sinus was fixed to the underlying bone. Abnormal mobility was present in mid-shaft of humerus and arm was short by 5 cm. The shoulder and elbow range of movement were decreased. Neurovascular examination was normal.

Q. What is the clinical diagnosis?

The clinical diagnosis is chronic osteomyelitis of right humerus with non-union of fracture shaft humerus with shoulder and elbow stiffness.

Q. Why do you say so?

It because of following reasons:

History
1. History of trauma with open fracture (open fracture is predisposed to infection)
2. Recurrent discharge from the fracture site

Examination
3. Underlying bone is thick, tender and irregular
4. Discharging sinus which is fixed to the underlying bone (Fig. 3.1)
5. Abnormal mobility at fracture site: signifies non-union.

Note: Points 3, 4 are hallmark signs of chronic osteomyelitis. Sinus may be absent as sometimes patient may present in quiescent phase of chronic osteomyelitis. However, underlying bone should be thickened, irregular and/tender.

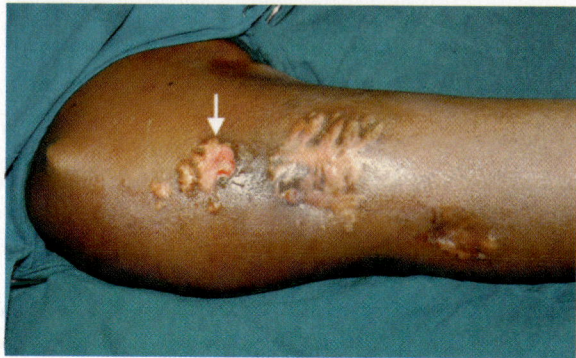

Fig. 3.1: Clinical picture showing discharging sinus over arm and multiple scars

Typical signs of chronic osteomyelitis
- Underlying thick, irregular and tender bone
- Discharging sinus fixed to underlying bone

Q. What is the reason behind infection of humerus?

Bone got infected because of *open fracture resulting in direct infection of the bone.*

Note: In case of open fracture where internal fixation by plate/nail is performed, chance of infection is high as implant acts as foreign body which in turn acts a nidus for infection. Hence, safer fixation modality of an open fracture would be an external fixator.

Q. How to investigate such a case?

1. **Complete blood picture**
   a. *Hemoglobin:* Normal or low (can be low because of anaemia of chronic disease, low appetite)
   b. *TLC:* Normal or high (high, if acute exacerbation)
   c. *DLC:* Normal or high neutrophil count (high if acute exacerbation)
   d. *ESR:* Elevated or normal
   e. *CRP:* Elevated or normal (high with acute exacerbation)
2. **X-ray** of the bone would reveal following findings (Fig. 3.2)
   a. Thick, irregular bone
   b. Periosteal reaction
   c. Sequestrum
   d. Involucrum
   e. Lytic areas
   f. Occasionally pathological fracture
   g. Deformity
3. **Sinogram:** To outline the sinus tract (Fig. 3.3)

Note: Performed only if sinus present

4. **Gram stain, culture and sensitivity of pus:** The pus collected from sinus opening at surface may grow bacterial contaminants, and may not represent real organism

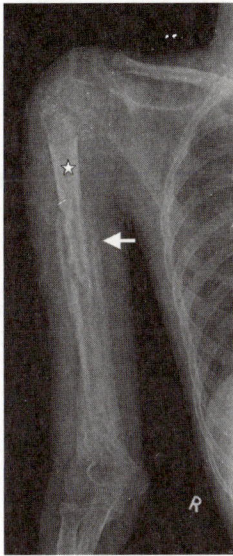

Fig. 3.2: Plain X-ray of humerus shows extensive sequestrum (star) and involucrum around sequestrum (arrow)

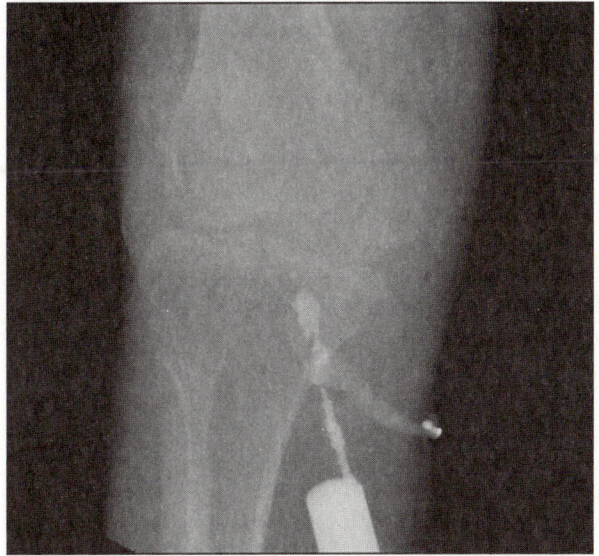

Fig. 3.3: Sinogram (different patient with OM of tibia) showing radiopaque dye being injected into the sinus outlining the sinus tract

causing infection. Hence, it is prudent to collect the pus from the depth of sinus/cavity especially during exploration of cavity during surgery as it would have minimal chance of contamination.

5. **CT scan:** If sequestrum is not visualized properly on a plain X-ray.
6. **MRI scan:** If there is associated soft tissue abscess
7. **Bone biopsy:** It is the most certain way of establishing the diagnosis especially if one is suspecting tubercular osteomyelitis.

Note: In general, bone scan or MRI scan is not done for the diagnosis of chronic osteomyelitis. Bone scan and MRI are helpful in the diagnosis of acute osteomyelitis in early phase (within 2–3 weeks of onset of infection) when X-ray is normal.

Q. What are the principles of treatment of chronic osteomyelitis?

The treatment of chronic osteomyelitis is always surgical. Medical treatment in form of antibiotic is started only after the surgery.

The fundamental of treatment of chronic osteomyelitis involves following principles.

1. Treatment of *dead tissues*
2. Treatment of *dead space*

Step 1: Treatment of dead bone, tissue
- Sinus tract excision
- Sequestrectomy
- Saucerisation

- Curretage
- Antibiotic impregnated bone cement may be added.

After step 1 of surgical treatment, antibiotic treatment (according to culture-sensitivity) is started and continued for 6–8 weeks. (2–3 weeks IV and 4–6 weeks oral).

Step 2: Treatment of dead space (after step 1)
- Bone grafting
- Myocutaneous/fasciocutaneous flaps

Q. What is the meaning of "treatment of dead tissues"?

It involves certain steps (Figs 3.4 to 3.7)
1. **Sinus tract excision**
2. **Sequestrectomy** (Fig. 3.5)
3. **Saucerisation:** The cavity of chronic osteomyelitis is often a "narrow mouth pitcher" shape cavity which must be converted into a "wide mouth saucer" like cavity so that infected purulent material must not pent up inside and should keep draining easily through a wide opening (Fig. 3.6).
d. **Curettage:** Curettage helps in converting infected, sclerosed margin to healthy bleeding edges which helps in healing by delivering antibiotics and immune cells in the curetted cavity via opened up blood vessels which were closed due to sclerosis.
e. **Antibiotic impregnated bone cement:** For prolonged local delivery of antibiotics (Fig. 3.7). Later, beads are removed after 4–6 weeks by re-surgery.

Note: There are substances available (absorbable calcium sulphate) which can be mixed with antibiotics like vancomycin/gentamycin and left in the dead space. These substances get absorbed and need not be removed unlike non-absorbable bone cement.

After the surgical treatment, **long-term antibiotic therapy is continued for 6–8 weeks according to culture and sensitivity reports.**

Note: If there is internal fixation device like plate/nail, it has to be removed in order to get rid of infection nidus. External fixation can be done if fracture is not yet united.

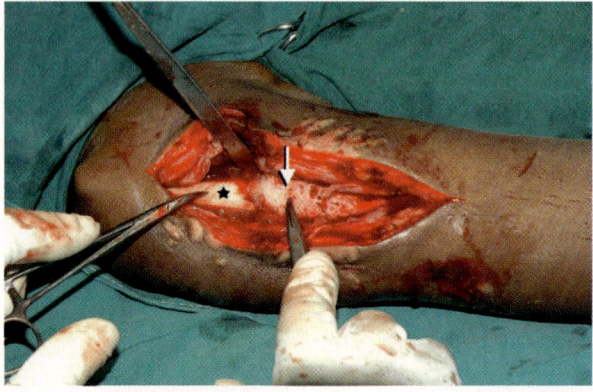

Fig. 3.4: Surgical exploration of osteomyelitic humerus shows sequestrum (star) and involucrum (arrow)

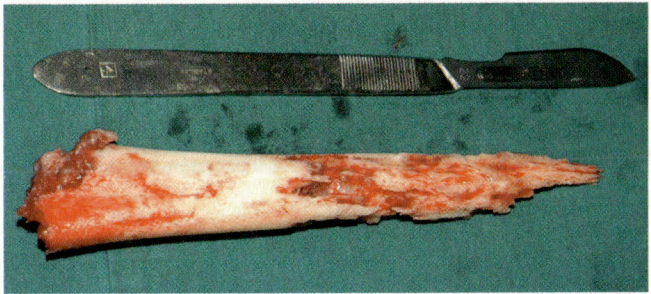

Fig. 3.5: Long diaphyseal sequestrum removed from the humerus

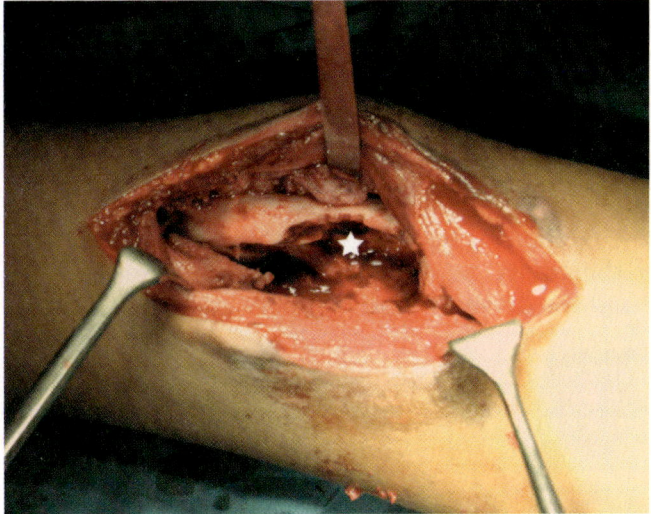

Fig. 3.6: Saucerisation of infected cavity (white star)

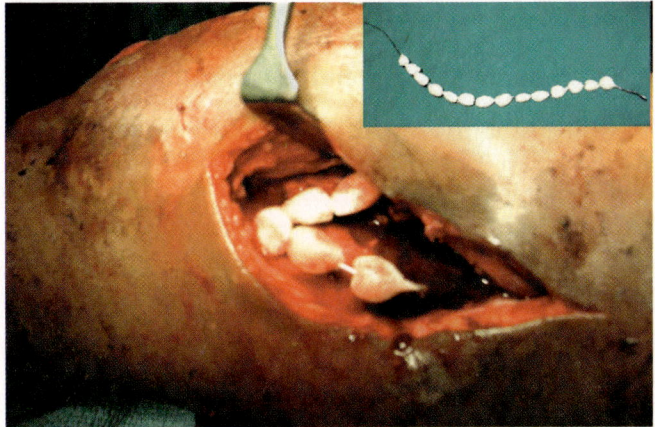

Fig. 3.7: Application of gentamicin beads into the cavity after saucerisation. Inset picture shows freshly prepared gentamicin beads from bone cement mixed with gentamicin loaded onto the stainless steel (SS) wire

Q. What antibiotic should be started after surgery, and how long it should be continued?

Broad spectrum antibiotic should be started immediately after surgery covering gram-positive (vancomycin/linezolid) and gram-negative (3rd generation cephaosporin) bacteria.

It should be switched to specific antibiotic after the C/S reports are ready.

The antibiotic therapy should be continued for 6–8 weeks (2–3 weeks IV, followed 4–6 weeks oral).

> Commonly, almost every student in reply to question of "how will you treat chronic osteomyelitis" invariably replies, I will give antibiotics. Remember! Antibiotic therapy is NOT a primary treatment of choice of chronic osteomyelitis. Surgery is the primary treatment of choice followed by antibiotics for 6–8 weeks.

Q. Why lone medical treatment is not preferred over surgical treatment in chronic osteomyelitis?

1. Sequestrum is avascular and acts as nidus of infection, and therefore resistant to any antibiotic treatment. Unless, sequestrum is removed surgically, antibiotics cannot make it sterile due to its avascularity.
2. In chronic osteomyelitis, the margin of infected cavity is sclerosed causing is poor vascularity of the cavity resulting in inadequate delivery of antibiotics and immune cells into the cavity which, hampers infection control/eradication.

   A thorough surgical debridement of local tissues, saucerisation and curettage of cavity helps in removing the infected granulation tissue, broadens the drainage area and increases the blood supply to the lesion (due to curettage of sclerosed margins of cavity) helps in eradicating the infection.

Q. What is the most optimal time of performing sequestrectomy and saucerisation?

The sequestrectomy and saucerisation is performed only after mature involucrum is formed all around the sequestrum. A **minimum of 2/3rd circumference** of cortical bone should have involucrum before sequestrectomy is performed.

Q. What will happen if sequestrectomy and saucerisation is performed prematurely?

If sequestrectomy and saucerisation is performed prematurely, i.e. without having adequate involucrum support, there is a chance of pathological fracture as the residual cortical bone would be inadequate to provide support and would not be able to endure the stresses over the bone.

Q. How to manage the large dead space created after saucerisation?

The dead space could result in re-infection and remains a potential risk factor for pathological fracture. Hence, it must be obliterated/filled by:

1. Once infection is controlled, "delayed open cancellous bone graft" **(papineau technique)** or "free vascular fibular graft" of the cavity can be performed after 3–4 weeks.
2. Filling or covering the space by myocutaneous fasciocutaneous flaps.

Q. What is the most appropriate way to stabilise a pathological fracture in chronic osteomyelitis?

External fixator should be used to stabilize the pathological fracture in chronic osteomyelitis.

Note: It is important to understand that an ***internal fixation device (plate/nail) should be avoided*** in case of chronic bone infection as an internal implant would invite ***formation of biofilm*** by the bacteria, and bacteria can thrive under the biofilm by avoiding the bactericidal/static effects of antibiotics. Thus eradication of infection becomes quite difficult in presence of an internal implant.

Note: Biofilm is an extracellular polymeric substance (EPS), a gooey substance secreted by the bacteria which is a network of sugars, protein and DNA. Biofilm enables a microbe to stick together on a surface. Layers and layers of EPS can form over each other and these biofilm layers.

Q. What are the complications of chronic osteomyelitis?

1. Acute exacerbations of infection
2. Pathological fracture
3. Growth disturbance (in children with open physis)
4. Deformity
5. Amyloidosis
6. Septic arthritis
7. Sinus tract malignancy (squamous cell carcinoma); usually after 15–20 years of persistent infection.

Q. Define sequestrum.

Sequestrum is a dead piece of bone surrounded by involucrum and infected granulation tissue in the body.

Q. What are the various types of sequestrum?

1. **Feathery:** Tuberculosis of ribs
2. **Sandy:** Tuberculosis of vertebra or Brodie's abscess
3. **Ring:** Amputation stumps/infected Steinmann pin tract
4. **Ivory:** Tibia in syphilis
5. **Black:** Open fracture due to bone exposure
6. **Diaphyseal:** Entire diaphyseal involvement

Note: In practice, "type of sequestrum" has no/minimal significance as diagnosis is not ascertained by the appearance of sequestrum. It is confirmed by the histopathology.

Q. Define involucrum.

Involucrum is the new bone formed around the sequestrum.

Note: Involucrum formation is the bone's response to re-strengthen the bone structure due to sequestered bone

Q. What happens if the involucrum formation is poor?

The affected bone remains susceptible for pathological fracture.

Q. How will you overcome the stiffness of the shoulder and elbow?

a. Physiotherapy

b. Surgical release of stiff joint if physiotherapy fails to optimize range of motion.

Note: Refer the chapter on stiff joint in trauma section (*see* page 47).

Q. How will you manage shortening in this patient?

Shortening in upper limb is well tolerated. So, it does not require any active treatment.

Q. In this case, the humerus fracture has not united. How to treat non-union in presence of infection?

In case of infected non-union of humerus or any other bone, there are two standard ways to treat infected non-union.

1. *Two stage procedure:* First, treat the infection along the lines of principles of treatment of chronic osteomyelitis. Once infection settles, one can treat the "aseptic nonunion" by open reduction, freshening bone edges, opening up of medullary canal and internal/external fixation with bone grafting.

2. *Single stage procedure:*

Using Ilizarov technique, whole infected segment is resected and infected necrotic tissues are thoroughly debrided followed by reconstruction of new bone with the principles of "compression-distraction osteogenesis" (Fig. 3.8).

Q. How to be sure that there is no infection anymore at the non-union site?

Clinically: Painless, no fever and no more active sinuses for at least several months.
Serology: ESR and CRP should remain normal for at least 6 months.

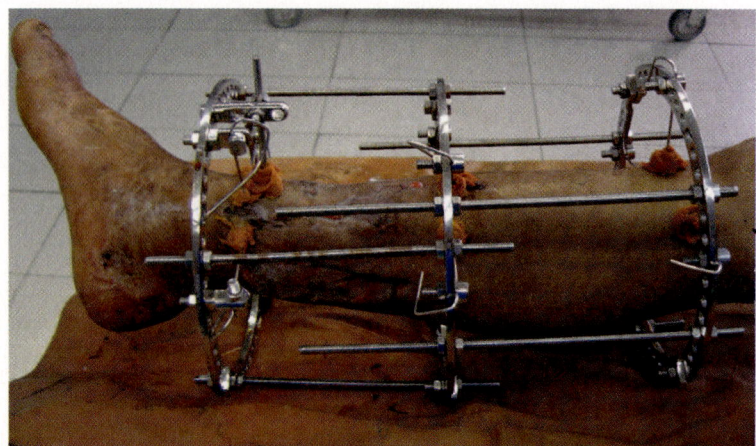

Fig. 3.8: Ilizarov's external fixator applied on the limb for the purpose of limb lengthening

Note: Principle of Ilizarov's technique: Compression-distraction osteogenesis

Q. Classify osteomyelitis?

A. *According to Route of Spread*

1. *Direct osteomyelitis:* Mostly, due to trauma and can happen in any region (metaphyseal/diaphyseal)
2. *Indirect or haematogenous osteomyelitis:* It occurs in metaphysis.

B. *Type of Infection*

Pyogenic/tubercular/fungal

C. *Duration of Infection*

1. *Acute:* <6 weeks
2. *Primary subacute:* 6–12 weeks—Brodies abscess, Garre's sclerosing osteomyelitis
3. *Chronic:* >12 weeks.

Q. Why hematogenous osteomyelitis occurs in metaphysis?

It occurs in metaphysis due to following reasons:

a. Hair pin loop configuration of metaphyseal vessels results in slowing down of the vascular flow and allows bacteria to multiply.
b. High cell turnover in metaphyseal region leading to availability of more dead cells for bacterial growth.

Note: While taking a case of a hematogenous osteomyelitis, always try to find the source of infection which may be UTI/RTI/GIT/skin, etc.

Q. Which osteomyelitis could occur in epiphysis?

1. Tubercular osteomyelitis
2. Direct osteomyelitis

Q. Which bacterial infection is the commonest cause of hematogenous osteomyelitis?

Staphylococcus aureus

Other bacterial infection of bone and special conditions

1. *Salmonella:* Sickle cell anemia. It can cause multifocal osteomyelitis
2. *E. coli:* Neonate
3. *Pseudomonas aerogenosa:* IV drug abuser, immunocompromised
4. *Brucella:* Drinking unpasteurised milk, those in contact with infected bovine/pig. The Brucella osteomyelitis can affect spine and mimic Pott's spine.

Q. What is Brodie's abscess?

- It is a primary subacute osteomyelitis of hematogenous origin which occurs due to organism of low virulence or in patients with strong immunity.
- It most commonly occurs in proximal tibia metaphysis. Rarely in distal tibia, fibula, radius, carpals or tarsals
- *Most common organism: Staph. aureus* (usually of low virulence)

Q. What is Garre's sclerosing osteomyelitis?

It is a primary subacute osteomyelitis of mandible due to low grade infection leading to peripheral bone deposition (proliferative osteomyelitis)

Common in mandible of children with dental caries.

Q. Usually, is there a sinus formation in Garre's osteomyeltis or Brodie's abscess?

No. Both are low grade infection characterized by bone thickening, periosteal reaction but no sinus formation.

Q. How do you confirm the diagnosis of Garre's osteomyelitis in mandible?

1. CT scan and MRI of the mandible
2. Orthopantomogram of mandible

Q. What is spina ventosa?

Tubercular osteomyelitis or tubercular dactylitis of the short tubular bones (phalanx, metacarpal, metatarsals) is known as spina ventosa.

TUBERCULOSIS OF THE KNEE

Common Presentation of Patient with Tubercular Arthritis of Knee

Case summary: A 42-year-old male patient case of pain and swelling in his right knee for 6 months. Pain was insidious in onset and was associated with gradually increasing swelling over the knee. Pain was activity related and at night as well. Morning stiffness was noticed lasting for 20–30 minutes. There was evening rise of fever with loss of weight and appetite. General examination revealed pallor. Rest of the systemic examination was normal. Local examination of right knee revealed flexion, posterior subluxation and external rotation deformity. Further, there was diffuse swelling, gross quadriceps wasting, synovial hypertrophy and joint effusion. Both joint lines (medial and lateral) were tender. Flexion movement was painfully restricted from 20 to 70°. Inguinal lymph nodes were palpable and enlarged. Neurovascular examination and hip-ankle were normal.

Q. What is the clinical diagnosis?

Chronic infective arthritis of right knee probably tubercular in origin.

Q. Why do you say that it is tubercular synovitis of knee?

It is because of following reasons:

History

1. Monoarticular involvement
2. Chronic (6 months)
3. History of evening rise of fever with loss of weight and appetite (observed in TB)
4. Presence of night pain and morning stiffness (indicates inflammation/infection)

Examination

5. Flexion, external rotation and subluxation of knee (typically seen in TB knee) (Figs 3.9 and 3.10)

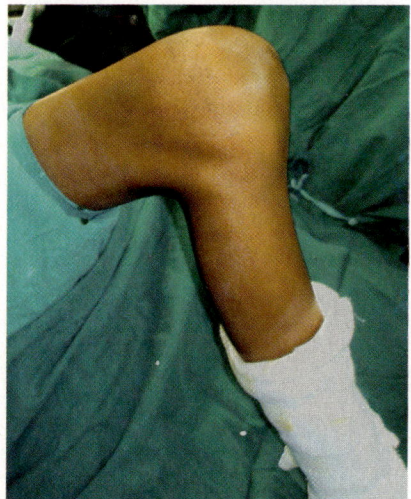

Fig. 3.9: Lateral view of right knee reveals flexion deformity and posterior subluxation of knee

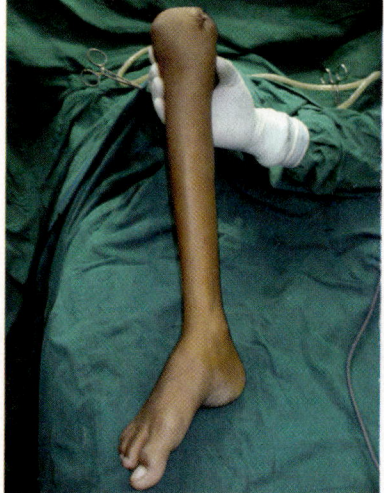

Fig. 3.10: Frontal view of knee reveals external rotation deformity of the leg

6. Joint line tenderness (joint line tenderness observed in arthritis)
7. Synovial hypertrophy (indicates synovial involvement)
8. Palpable and enlarged inguinal lymph nodes (indicates infectious etiology)

Q. What is the relevance of family history in patients with suspected tuberculosis?

Patients can acquire TB of the musculoskeletal system through contact with those who are suffering with TB in family or neighborhood.

Q. What is the relevance of past history in this patient?

Past history of tuberculosis is vital in such patients as **musculoskeletal tuberculosis is always secondary** to a primary focus in body, covert or overt, present or in past. Current patient does not give any history suggestive of tuberculosis of lungs/lymph node/genitourinary/abdominal.

Q. How do you explain tuberculosis in the knee joint when there is no such past history?

Asymptomatic tuberculosis in past is a known entity especially in lungs and lymph nodes. Patient may get subclinical infection with no symptoms.

Q. What are the pathological stages of tuberculosis of knee?

There are three stages:
1. Stage of synovitis
2. Stage of arthritis
3. Stage of deformity or triple dislocation

Q. What is the typical deformity in a tubercular knee?

The typical deformity is known as **triple dislocation/triple deformity.**
   It is characterized by *flexion, posterior subluxation and external rotation deformity* of the knee.

> Note: It is a **misnomer** as there is no triple dislocation

Q. What is the relevance of examining the popliteal fossa in such a case?

In patients with chronic inflammatory, degenerative (OA) and infective disorders, there could be presence of Baker's cyst in popliteal fossa.

> Note: Baker's cyst is more common in rheumatoid arthritis or osteoarthritis.

Q. Can it be pyogenic infection of knee?

Very unlikely, as the duration is 6 months and this is too long duration for septic arthritis. Septic/pyogenic infection of a joint is usually an acute condition which presents within few days to 2–3 weeks. Moreover, patients with septic arthritis would complain of high fever with chills. Locally, the knee would be very warm, gross

> Often in exams, answer to the question on triple deformity is description of CTEV!! Remember, both are completely different entity.

effusion, exquisitely tender and the range of movement would be grossly restricted and painful (pseudoparalysis). Occasionally, pyogenic arthritis can present in subacute phase, i.e. after a few weeks known as subacute septic arthritis.

Q. How would you manage this patient with TB knee?

1. *CBP:* Low hemoglobin, may reveal lymphocytosis, normal counts
2. *ESR:* Raised
3. *Mantoux test:* More helpful to rule out TB rather than establishing the diagnosis
4. *X-ray of the knee:* AP, lateral view (Fig. 3.11). It may show following findings
   a. Periarticular osteopenia (common in inflammatory and infective pathologies)
   b. Osteolytic cavities in the bone
   c. Decreased and irregular joint space (indicates cartilage destruction and arthritis)
   d. Deformities, subluxation
5. *MRI of the knee:* To look for synovial hypertrophy, cystic cavities in bone, effusion, periarticular abscess
6. *Synovial fluid aspiration:* It can be sent for
   a. *AFB* staining and culture
   b. *CB-NAAT (cartridge based nucleic acid amplification test)/Genexpert:* It is a real time PCR technique which can detect MTB in sample within 2–3 hours. It also provides information regarding 'resistance against rifampicin', if any.
   c. *LPA (line probe assay):* It is a rapid PCR based technique used to detect MTB as well as 'resistance against rifampicin and isoniazid'
7. *Synovial biopsy (open/arthroscopic):* It is the confirmatory investigation. Histopathologic examination of synovium and affected bone confirms the diagnosis by demonstrating the classical "caseating tubercular granuloma". The synovial samples can also be sent for AFB stains, CBNAAT, LPA.
8. *Other investigations to detect the source of primary TB:* Sputum examination, chest X-ray/abdominal and pelvis USG or CT scan/urine examination, bronchoscopy.

> Note: Narrowed joint space is hallmark of any arthritis due to cartilage damage (degenerative/inflammatory/infective/ traumatic).

> Note: Remember to tell the finding which are present on X-ray rather than all the finding you remember theoretically.

Q. Describe a classical tubercular granuloma.

A classical tubercular granuloma is characterized by **central caseating necrosis** surrounded by **Langhans' giant cells**, macrophages and epithelioid cells.

Q. How will you treat your patient?

The treatment of tubercular arthritis comprises several methods.
1. *General measures*
   a. Improve nutrition, correct anemia,
   b. Analgesic for pain control
   c. Traction/splint to prevent or correct a deformity

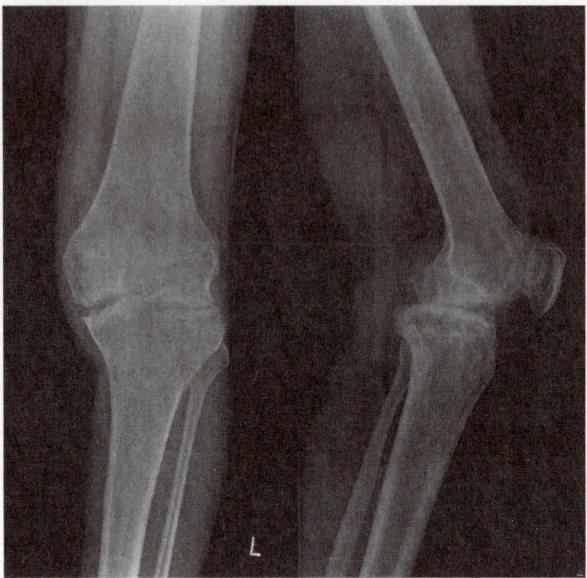

Fig. 3.11: X-ray of the knee reveals reduced joint space in medial and lateral compartment. Irregular joint margins indicating destructions of bone and cartilage and subchondral lytic lesion in tibia (seen on lateral X-ray)

2. *Antitubercular medications:* Daily antitubercular treatment (ATT) for 12–18 months depending upon the region and considerations by surgeon according to response of treatment.
   a. Isoniazid (INH): 5 mg/kg/day
   b. Rifampicin (RIF): 10 mg/kg/day
   c. Ethambutol (ETM): 15 mg/kg/day
   d. Pyrazinamide (PYZ): 20 mg/kg/day

> **Classical side effects of ATT**
> 1. INH—peripheral neuropathy
> 2. Rifampicin—hepatotoxicity
> 3. Ethambutol—optic neuritis
> 4. Pyrazinamide: Hyperuricemia leading to gout

   In addition, pyridoxine is added to prevent INH induced neuropathy
   Current ATT regime: Intensive phase of 2 months: All four drugs (INH, RIF, ETM, PYZ). Maintenance phase of 10–16 months: INH, RIF, ETM.
3. **Physiotherapy**
   a. Quadriceps strengthening exercise
   b. Initially, the painful joint could be provided rest in a knee brace or above knee cast for 3–4 weeks. Later, mobilization of the stiff joint is initiated.
   c. Traction may be used in the stage of synovitis/early arthritis to correct flexion deformity
4. **Orthotic devices:** Walking stick/axillary crutch
5. **Surgical:** Depends upon pathological stage
   a. *Early stages of disease (synovitis or early arthritis) requires arthroscopic synovectomy of knee:* The aim is to resect hypertrophied inflamed infected synovium which is responsible for pannus formation. Pannus destroys the cartilage. By removing the hypertrophic inflamed and infected synovium along

with pannus, cartilage is protected in early stages of disease, thereby preventing the disease progression into the stage of arthritis. But once the arthritis is established, this procedure is not useful. Also, the bony lesions are curetted, cold abscess can be drained.

Also, synovectomy is helpful for taking synovial biopsy for histopathological diagnosis of TB, CBNAAT and LPA.

b. *Late stages of disease with established arthritis along with or deformity:* Established tubercular arthritis finally ends up in fibrous ankylosis. There are multiple options of treatment of such a joint
   1. *Arthrodesis of joint (knee) in sound position:* Arthrodesis of knee in extension would provide a painless and stable joint, albeit no movement.
   2. *Joint replacement:* It would provide a painless, stable and mobile joint.

Q. What can be done for triple deformity?

a. Arthroscopic debridement and release of adhesion can correct the deformity in very early stages of triple deformity. The knee may regain quite functional movements with appropriate rehabilitation if joint cartilage was still preserved.
b. Later stages of triple deformity with major cartilage destruction require "biaxial traction" to correct the deformity (Fig. 3.12) followed by arthrodesis of the knee joint into the sound position (Fig. 3.13).

Q. What is the end stage result of tubercular arthritis?

The end stage of **tubercular arthritis** is *fibrous ankylosis* with deformity of the joint.

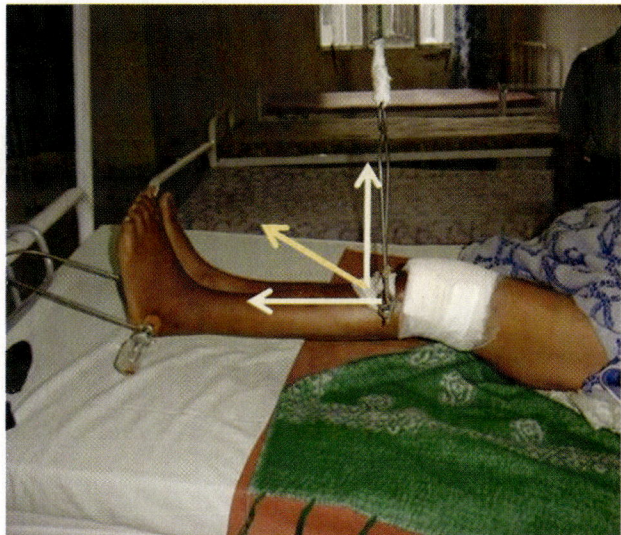

Note: In biaxial traction, skeletal traction is applied through calcaneum and upper tibia which provides traction in longitudinal and vertical direction giving a resultant vector which reduces flexed and subluxed knee. Alone longitudinal traction through calcaneum will further sublux the knee posteriorly.

Fig. 3.12: Biaxial traction (white arrows) applied in case of tubercular knee (yellow arrow marks resultant vector)

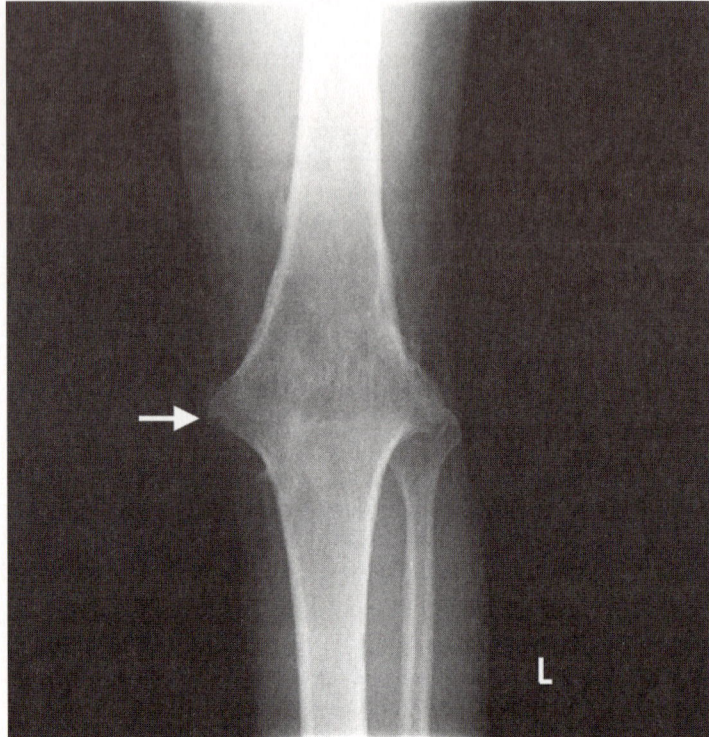

Fig. 3.13: Radiograph of an arthrodesis knee showing trabeculae crossing the former joint line (white arrow)

Note: In two situations, the sequalae of a tubercular joint is bony ankylosis.
1. Pott's spine: The tuberculosis of vertebra ends up in bony ankylosis with adjacent vertebra.
2. TB of peripheral joint with super-added pyogenic infection

Q. What is the treatment of septic arthritis?

Septic arthritis needs immediate arthroscopic or open debridement of joint followed by antibiotics (2 weeks of IV antibiotics and then 4–6 weeks of oral antibiotic) according to culture and sensitivity of the pus.

Q. Which is the commonest bacteriological cause of septic arthritis?

Staph. aureus is the commonest cause.

Q. What is the end stage local complication of septic arthritis?

Septic arthritis leads to *bony ankylosis*.

Q. How would you treat bony/fibrous ankylosis?

Fibrous/bony ankylosis is treated by arthrodesis in sound position once infection has clinically and serologically settled.

Q. Can total knee replacement be performed after ATT course is over in case of tubercular arthritis of the knee with painful fibrous ankylosis?

Note: There are three situation with respect to joint replacement and tuberculosis of the concerned joint.

1. Once must avoid replacement of a 'tubercular joint' with ongoing ATT.
2. Total joint replacement (TJR) of a joint can be performed with past history of TB in that joint once the ATT course is over. Further, one must rehabilitate the joint and wait for normalised ESR to proceed with TJR if the concerned joint function is grossly compromised in terms of pain and movements.
3. If a joint is found to be infected (co-incidentally detected in synovial biopsy) with *Mycobacterium tuberculosis* after the replacement is performed, there is no need to worry. One must start standard ATT for such a total joint replaced 'tubercular' joint and complete the ATT course.

Please note: Unlike the pyogenic infection of a prosthetic joint wherein the prosthetic component removal is almost mandatory after the TJR, the component removal is not mandatory in joints infected with MTB. It is because that the biofilm formation tendency is minimal in MTB as compared to pyogenic organisms. A resistant biofilm of pyogenic organism is impregnable to antibiotics which mandates the removal of prosthetic components to cure the local infection.

Q. Is it safe to perform joint replacement in a joint with past history of septic arthritis?

Total joint replacement in a joint with past history of septic arthritis carries high chance of recurrence of infection even if it is done after many years. However, it can be attempted after few months to years of treated pyogenic infection with normal ESR and CRP, where aspiration of joint is negative for bacteriology and tissue culture and frozen section is negative. If TJR cannot be done, arthrodesis in functional position is other alternative.

Note: By and large, joint replacement should be avoided in case where there is recent history of pyogenic infection in and around joint.

4

Arthritis

OSTEOARTHRITIS

Common Presentation of Patient with Osteoarthritis of Knee

Case summary: A 55-year-old man case of pain in his both knees while walking, squatting, and sitting cross legged since 5 years with increased pain since 4 weeks. There is minimal pain at rest and no morning stiffness. There is no history of fever, loss of weight or appetite. There is no other joint involvement. General and systemic examination is normal, BMI is 33. Local examination revealed bilateral genu varum and flexion deformity. Bilateral medial joint line is tender, crepitus is present and movements are painfully restricted. Neurovascular examination is normal.

Q. What is the clinical diagnosis?

The clinical diagnosis is bilateral osteoarthritis of knee with genu varum and flexion deformity (Fig. 4.1).

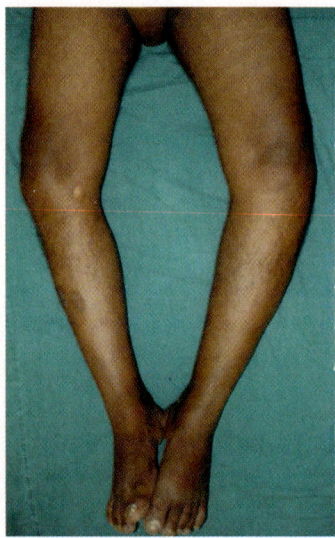

Fig. 4.1: Clinical picture of osteoarthritis of knee with bilateral genu varum

Q. Why do you say that it is OA of the knee?

It is because of following reasons:

History
1. **Older patient:** Primary OA is a degenerative process which frequently occurs after 50–55 years
2. **Weight bearing joint:** Non-weight bearing upper limb joints undergo arthritic changes much later in life (65–70 years)
3. **Mechanical pain:** Pain which occurs on loading the affected structure

Examination
4. **High BMI:** Indicates obesity (increased loads on the joint)
5. **Medial joint line tenderness*:** Joint line tenderness indicates arthritis of the joint
6. **Crepitus*:** Indicates irregular joint surface due to loss of cartilage
7. **Painful** and **restricted** range of motion*

*These are three important clinical signs for OA knee

Q. Why BMI assessment is important in patients with OA knee?

BMI should be assessed because primary OA is common in obese patients.

Obesity is an epidemic in the world, which is now a leading cause of osteoarthritis of knee.

Q. Why it cannot be rheumatoid arthritis (RA)?

It cannot be RA because of following reasons:
1. RA is quite uncommon to start at the age of 60 years (RA is common between 20 and 40 years).
2. RA is more common in **females**
3. In RA, **small joints of hand and feet** are commonly involved
4. History of **morning stiffness** in RA >60 minutes
5. Bilateral genu varum deformity goes more in favor of osteoarthritis whereas **genu valgum is seen more commonly in RA**
6. No classical deformity in hand or feet

Q. Is it a post-traumatic secondary OA?

No. Because there is no history of trauma

Q. Why it cannot be TB of knee or any other infection of knee?

No. It cannot be TB of knee joint in this patient because of following reasons.
1. Patient has presented with bilateral knee pain of mechanical nature which is typical of OA. In TB, it is rare to have bilateral involvement. Also in TB, pain is felt more at the night (due to infection and inflammation).
2. TB of the knee or any other part of the musculoskeletal system is **always secondary** to primary lesion elsewhere in the body. There is no past history of TB.

3. There is **no history of systemic features** (fever, weight loss, loss of appetite)
4. Also, history is of long duration, i.e. five years. In infective condition, the duration would be shorter (a few weeks to a few months)
5. Often, TB of knee presents with **classical triple deformity** (flexion, external rotation and posterior subluxation)

Q. In cases of OA, what should popliteal fossa be examined for?

Popliteal fossa must be examined for presence of Baker's cyst (Fig. 4.2).

Note: Baker's cyst is usually secondary to a primary pathology in the knee like OA/Chronic meniscal tear/rheumatoid knee. Once the primary pathology is treated, Baker's cyst often subsides naturally.

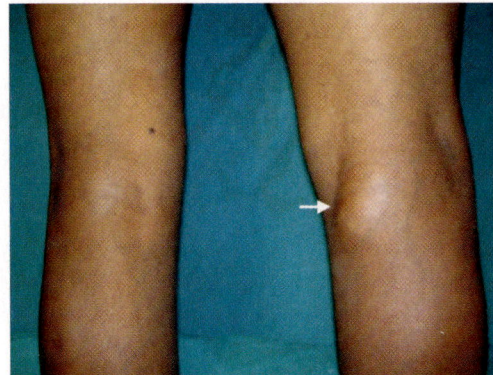

Fig. 4.2: Clinical picture of Baker's cyst (white arrow) in the popliteal fossa

Q. How would you manage this patient?

X-ray of the knee, anteroposterior and lateral view.

Q. What are the classic findings on a plain X-ray of the knee in patients with OA knee?

X-ray of knee would reveal following findings (Fig. 4.3):
1. Narrowed joint space, mostly medial
2. Osteophytes
3. Subchondral sclerosis
4. Subchondral cyst
5. Prominent tibial spine
6. Deformity
7. Loose body

Q. Is there a role of serological investigation in OA knee?

In general, serological investigations are not done for confirmation of the OA knee except when some other inflammatory, metabolic or infective arthritis is a differential diagnosis or patient is being planned for any surgical intervention.

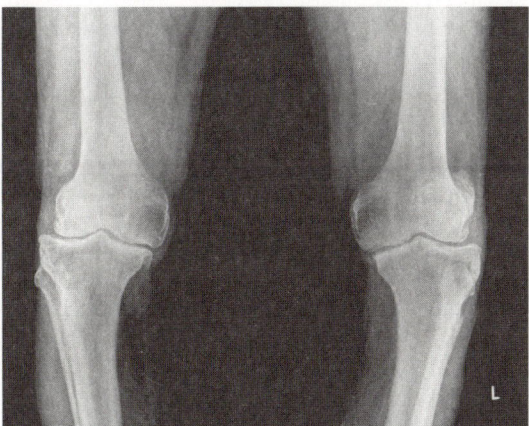

Fig. 4.3: Plain radiograph of knee with OA showing reduction in joint space, osteophytes and varus deformity

---

Difference between X-ray of primary OA and rheumatoid of 'any joint'

A. Primary OA
- Osteophytes are remarkable.
- No periarticular osteopenia.
- Knee OA shows predominantly medial compartment joint space reduction

B. Rheumatoid arthritis or other inflammatory arthritis
- Osteophytes are absent/minute
- Periarticular osteopenia.
- Knee rheumatoid shows symmetrical joint space reduction or more reduction of lateral compartment.

Q. How will you treat this patient?

The treatment of OA knee comprises several methods.

1. *General Measures*

a. *Weight loss:* A **very important measure** in obese patients
b. *Activity modification:* **Avoid/minimize** stair climbing, sitting cross legged and squatting as it exacerbates pain
c. Preference to Western toilet as it will avoid squatting induced deep flexion

2. *Medications*

a. Analgesics
b. **Intra-articular steroids** for **acute exacerbations**
c. Intra-articular **hyaluronic acid injection**

3. *Physiotherapy*

a. Moist heat

b. Short wave diathermy/local ultrasound therapy/TENS

c. **Quadriceps strengthening exercise:** It is the single **most important measure** which helps in improving functional outcome in OA knee.

4. Orthotic Devices

a. **Walking stick** on affected side (**unloads** painful joint)

b. **Lateral border shoe raise** (transfers the weight from medial to lateral compartment of knee, hence reduces pain)

c. **Unloader braces:** 'G2 unloader brace' shifts body weight from medial to lateral compartment of the knee and hence **unloads painful medial compartment** and reduces pain. Frequently, a simple knee cap too helps in reducing the pain of OA knee.

5. Surgical

a. **Arthroscopic debridement of the knee:** It is indicated in mild to moderate OA with minimal deformity. The purpose is to remove loose bodies, cartilage flaps, and hypertrophied synovium.

b. **High tibial osteotomy (HTO):** It is a preferred option in young adults with OA knee predominantly affecting the medial compartment of knee with varus deformity and minimal flexion deformity.

In HTO, the osteotomy performed just above the level of tibial tuberosity converts a varus deformity into a 5–7° valgus which helps in weight transfer from worn out medial compartment to normal lateral compartment.

c. **Unicompartment replacement:** Option in OA of medial compartment in young adults.

d. **Total knee replacement:** Currently, it is the best option in severe OA (Fig. 4.4). However, it should be reserved in patients who are elderly.

e. **Arthrodesis of the knee:** Very rarely performed for OA knee.

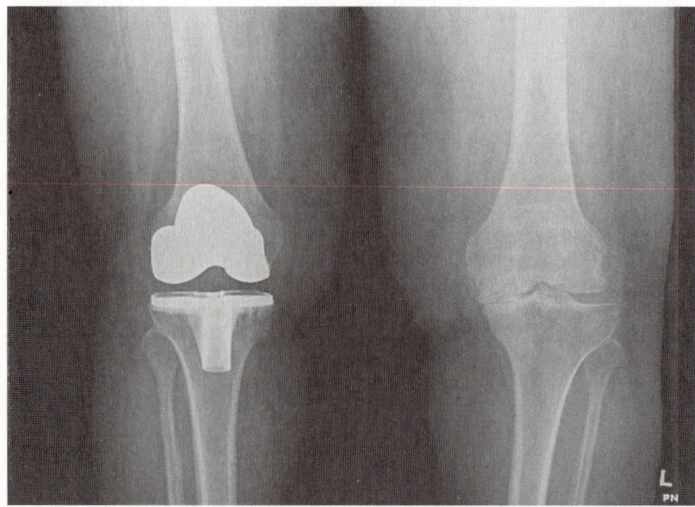

Fig. 4.4: Plain radiograph of total knee replacement of knee joint (right side)

Note: Excision arthroplasty which is also a method of treating an arthritic joint, is NOT performed in the arthritic knee as it will render the knee joint very unstable. In lower limb, excision arthroplasty is classically performed for tubercular arthritis of hip (k/a Girdlestone arthroplasty) where diseased head and neck of femur is removed.

Q. Is osteoarthritis an inflammatory disorder as term carries 'itis' in that? Then, how do we define OA?

No. Traditionally, primary OA is not considered to be an inflammatory disorder and 'itis' in the term 'osteoarthritis' is considered to be a misnomer!

Since walking induced weight bearing increases pain in OA knee, often students mention that the "patient should not walk". Not only it sounds funny but also is wrong concept as human beings ambulate only by walking and not by flying!

Q. Define osteoarthritis/Osteoarthrosis?

OA is a disease of wear and tear resulting in loss of hyaline cartilage of the joint followed by reactive bone formation in form of osteophyte.

Note: Recent researches point out that primary OA could be a result of underlying low grade inflammatory disorder.

Q. What is the other name of osteoarthritis?

It is also known as **osteoarthrosis. (Pathologically, correct term!)**

Q. Are there any predisposing factors for OA knee?

Yes. There are a few to names!
a. Obesity
b. Females (slightly more prone but cause not established)
c. Certain occupation which require repeated squatting and prolonged sitting cross leg.

Q. What is secondary OA?

Secondary OA means that there is a known predisposing factor, e.g. preceding trauma/infection/inflammation to the joint damaging the hyaline cartilage resulting in OA (unlike primary OA wherein no cause can be ascertained).

Q. What is a Baker's cyst?

Baker's cyst is an **outpouching or herniation** of synovial membrane through a **naturally occurring rent** in posterior knee capsule. It arises between medial head of gastrocnemius and semimembranosus tendon.

Note: Baker's cyst is an indication of **intra-articular pathology**. So, treatment is **always** directed toward detection and treatment of primary intra-articular knee pathology. Alone excision of Baker's cyst may not relieve pain.

Why does a Baker's cyst arise?

Baker's cyst is herniation of synovial membrane. So the question is why does it herniate at all?

Several pathologies in the knee chronically irritate the synovial membrane (inflammation of synovium, chronic meniscal tear, multiple loose bodies or cartilage flakes of osteoarthritis or infection resulting in excess production of synovial fluid. Beyond a point, this excess fluid cannot be accommodated in the knee joint resulting in synovium herniation though natural posterior capsular rent to accommodate excess fluid.

Q. Is it a true cyst?

It is **not a true cyst**. It is a knee synovial outpouching through the rent in the posterior capsule.

Q. What are the symptoms and sign in a patient with Baker's cyst?

Symptom
- Pain and swelling at the back of knee (popliteal fossa)
- Pain in the knee

Sign
- Firm and prominent swelling in the popliteal fossa in an extended knee, while soft and less prominent swelling in a flexed knee (Foucher's sign).
- Knee may have features of arthritis, meniscal tear, synovitis, etc. indicating a primary pathology in the knee.

Q. Which investigation can confirm the diagnosis of Baker's cyst?

USG of popliteal fossa and MRI of the knee.

Q. Which is a better investigation, USG or MRI?

MRI, as it would also detect intra-articular pathology of the knee along with Baker's cyst.

Q. What is the treatment of Baker's cyst?

1. The treatment of Baker's cyst should always **aim at detection and treatment of intra-articular pathology first** with medical and/or surgical options.
   Once intra-articular problem is treated appropriately, **Baker's cyst may subside** at its own or may decrease in size and become asymptomatic.
2. In case, the Baker's cyst remains symptomatic despite the treatment of intra-articular pathology:
   a. **Open or arthroscopic excision of Baker's cyst** could be performed.
   b. Occasionally, **aspiration of the cyst and intracystic injection of steroid** may help in resolving the cyst.

Baker's **cyst excision** is **reserved** for cases where symptoms have failed to resolve even after treating intra-articular pathology adequately.

Q. What is the differential diagnosis of Baker's cyst?

Most common differential diagnosis of Baker's cyst is semimembranosus bursa.

Baker's cyst	Semimembranosus bursa
Below the joint line	Above the joint line
Midline swelling	Located medially

Q. What is the complication of Baker's cyst?

Baker's cyst can rupture or get infected (known as complicated Baker's cyst)

Q. What is the differential diagnosis of ruptured Baker's cyst?

Ruptured Baker's cyst very closely mimics deep vein thrombosis of calf veins as leaked fluid after rupture of Baker's cyst irritates muscles of the calf. It causes pain and swelling of calf mimicking symptoms and signs of DVT (Moses' and Homans' sign of DVT).

It is extremely important to rule out DVT in case of ruptured Baker's cyst as former is a life-threatening condition. Similarly, the differential diagnosis of DVT is ruptured Baker's cyst!

Q. Is there any pertinent history or clinical finding which could suggest the existence of Baker's cyst before it ruptured?

Patients may give a history of popliteal fossa pain and swelling before the onset of calf swelling. They say that after the onset of calf swelling, the popliteal fossa swelling has disappeared!

RHEUMATOID ARTHRITIS

Common Presentation of Patient with Rheumatoid Arthritis

A 36-year-old female patient case of pain and swelling in her both knees for one year. She experiences pain while walking, at night while taking rest and experiences morning stiffness which lasts more than an hour. She also complains of pain and swelling in her small joints of hand and wrist along with malaise and generalized weakness with occasional history of fever. General examination revealed pallor. Local examination of both knees revealed swelling, effusion with mild genu valgum and flexion deformity. Lateral knee joint line was tender. Crepitus was present and movements were painfully restricted (ROM 10–80° flexion). There were typical deformities in wrist and hand.

Q. What is the clinical diagnosis?

The clinical diagnosis is rheumatoid arthritis of both knees with genu valgum and flexion deformity.

Q. Why do you say so?

It is rheumatoid arthritis (RA) because of following reasons.

History

1. **Female** sex: RA is more common in females by ratio of 4:1
2. **Young** age: RA is common in younger patient (20–40 years). Although it can be seen in older age group too.
3. Pain and swelling in **small joint** of hand and wrist (MCP, PIP) with involvement of knees
4. **Symmetric** involvement of joints (both wrist and hand and knees)
5. **Morning stiffness** lasting for an hour
6. Presence of night pain (indicates inflammation)

Examination

7. Lateral joint line tenderness (joint line tenderness indicates arthritis for any joint)
8. Presence of genu valgum (favors rheumatoid arthritis)
9. Painfully restricted range of motion
10. Typical deformities of wrist and hand

Q. What are the deformities in wrist and hand?

Following deformities are present (Figs 4.5 to 4.8).

1. Swan-neck deformity of finger
2. Boutonniere deformity of finger
3. Z deformity of thumb
4. Volar subluxation of MCP
5. Volar wrist subluxation
6. Radial deviation of wrist
7. Ulnar deviation of fingers at MCP joint

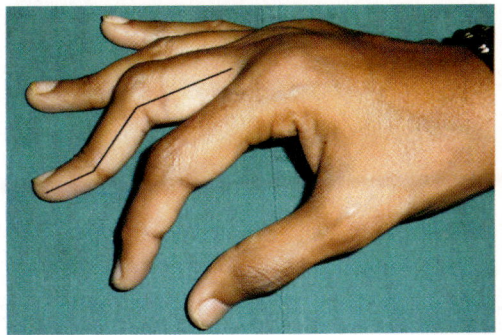

Fig. 4.5: Clinical picture of classic Bouton-niere deformity in middle finger (black line)

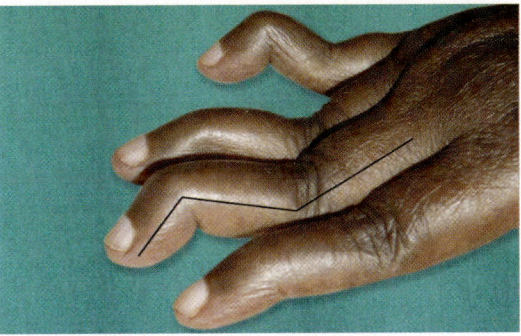

Fig. 4.6: Classic swan-neck deformity in all fingers (black line)

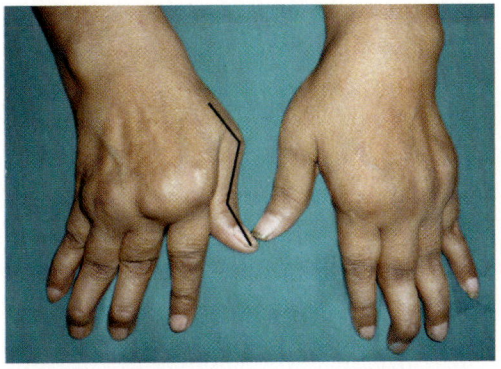

Fig. 4.7: Classic Z deformity of thumb (black line). Also note radial deviation of left wrist and ulnar deviation of right fingers at MCP joints

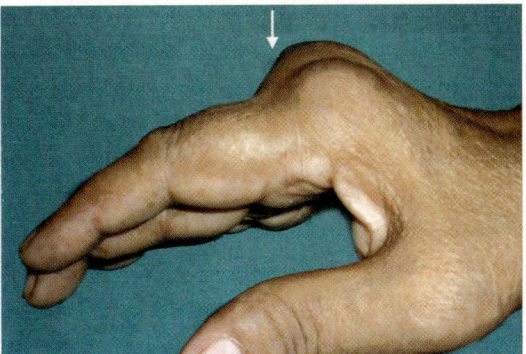

Fig. 4.8: Volar subluxation of MCP joint (white arrow shows subluxed MCP)

Q. Which joints are involved in hand in RA?

1. Wrist
2. Metacarpophalangeal (MCP) and proximal interphalangeal (PIP) joint of finger

Q. What deformities are seen in foot?

a. Claw toes
b. Hallux varus/valgus (Fig. 4.9)

Q. What is the role of family history in such cases?

Many inflammatory disorders like RA, SLE may have positive family history. RA is more common on maternal side.

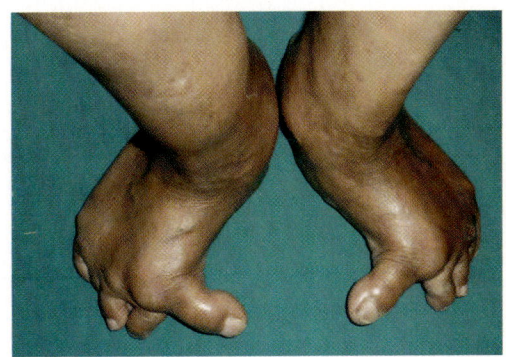

Fig. 4.9: Bilateral hallux varus deformity of foot

Q. What else did you ask in history?

Since this is a case of polyarticular arthritis, following history was taken to rule out other causes.

a. *Skin lesions:* Psoriasis, extensive dermatitis. Psoriasis is associated with sero-negative spondyloarthropathy, and any form of extensive dermatitis can cause gout due to high turnover of skin cells
b. *Facial malar rash:* Systemic lupus erythematosus (SLE)
c. *Current symptoms preceded by diarrhea or dysentery:* Reactive arthritis
d. *Altered bowel habits with diarrhea and constipation:* Inflammatory bowel disease
e. *Small joint of foot and ankle:* Gout
f. *Conjunctivitis, urethritis and arthritis:* Reiter's disease
g. *Low back pain with morning stiffness of back* indicates spondyloarthropathy.

Q. Why it cannot be tuberculosis or any other infection of the knee?

No. Unlikely to be TB of knee joint in this patient because of following reasons
1. TB of the knee or any other part of the musculoskeletal system is always secondary to primary lesion elsewhere in the body. There is no past history of TB in this patient.
2. Current patient has polyarthritis whereas TB is usually monoarticular.
3. Also, the history is chronic, i.e. one year whereas in chronic infective condition, the duration would be shorter (a few weeks to a few months)
4. Although history of occasional fever is present but TB is quite consistently characterised by evening rise of temperature.

Q. Which deformity of the knee, varus or valgus, is common in the rheumatoid arthritis?

Genu valgum deformity is more common in rheumatoid arthritis of knee. (Genu varum is common in OA.)

> Note: **Genu varum is more common in primary OA of knee** as the cartilage wear pattern follows the mechanical axis of the joint which falls in the middle of the knee joint or slightly medial resulting in more wear in the medial compartment causing varus deformity. **Genu valgum is more common in Rheumatoid or other inflammatory disorders as it is a disease which uniformly affects both medial and lateral compartment.** Thus the symmetric wear of the joint follows anatomical axis wear pattern which is in valgus, and hence the deformity. Further, an associated flat 'pronated' foot (due to dysfunctional or ruptured tibialis posterior tendon, arthritic and deformed foot joints) aggravates the valgus deformity.

Q. What is the relevance of popliteal fossa examination in case of RA?

Often, there can be a Baker's cyst in popliteal fossa.

Q. Was there any synovial hypertrophy? Is it more common in rheumatoid or osteoarthritis?

Synovial hypertrophy was present in this case and is more common in rheumatoid as it primarily affects synovium.

Q. Did you examine the extensor aspect of forearm and what you looked for?

Extensor aspect of forearm was looked for rheumatoid nodules.

Q. What is the significance of presence of Rheumatoid nodules?

Presence of rheumatoid nodules indicates the severity of disease.

Patients with rheumatoid nodule have high titers of RA factor.

Q. What are the criteria to diagnose rheumatoid arthritis?

RA is diagnosed based upon the criteria laid by the **American Rheumatologist Association**.

1. Morning stiffness >1 hr
2. Arthritic involvement of 3 or more joints
3. Arthritis of wrist and hand (MCP, PIP) joints
4. Symmetric involvement on both sides of the body
5. Rheumatoid nodules
6. RA factor positive
7. Radiological changes typical of RA (periarticular osteoporosis) must be present over PA view of hand

To diagnose RA
a. Criteria 1–4 must be present over 6 weeks
b. At least 4 out of 7 criteria must be present.

Q. Does rheumatoid arthritis has a genetic basis?

Yes. It is associated with HLA-DR4 and HLA-DW4

Q. What are the pathological stages in rheumatoid arthritis?

There are three pathological stages in rheumatoid arthritis (generally, common for all inflammatory arthritis; SAD)

1. *Stage of synovitis:* Synovial inflammation, effusion and ends with pannus formation
2. *Stage of arthritis:* Persistent inflammation causes joints and tendon destruction. Pannus creeping over the cartilage chokes the cartilage and various inflammatory proteolytic enzymes in synovial fluid destroy the cartilage resulting in arthritis
3. *Stage of deformity:* End stage of joint disease due to:
   • Articular cartilage destruction
   • Capsular stretching
   • Tendon rupture

Q. Pathologically, which structure(s) are involved in rheumatoid arthritis?

Musculoskeletal (MSK) system: In MSK system, RA involves the *synovium* which is in the *joints* and surrounds the *tendons*. Hence, joints and tendons are involved in RA.

Extra-articular tissues: Rheumatoid nodules, lymph nodes, vasculitis, muscle weakness and visceral disease (lung, heart, kidney, GIT and brain)

Note: Extra-articular tissue involvement in RA indicates severity of the disease.

Q. What is the systemic involvement observed in patients with RA?

RA is a systemic disease which can involve any system (CVS, RS, CNS, eye and hematopoietic system). The systemic involvement may manifest as:
a. *Sjögren's syndrome:* Dry eyes and mouth. Most common extra-articular manifestation
b. Vasculitis, pericarditis
c. Felty's syndrome (RA with spenomegaly with leucopenia)
d. Pulmonary disease: Lung fibrosis
e. Neurological: Nerve entrapment, mononeuritis multiplex
f. Cardiac: Pericarditis, valvular heart disease, conduction abnormality
g. Ocular: Keratoconjuctivitis, scleritis
h. Hematologic: Anemia

Q. How would you manage this patient?

1. *X-ray* of the knee and other involved joints, anteroposterior and lateral view
2. *CBP:* Low Hb. TLC and DLC usually normal unless there is acute infection.
3. *ESR, CRP:* Raised in untreated RA cases
4. *RA factor:* Sensitivity—70%, specificity—82%
5. *Anti-CCP antibody:* Sensitivity—70%; specificity—95%

Q. Why patients with RA are anemic?

Anemia in patients with RA is due to anemia of chronic disease and also drug related.

Q. What is RA factor?

RA factor is IgM antibody against Fc fragment of IgG antibody. Only 60–70% cases of RA will have RA factor positive whereas 30% cases of RA are RA factor negative.

It can be false positive in elderly. With very low titre, one must interpret RA factor carefully.

Q. What is the significance of anti-CCP positive status in rheumatoid arthritis?

If RA factor is negative, positive anti-CCP status confirms rheumatoid arthritis. However, if the RF is positive, anti-CCP does not seem to add any valuable information.

If both are positive, it indicates severity of disease.

Q. What are the possible differential diagnosis of rheumatoid arthritis?

Any condition which present as polyarthralgia or polyarthritis is a possible differential diagnosis such as:
1. *SLE:* Presents with painful swelling of small joints of hand and feet. However, it is "non-deforming" unlike RA. Further; ANA (highly sensitive) and anti-dsDNA

antibody (highly specific) are positive which are not seen in RA. Also, the X-rays will not show bony erosions.

2. *Psoriatic arthritis:* Involves small joints of hand and feet but mostly DIP joints are involved and less symmetrical. Further, there is associated psoriasis.
3. *Gout:* Occasionally, gout can be polyarticular. But, it is associated with high serum Uric acid levels, tophi and joint aspirate would reveal gouty crystals.
4. *Parvovirus B-19 infection:* May present as polyarthralgia in people who regularly interact with children (teachers).
5. *Others:* Reiters', viral arthritis

Q. What is commonly observed in the plain X-ray of a rheumatoid joint (knee in this case)?

X-ray of knee would reveal following findings (Fig. 4.10)
1. Symmetrical narrowing of both joint spaces
2. Periarticular osteoporosis
3. Juxta-articular bone erosions
4. Deformity

Note: Narrowed joint space is hallmark of arthritis due to cartilage damage (degenerative/inflammatory/infective).

Difference between X-ray rheumatoid arthritis *vs* primary osteoarthritis of 'any joint'

Rheumatoid arthritis or other inflammatory arthritis:
• Osteophytes are absent/minute
• Periarticular osteopenia
• Rheumatoid shows symmetrical joint space reduction

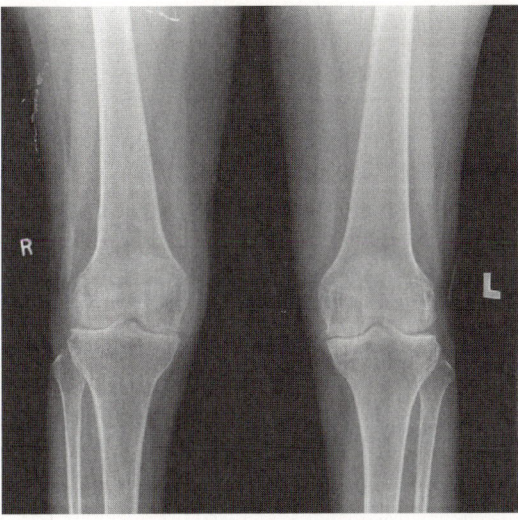

Fig. 4.10: X-ray of both knee reveals symmetrical reduction in medial and lateral joint space, absent osteophytes, periarticular osteopenia and juxta-articular bone erosions

Primary OA:
- Osteophytes are prominent
- No periarticular osteopenia
- May show asymmetric joint space reduction according to weight bearing pattern

Q. How will you treat your patient?

The treatment of rheumatoid arthritis is multifacetal. Various comprehensive measures are deployed to manage RA.
- **General measures**
- **Physiotherapy and orthotics**
- **Medical management**
  a. NSAIDs
  b. Steroids: Oral, injectable
  c. DMARDs: Conventional, biologic agents
- **Surgical treatment**

A. *For joints and bones*
  a. Synovectomy: Open/arthroscopic
  b. Total joint replacement
  c. Arthrodesis
  d. Resection arthroplasty
  e. Osteotomy

B. *For soft tissues*
  a. Capsule: Capsulotomy, capsulectomy
  b. Tendons: Tenosynovectomy, debridement, tendon repair, and tendon transfer

1. *General Measures*

a. *Activity modification:* **Avoid/minimize**—stair climbing, sitting cross legged, squatting, etc. to avoid pain and possibly prevent further damage to the knee cartilage.
b. Improve nutrition
c. *Blood transfusion:* If severe anemia
d. *Prevent osteoporosis:* Patient with RA are prone for osteoporosis due to various causes like:
   - Less mobility due to disease
   - Postmenopausal status
   - Steroid treatment hence, they must be given
     i. Daily appropriate dose of calcium, vitamin D
     ii. Improve mobility, exercises
     iii. Steroids must be given for short course if possible
e. *Stop smoking:* Smoking is a risk factor and disease improves on quitting smoking
f. *Minimise or stop alcohol intake:* Concomitant liver damage due to alcohol may add up the liver damage due to DMARDs especially MTX.

2. Physiotherapy

a. Moist heat/cold pack (over the involved joint)
b. Short wave diathermy, local ultrasound therapy
c. Improve strength and endurance of muscles, stretching of muscles
d. Mobilization of stiff joints.

3. Orthotic Devices

a. Walking stick, knee brace
b. Various orthosis/splints for wrist and hand to prevent deformity

4. Medical Treatment

The aim of medical treatment is reduce pain, inflammation and minimize further damage in various joints and soft tissues (tendons, organs) by preventing or slowing down the progression of RA. This is achieved by controlling inflammation as rapidly as possible.

The treatment is always started with:

- **One or two DMARDs + NSAID ± Steroids.**

Methotrextae and hydroxychloroquine are the two most common DMARDs used in RA. Steroids can be added as adjunct to control severe pain and inflammation while DMARDs start acting in 4–6 weeks. Steroids are rapidly tapered off to avoid the potential side effects.

If the DMARDs fail to achieve the satisfactory response in few weeks, it is wise to add biologic DMARDs to control the disease.

Various medication used are:

a. *DMARDs:* **Most useful** in **preventing progression of synovitis stage**, may be of less use in arthritis or deformity stage but will prevent progress in other joints which are not yet involved or are in synovitis stage.
b. *NSAIDs:* To reduce pain and inflammation
c. *Intra-articular steroids:* In patients with exacerbation of disease (RA) in a single joint.

> Single joint exacerbation in rheumatoid arthritis should *always* be taken as septic arthritis unless proved otherwise. Hence, septic arthritis should be *ruled out* before injecting the steroid into the joint.

d. *Oral corticosteroids:* Usually, it is administered as an adjunct along with DMARDs for short course to control pain and inflammation especially in severe form of RA as DMARDs may take few weeks (4–12) to provide relief.

DMARDs are most useful drugs in the management of RA and act by preventing or retarding the progression of the disease. It is classified as:

 i. *Traditional non-biological DMARDs:* Regular use: Methotrexate, hydroxychloroquine, leflunomide, sulphasalazine, rarely used (in very severe disease): Cyclosporine, azathioprine
 ii. *Biological DMARDs:* Etanercept, infliximab, adalimumab, abatacept

Both types of DMARDs are best effective in "stage of synovitis and inflammation" and act by substantially reducing synovitis which helps in preserving the cartilage integrity and function, and thereby preserving and improving joint function.

The DMARDs act after 4–6 weeks of administration. Successful DMARD therapy may eliminate the need for other anti-inflammatory or analgesic medications; however, until the full action of DMARDs takes effect, anti-inflammatory or steroids may be required as adjunct therapy to reduce pain and swelling.

Musculoskeletal complications of steroids
- Osteoporosis
- Avascular necrosis of head of femur
- Tendon rupture (e.g. if injected close to tendon like tendo Achillis)

Potential side effects of conventional DMARDs are:
- *Methotrexate:* Upper GI effects*, liver disease, interstitial pneumonitis
- Chloroquine: Upper GI effects*, retinal and corneal damage
- Sulphasalazine: Upper GI effects*, neutropenia, bone marrow suppression
- Leflunomide: Upper GI effects*
  *Common upper GI effects could be: Nausea, vomiting, loss of appetite

Potential Side effects of Biologic DMARDs are:
- Potentially severe infections, possible lymphoma

5. Surgical Management of Rheumatoid Joints

a. Arthroscopic or open synovectomy of the involved joints

Note: Synovectomy should be answered only if there is synovitis of the involved joint.

Aim of synovectomy: In the stage of synovitis, the synovium is inflamed and hypertrophied. There is pannus formation over the cartilage and altered synovial fluid contains lysosomal enzymes. The cartilage of the joint undergoes damage as pannus chokes the cartilage and lysosomal enzymes destroy the cartilage. During synovectomy; hypertrophied, inflamed synovium is resected and pannus is removed. Hence; by removing the hypertrophied inflamed synovium and pannus, the choking effect of pannus and destructive effect of lysosomal enzymes over the cartilage is avoided resulting in protection of the joint cartilage in early stages of disease; thereby preventing the disease progression into the stage of arthritis. But, once arthritis is established, this procedure is not useful for that joint.

b. **Total knee (or joint involved) replacement:** Performed in stage of arthritis and deformity.

c. **Arthrodesis:** Performed in arthritic or unstable joints where replacement is not feasible or possible.

d. **Resection/interposition arthroplasty:** It is rarely performed in upper limb joints like elbow. It is not recommended in lower limb joints.

e. **Osteotomy:** For bony deformities, arthritis

Other procedures for soft tissue pathology

f. **Capsulotomy/capsulectomy** for stiff joint

g. *Soft tissue release* for stiff joint

h. *Tendon transfer/tendon repair* for tendon rupture

Q. Which conventional DMARD cannot be given if patient is planning conception or is pregnant? What are the alternatives?

Methotrexate (MTX) cannot be given if patient is planning conception or is pregnant. If patient is planning pregnancy, MTX must be avoided as there is risk of teratogenicity with the usage of drug.

In such a case, hydroxychloroquine, sulphasalazine and steroids can be used with caution.

Q. When to add biological DMARDs?

Biological DMARDs are added only:

1. When there is severe form of RA which does not respond to conventional DMARDs tried for at least 3–4 months.
2. Initial presentation is quite severe with systemic involvement like pleural disease, interstitial lung disease, pericarditis

Q. Can there be involvement of spine in RA?

Yes, but only cervical spine. Rest of spine involvement is not common.

a. Atlantoaxial subluxation

b. Subaxial subluxation

c. Basilar invagination

Q. Is osteoporosis common in patients with RA?

Yes. Osteoporosis is quite common in patients with RA. Hence, a long term supplementation with calcium and vitamin D should be continued.

Q. What are the complication of RA?

- Fixed deformities
- Muscle weakness
- *Infection:* Especially one who are on steroids
- *Spinal cord compression* especially if there is cervical spine involvement
- *Amyloidosis* can present with renal failure

Q. What is the prognosis of patients with RA?

Patients with high titres of RA factor and Anti-CCP antibody, joint erosions, vasculitis, rheumatoid nodules, cardiac or other systemic features carry bad prognosis.

10%—improve steadily

60%—remissions and exacerbations

20%—severe joint erosion with five years

10%—completely disabled

Q. What is arthritis mutilans?

It is a **severe form** of arthritis of **hand joints** characterized by severe destruction of joint and instability. It is seen in **psoriatic and rheumatoid arthritis.**

Various surgical options for any arthritic joint

1. **Arthroscopic debridement:** It is helpful in early stages of arthritis. It removes hypertrophied synovium, cartilage debries, loose bodies, etc.
2. **Realignment osteotomy:** It is helpful in early-mid stages of arthritis wherein some part of joint is 'uninvolved' When a part of joint is uninvolved in early arthritic stages, realignment osteotomy brings the uninvolved part in weight bearing axis and unloads damaged arthritic part reducing pain and improved function.
3. **Unicompartment replacement:** It is a good option for arthritis in young individuals. Only the involved part of the joint is replaced.
4. **Total joint replacement:** Best option in severe arthritis of the joint. It provides painless, stable and a mobile joint (avoided in postseptic arthritis).
5. **Arthrodesis:** When replacement is not an option (e.g. after the septic arthritis), the joint could be fused. It provides stable and a painless joint but movements at the joint are lost.
6. **Resection arthroplasty:** Occasionally arthrodesis may not be a good option especially when movements are required for performing certain activities. Resection arthroplasty removes the damaged articular surface and provides painless, mobile joint but 'joint' remains unstable.
   It can be done in upper limb but avoided in lower limb as it causes instability, and stability is profound requirement in lower limb for ambulation.
   (Note: Read Girdlestone hip resection arthroplasty in TB hip section)

Q. Classify arthritis?

The arthritis classification is given in Flowchart 4.1.

Flowchart 4.1: Arthritis classification

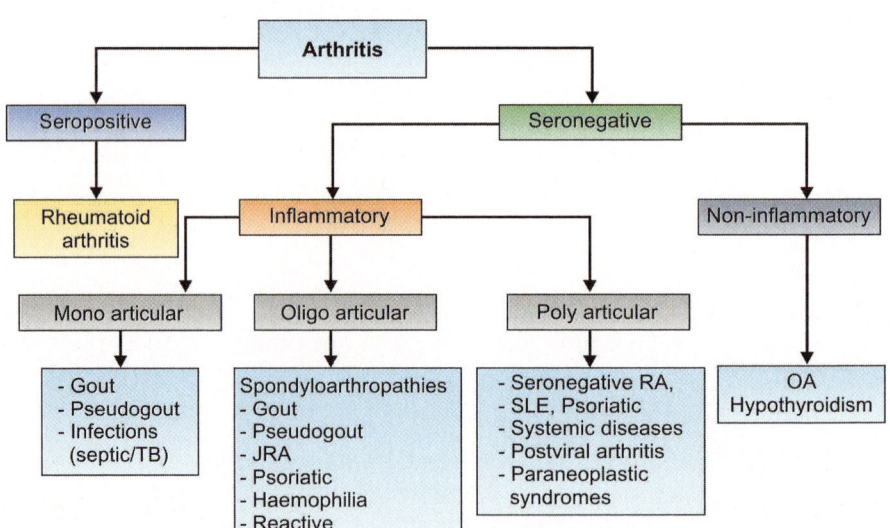

Painful Hip

HIP PAIN

Common Presentation of Child with Synovitis of the Hip Joint

Case summary: An 8-year-old boy was brought to the hospital with painful limp since one month. The limp was insidious in onset and non-progressive. The child was able to walk despite pain. No history of night cry, cough, expectoration, fever, loss of weight and loss of appetite. All developmental milestones were normal. No family or past history of tuberculosis. General and systemic examination were normal. On examination of the hip, no deformity of both hip joints was noted. Tenderness was present on left side hip joint. Left side abduction and internal rotation of the hip joint were painful and terminally limited. There was no limb length discrepancy. Examination of distal limb and spine were normal.

Q. What is the clinical diagnosis?

The clinical diagnosis is left side synovitis of the hip joint for that I like to put differential diagnosis
- First—tuberculosis of the left hip joint
- Second—Perthes' disease left
- Third—transient synovitis of left hip

Q. Justify your clinical diagnosis (synovitis of the hip joint).

It is because:
1. Child presented with painful limp
2. Tenderness over the left anterior hip joint line
3. No fixed deformity of hip joint
4. Limitation of passive abduction and internal rotation
5. Terminal restriction of the range of motion of hip joint
6. No true shortening (supratrochanteric)

Q. Why do you put first differential diagnosis as tuberculosis of the hip joint?

Tuberculosis is very common in Indian of all the age groups (endemic). After spine, the hip joint is the most common site of involvement for tuberculosis (15%). Synovitis of the joint is the first stage of the tuberculosis so I have put the first differential diagnosis as tubercular synovitis of the hip joint (first stage).

Q. What are the point not favoring tuberculosis of the hip joints?

There is no associated history of constitutional symptoms, chest TB or history of exposure to tuberculosis from closed relatives or neighbours. Further, there is no history of TB of any other system of body (gastrointestinal, urinary tract) or neck node swelling in the past. There is no history of night cry.

Q. What is the importance of pulmonary or extrapulmonary TB even if bone and joint TB is suspected?

Osteoarticular tuberculosis is **always secondary** involvement. One has to **screen and suspect primary** sites of tuberculosis.

Q. What are primary sites of tuberculosis?

Pulmonary, gastrointestinal tract, urogenital system, skin and cervical lymph nodes are primary sites of tuberculosis.

Q. How do you justify Perthes disease as a differential diagnosis?

Perthes disease is very common in south-west coastal region of India. If the child presents from this region, we must consider Perthes' disease as one of the differential diagnosis in case of limp with or without painful hip. The **key clinical features of the Perthes'** disease are **restriction of abduction and internal rotation** of the **hip joints** with terminal painful range of motion.

Q. What are the points, not favoring the Perthes' disease?

Perthes' disease is **very common in south-west coastal** region. It is **quite uncommon in rest of India.** If the child presents outside the south west-costal region or those with constitutional symptoms, it might not favour Perthes' disease.

Q. What do you mean by transient synovitis of the hip joint?

Transient synovitis of the hip joint is **benign, self-limiting condition** of children between **3 and 10 years of age** which is **diagnosed after exclusion** of other hip diseases. It is one of the common pathology of the hip, so I have put the third differential diagnosis of the synovitis of the hip joint.

Q. Why have you not put septic arthritis of the hip joint as a differential diagnosis?

I do not suspect septic arthritis of the hip joint because:
1. The onset is not acute
2. All symptoms are not very severe (pain is very severe in septic arthritis)
3. Child is able to weight bear
4. No history of high grade fever
5. Only terminal range of motions are restricted whereas septic arthritis leads to pseudoparalysis implying severe pain restricting all movements severely at the hip almost mimicking paralysis.

Q. How do you confirm your diagnosis?

We can confirm the diagnosis with

a. Plain radiograph AP of pelvis with both hips and lateral views of hip
b. Blood counts
c. ESR
d. Mantoux test, chest X-ray, or screening other areas (GIT, urinary tract) if TB suspected
e. Hip synovial biopsy in case of TB hip

- Characteristic radiological features would differentiate all three conditions easily.
- High lymphocyte count and ESR would help to diagnose tuberculosis.
- Pulmonary chest radiograph and Mantoux test would also be required with child with high ESR or when we suspect tuberculosis of the hip joint.

Q. What are the radiological findings in Perthes' disease?

Sclerosis and **collapse** of the **capital femoral epiphysis** are two cardinal radiological features of Perthes' disease (Fig. 5.1).

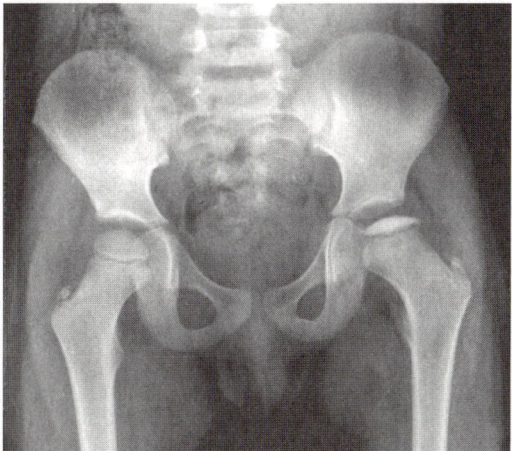

Fig. 5.1: Plain radiograph of pelvis with both hips of skeletally immature child shows left side dense epiphysis of proximal femur with reduction of the height of epiphysis suggestive of Perthes' disease

Septic arthritis is characterized by:
- Acute onset, severe pain around the hip joint with pseudoparalysis of the limb
- Acute constitutional symptoms like: Fever, chills
- Any attempt of hip movement is very painful

Full name of Perthes' disease is "Legg-Calé-Perthes disease"!
Once in MBBS exam, a question was asked as "what is Legg-Calvé-Perthe" disease?
A student wrote; it is a disease of leg and calf, another one wrote disease of calves!!

Q. What are the important classifications for Perthes' disease?

Caterall's, modified Elizabethtown and Herring's classification.

Q. What are the radiological features of tuberculosis of the hip joint?

Osteopenia (due to reactive hyperemia) and local bone destruction lytic lesion) are commonest radiological features of tuberculosis of the hip joint.

Radiological type of TB hip
1. Normal type
2. Perthes type
3. Pestle and Mortar type
4. Wandering acetabulum
5. Atrophic type
6. Protrusio acetabuli
7. Dislocated type

Q. What are the radiological features of transient synovitis of the hip joint?

The bone and joint are normal in plain radiograph in transient synovitis of the hip joints.

Q. What do you mean by Perthes disease?

Perthes disease is **self-limiting idiopathic avascular necrosis of the capital femoral epiphysis**.

Q. What do you mean by self-limiting avascular necrosis in Perthes' disease?

Avasularity of the femoral head is **followed by revascularization** in Perthes' disease **irrespective of the treatment,** so it is called self-limiting avascular necrosis.

Q. Why should we treat Perthes' disease, if it is self-limiting disease?

The prime aim of treating Perthes' disease is to prevent secondary osteoarthrosis of the hip by preventing the femoral head from getting deformed.

   Influencing the rate or completeness of revascularization of the avascular epiphysis is not the aim of the treatment. None of the currently available treatment modalities appreciably influence the revascularization process.

Q. How do you treat Perthes' disease?

Perthes disease can be treated with **non-operative or operative containment methods** with weight relief.

Q. What do you mean by containment?

Reposition of the extruded part of the epiphysis into the acetabulum to enable the femoral head to mould into a "**normal spherical shape**" is called containment.

Q. How can you achieve containment of femoral head?

Containment of femoral head is achieved by:

Conservative
- Braces which keep limb in abduction and internal rotation is applied
- Bilateral above knee cast (broomstick cast) which can keep lower limb in abduction and internal rotation.

Surgical
- Varus derotation osteotomy of femur (Fig. 5.2)
- Pelvic osteotomy

Q. What are the prognostic factors for Perthes' disease?

Various factors affect the outcome.
1. Age of onset of the disease
2. Extent of the involvement of the head
3. Extrusion of the femoral head
4. Stage of the disease
5. Range of the motion

Q. How do you treat transient synovitis of the hip joint?

Transient synovitis can be treated with
1. A few days of rest and above knee skin traction
2. NSAIDs.
   It is self-limiting benign condition.

The approach to the case would be a bit different if this patient was an adult. Perthes' disease and transient synovitis *does not occur in adults*.
Diagnosis and management changes!!

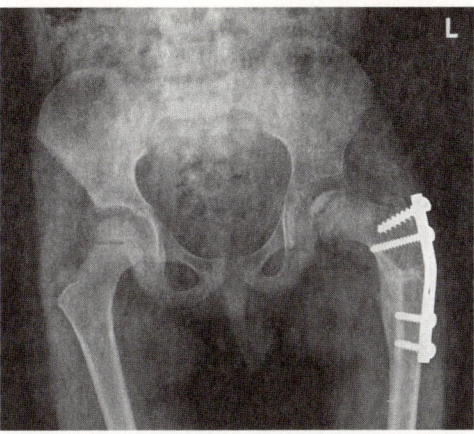

Fig. 5.2: Plain radiograph of Perthes' disease showing well contained femoral head treated with varus derotation osteotomy

Q. What are the clinicopathological stages of tuberculosis of the hip joint?

There are three clinicopathological stages of tuberculosis of hip
- *1st stage:* **Stage of synovitis**—stage of apparent lengthening/abduction deformity
- *2nd stage:* **Stage of arthritis**—stage of apparent shortening/adduction deformity
- **3rd stage: Stage of late arthritis or deformity**—stage of true shortening

Q. What is the treatment of tuberculosis of the hip joint?

Tuberculosis of the hip joint can be managed according to stage of presentation. All efforts must be instituted to salvage the normal hip joint.
1. *Early stage (synovitis)*
   - ATT for 9–12 months
   - Above knee traction and supervised mobilization
   - Occasional synovectomy (open or arthroscopic)
2. *Stage of arthritis*
   - ATT, traction followed by mobilization.
   - Salvage surgeries
3. *Advanced arthritis/deformity:*
   - ATT
   - Salvage surgeries, arthrodesis
   - Total hip replacement

Q. Name standard 1st line ATT drugs, dosage and major side effect

1. *Isoniazid (H):* 5 mg/kg/day; Peripheral neuropathy*, hepatitis
2. *Rifampicin (R):* 10 mg/kg/day; Hepatitis
3. *Ethambutol (E):* 15 mg/kg/day; Optic neuritis, hepatitis
4. *Pyrazinamide (Z):* 20 mg/kg/day; Gout
   *Pyridoxine is recommended to prevent peripheral neuropathy of INH.

Q. What is the current ATT regime using 1st line drugs recommended for Musculoskeletal TB?

The current ATT regime is as follows:
Intensive phase: 0–2 months: All four drugs (HREZ) + 10 mg pyridoxine
Maintenance phase: 2–12 months: HRE + 10 mg pyridoxine

Patient are followed every 2 months to
1. Assess the clinical improvement and to look for any side effect of the drugs.
2. CBP, ESR is performed to check whether disease is responding to ATT or not.
3. LFT is performed to assess the hepatotoxic effect of ATT.

Q. Name 2nd line ATT drugs?

The 2nd line ATT drugs are used in case of resistance or intolerance to 1st line drugs.
1. *Fluoroquinolones:* Levofloxacin, moxifloxacin
2. Linezolid

3. Clofazimine
4. Thioacetazone, ethionamide, PAS
5. Streptomycin, amikacin

Q. Can you name any salvage surgery in tuberculosis of hip?

1. Girdlestone excision arthroplasty of hip.
2. Pelvic support osteotomy

Q. What is Girdlestone excision arthroplasty?

In **Girdlestone hip excision arthroplasty**, diseased head and neck of femur is excised. Following this, limb is kept in traction for a few weeks and later limb is mobilized.

Q. What is the advantage and disadvantage of Girdlestone procedure?

Advantage: Painless and mobile hip
Disadvantage: Unstable gait with shortening of limb.

Q. In which case, it would be advisable to perform Girdlestone procedure?

In case where person need to squat and sit cross leg either in order to perform his activities of daily living or occupation would be benefitted by this surgery. For example Cobbler, blacksmiths.

Q. What are the other surgical options for a tubercular hip arthritis?

Other options are:
a. Arthrodesis
b. Total hip replacement (THR)

Pelvis support ostetotomy is preferred in children where, arthrodesis and THR are not advised.

> **Surgical options for an arthritic joint**
> 1. Total joint replacement
> 2. Realignment osteotomy
> 3. Arthroscopic debridement
> 4. Arthrodesis
> 5. Excision arthroplasty

Q. Is it possible to perform total hip replacement (THR) in a treated case of TB hip?

Yes, it is possible to perform THR in such situations as chance of biofilm formation in tubercular infection is minimal. So, infection can be treated even in presence of implant.

Q. What are the prerequisites, position, contraindication and complication of hip arthrodesis?

Prerequisite: Normal ipsilateral knee, contralateral hip and spine.

Position of hip arthrodesis:
Flexion: 20–25°
External rotation: 0–15°
Adduction: 0–5° (avoid abduction as it increases pelvic obliquity resulting in low back pain)

Contraindication of hip arthrodesis:
Active infection, other hip arthritis, Limb-length discrepancy >2.0 cm, degenerative changes in lumbar spine, contralateral hip and ipsilateral knee, severe osteoporosis, contralateral total hip arthroplasty (increases the failure rate of existing total hip arthroplasty)

Complications: Ipsilateral knee, contralateral hip and lumbar spine arthritis.

Q. What is arthrodesis?

Arthrodesis means "surgical fusion of joint".

Q. What is the indication of arthrodesis?

Arthrodesis can be performed in arthritic joints of various etiologies (traumatic, degenerative, failed replacement and neuropathic joint).

Q. What are the advantages and disadvantages of arthrodesis?

Arthrodesis leads to **painless, stable but stiff joint**. So patient experiences no pain but loses all movement at that joint.

Other major disadvantage is that the stress arising from arthrodesis joint is transferred to adjacent joint resulting in degenerative changes in few years.

Q. Which is the best treatment of an arthritic joint?

Best treatment option for an arthritic joint is to achieve a painless, stable and mobile joint. And, this can be achieved by **total joint replacement**.

Q. What is the absolute contraindication of total joint replacement?

Active pyogenic infection in the joint is the **absolute contraindication** of joint replacement.

However, total joint replacement can be performed in the joint with past history of infection if there is no current clinical, serological or tissue evidence of infection. However, the risk of reactivation of infection always persists!!

Q. Is joint replacement contraindicated in tuberculosis of joints too?

It should be avoided in active tuberculosis. However, it can be performed in a treated case of tuberculosis of the said joint after complete clinical and serological improvement. The risk of reactivation of infection is low as *Mycobacterium tuberculosis* has very little tendency to form biofilm. So, even if there is reactivation of infection, it can be treated with standard ATT.

Never mention joint replacement for an infective arthritis!! It is a viva disaster!

Q. Generally, all arthritis are painful. Which is a painless arthritis?

Neuropathic arthritis or Charcot's arthropathy is characterized by **painless, massive destruction** of joint.

Q. What are the common causes of Charcot's arthropathy?

Following are the common causes:

1. **Syringomyelia:** Especially in upper limb; due to syrinx in cervical region of spinal cord
2. **Diabetes mellitus:** Currently, the most common cause of Charcot's arthropathy in lower limbs (ankle and foot)
3. Hansen's disease

Other causes:

4. Tabes dorsalis in syphilis (rare cause, common in past!)
5. Meningocele, meningomyelocele
6. Spinal cord injury
7. Alcoholic neuropathy
8. Congenital insensitivity to pain

Q. Is Charcot's arthropathy always painless?

Classical Charcot's is theoretically considered to be painless but there can be **mild pain in 75% cases**. However, amount of destruction and arthritis of joint does not corroborate with pain. Usually destruction of joint is quite severe and pain is less.

Q. What is the clinical feature of Charcot's arthritis?

Charcot's arthritis is characterized by painless, gross destruction of joint rendering it very unstable.

In Charcot's arthropathy, joint reveals grossly exaggerated movements in various planes due to massive destruction of bone and soft tissues.

Q. Which is the commonest clinical condition in which you see Charcot's arthropathy?

Currently **diabetes mellitus** is the **most leading cause** of Charcot's arthropathy. It affects the **small joint of foot and ankle.**

Charcot's arthropathy was described by a French neurologist, Jean- Marie-Charcot. He is regarded as father of modern neurology.

One must remember that **early stages of Charcot's arthropathy are painful and can mimic cellulitis** of foot and ankle which is very common presentation in diabetes mellitus. In other words, one must keep Charcot's arthropathy in mind while treating diabetic foot.

Q. What leads to neuropathic/Charcot's arthropathy?

Any condition which causes loss of:
1. Pain and peripheral sensation
2. Proprioception
3. Fine motor control

Q. What are the investigation in neuropathic joint shows?

a. *Plain X-ray of the joint:* Classical description of a neuropathic joint included 6 "Ds" (Fig. 5.3).
   1. *Distended joint:* Due to effusion
   2. *Disorganized*
   3. *Destruction* of bone and joint surface
   4. *Density increase* of bones
   5. *Debris:* Bone destruction causes debris
   6. *Dislocation:* Destroyed articular surface causes dislocated joints
b. *Bone scan:* Helpful in early detection of Charcot's joint especially to differentiate with osteomyelitis.

Q. What is the management of Charcot's arthropathy?

• Management is usually **conservative, and treat the underlying condition**
• Orthosis is a good option to stabilise the joint, and rarely arthrodesis of the joint could be attempted.
• **Joint replacement results in failure.**

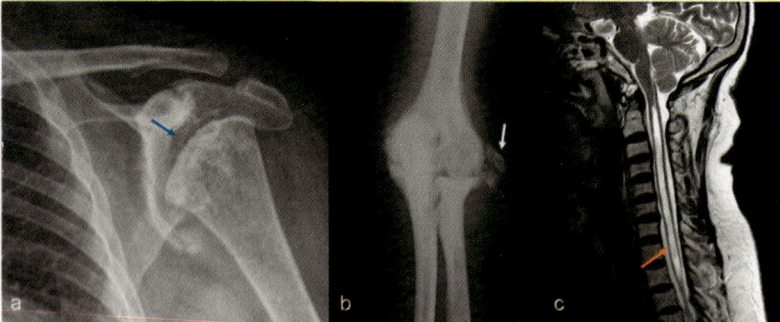

Figs 5.3a to c: (a) is plain X-ray of left neuropathic shoulder joint showing grossly disorganized and damaged joint (blue arrow), (b) shows neuropathic elbow joint radiograph with dense sclerosis and debris (white arrow), (c) shows sagittal section of cervical spine MRI revealing syringomyelia (dilated central canal, orange arrow) from C2 to T2 vertebra

6

Metabolic Diseases

RICKETS AND VALGUS KNEE DEFORMITY

Common Presentation of Rickets with Genu Valgum Deformity

Case summary: A 7-year-old child was brought to an orthopedic OPD with painless progressive deformity in the legs. Child was apparently all right till 6 years of age when parents noticed a progressive deformity around knee and leg where both legs were moving away from body. Parents also noticed a symmetric swelling just above both the wrist joint. Child also complained of gradual onset of fatigue. On general examination, child appeared to be malnourished. Local examination revealed bilateral genu valgum deformity. There was no bony or soft tissue tenderness around knee joint. The valgus deformity of both knees was totally correctable with knee completely flexed. Intermalleolar distance was 15 cm. There was bilateral distal radius metaphyseal broadening.

Q. What is the clinical diagnosis?

The clinical diagnosis is bilateral genu valgum most likely due to nutritional rickets (Fig. 6.1)

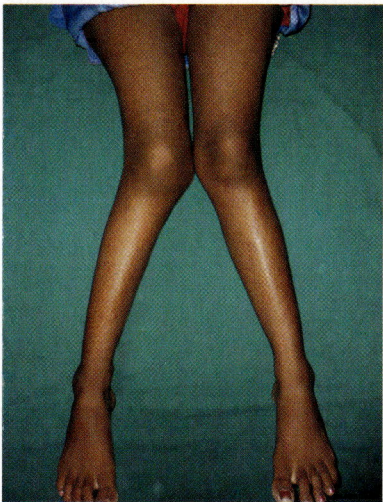

Fig. 6.1: Clinical photograph of a child with bilateral genu valgum

Q. Why do you say so?

It is so because of

1. Growing child
2. Features of malnourishment
3. Progressive bilateral genu valgum
4. Broadening of the distal end of radius (metaphysis)

Q. What other history is important in suspected rickets?

1. *Diet:* Diet poor in calcium or vitamin D (nutritional rickets)
2. *Past history of local infection/trauma/surgery:* Suggest physeal damage resulting in unilateral deformity
3. *Family history of:* Skeletal dysplasia
4. *Chronic bowel/liver disorder:* It could result in malabsorption syndromes leading to poor absorption of calcium/Vit D
5. *Chronic skin disorder:* Dermatitis/other exfoliating skin disorder leading to poor Vit D synthesis in skin
6. *Chronic drug intake:* Loop diuretics, Antacids, corticosteroids or antiepileptic drugs (phenytoin sodium, phenobarbitone)
7. *Chronic renal disorder:* Renal tubular acidosis can cause vitamin D resistant rickets

Q. What are the clinical features of rickets?

General

- Delayed milestones
- Features of malnutrition
- Bone pain, muscle weakness
- *In severe cases:* Carpopedal spasm, tetany, hypocalcemic seizures

Head

a. Frontal bossing
b. Ping-pong skull
c. Flat occiput
d. Delayed closure of frontanelle
e. Poorly developed malar prominences
f. Square shape head (caput quadratum)
g. Poor dentition

Spine

a. Cat back deformity (mobile kyphosis)

Chest

a. Harrison's sulcus (a depression over the lower part of chest due to rib deformity arising out of pull from the diaphragm)
b. Rachitic rosary (painful swelling of the costochondral junction)

c. Pigeon's chest (pectus carinatum)

d. Pectus excavatum

Abdomen

a. Pot belly (abdomen appears protuberant due to loss of tone in abdominal muscles)

Upper Limb

a. Broadening of wrist (actually, it is distal radius metaphyseal widening which gives an appearance of broad wrist).

Pelvis

a. Triradiate pelvis

b. Coxa vara

Lower Limb

a. Genu varum/genu valgum

b. Double malleoli sign at ankle (it is due to broadened distal tibial metaphysis which gives an appearance of double malleolus, i.e. another malleolus above the normal ones).

Q. In this patient, the genu valgum deformity is contributed by which bone, femur/tibia?

Knee flexion-extension helps in determining the location of the deformity. If the genu valgum or varum deformity.

a. **Disappears with knee flexion:** The bony deformity is in femoral condyles

b. **Remains same with knee flexion:** The bony deformity is in tibial plateau

c. **Decreases with knee flexion but not completely:** The deformity is partly in femur and partly in tibia.

Q. Why it is important to know that which bone is contributing to the deformity?

It is important to know because if deformity needs operative correction, the deformed bone should be operated upon and not the normal one.

Q. What are the causes of bilateral genu valgum or varum?

Bilateral deformity (varum or valgum) could be:

- **Physiological** or due to causes which have systemic influence such as:
  - Skeletal dysplasia
  - *Metabolic:* Nutritional rickets, renal rickets
  - *Inflammatory:* Rheumatoid arthritis
  - *Neuromuscular:* Cerebral palsy

Q. What are the causes for unilateral genu valgum or varum?

Unilateral deformity is a result of those causes which have local influence on skeleton such as:

a. **Injury to physis:** Due to trauma, infection

b. *Proximal metaphyseal fracture* (Cozen fracture)

c. *Tumors:* Fibrous dysplasia, osteochondroma

> Note: Unilateral deformity is always pathological whereas bilateral could be a physiological variation.

Q. What is the normal physiologic variation in knee alignment?

At birth, normal knee alignment is *genu varus (10–15°)*. As the child starts walking, varus may increase till 2 years. Physiological genu varum improves after 2 years of the age and then *physiological valgus* starts appearing around 3 years of the age. Physiologic valgus presents between 4 and 6 years of age (10–20°). It attains *'neutral' adult leg alignment* around 7 years of the age.

Easy to remember: "Varus-neutral-valgus-neutral"

Q. Is it normal physiologic valgus in this patient?

No, because it is associated with other signs of rickets.

Q. What are the characters of physiologic valgus?

The characteristics of **physiologic valgus** are:

a. Age between 3 and 6 years

b. Bilateral symmetrical

c. Normal growth

d. Absence of features of malnutrition.

> **Clue to abnormal valgus**
> 1. Increasing valgus even after 7 years or valgus <2 years of age
> 2. Short stature
> 3. Unilateral valgus
> 4. Presence of pathologic features like rickets, malnutrition

Q. Is there any classification for severity of genu valgum?

Severity of genu valgum is assessed by measuring intermalleolar distance (IMD), and is classified into three groups. Both knees touch each other while assessing IMD.

- **Mild deformity:** IMD 8–10 cm
- **Moderate deformity:** IMD 10–15 cm
- **Severe deformity:** IMD >15 cm

Severity of genu varum is assessed by measuring **distance between two medial femoral condyles of right and left knee** while both ankles touch each other.

Grade 1: 5–7.5 cm

Grade 2: 7.5–10 cm

Grade 3: >10 cm

Q. How would you investigate a patient with rickets?

1. *X-ray of the long bones*
2. *Serum calcium (Ca), phosphorus (P):*
   In hypocalcemic rickets (HCR): Both low
   In hypophosphatemic rickets (HPR): Calcium normal, phosphate low
3. Serum alkaline phosphatase **(ALP):** Always high in all forms of rickets
4. Serum parathormone **(PTH):** High in HCR; normal in HPR
5. **Urinary calcium and phosphorus:**
   HCR: Low calcium, high P
   HPR: Normal calcium, high P
6. Renal function test **(RFT):** High serum urea, creatinine in renal rickets
7. Liver function test **(LFT):** Liver and biliary tract disease can cause abnormal vitamin D metabolism
   HCR: Hypocalcemic rickets
   HPR: Hypophosphatemic rickets
   Table 6.1 outlines the serological investigations performed in rickets.

Q. What will be the X-ray findings in nutritional rickets?

1. Physeal widening, cupping, fraying (Fig. 6.2)
2. Metaphysis splaying
3. Thinned out epiphysis
4. Osteopenia

Table 6.1: Rickets investigation									
Type of rickets		*Ca*	*P*	*ALP*	*PTH*	*25 HCC calcidiol*	*1, 25 DHCC calcitriol*	*Urine calcium, phosphate*	*Serum urea, creatinine*
Hypocalcemic rickets (HCR)	Nutritional rickets	↓	↓	↑	↑	↓	Normal or high in HCR as a result of PTH stimulation	*In HCR rickets:* Urinary calcium is low and phosphorus high	High in renal disorders resulting in rickets
	Type 1 Vit D dependent rickets	↓	↓	↑	↑	↓			
	Type 2 Vit D dependent rickets	↓	↓	↑	↑	↑			
Hypophos-phatemic rickets (HPR)		N	↓	↑	N	N	Normal	*In HPR rickets:* Urinary calcium is normal, phosphorus is high	

Ca: Calcium; P: Phosphorus; ALP: Alkaline phosphatase; PTH: Parathormone; 25HCC: 25 hydroxycholecalciferol; DHCC: Dihydroxycholecalciferol

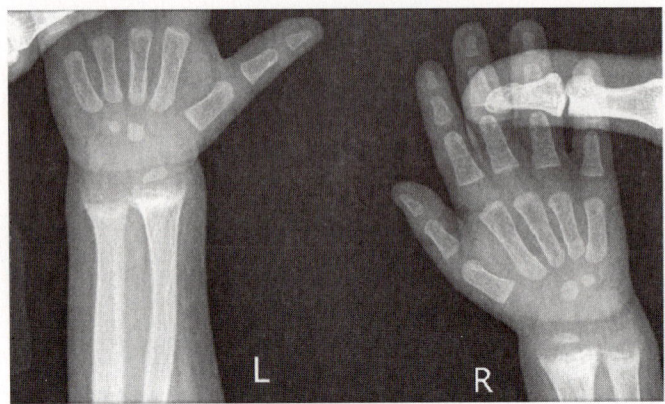

Fig. 6.2: Plain X-ray of wrist shows typical features of rickets; metaphyseal widening, cupping and fraying

Q. How will you treat nutritional rickets?

The goal of the treatment of nutritional rickets are:
1. Medical treatment of rickets by—
   a. Single 6,00,000 unit of vitamin D, oral or intramuscular.
   b. Oral calcium supplementation
   c. Dietary calcium via milk, cheese, etc.
2. Treat deformity

Knee deformity correction
a. Mild deformity: Reassurance, remodels with time
b. Moderate deformity: Observation, braces
c. Severe deformity:
   i. Corrective osteotomy: Age near skeletal maturity
   ii. Hemiepiphysiodesis: Age <10 years

Q. When would you do the corrective osteotomy?

Corrective osteotomy must be performed when there is evidence of:
a. Radiological healing of rickets: Zone of calcification (Fig. 6.3)
b. Most importantly, when **ALP returns to normal** indicating return of normal bone physiology.

Q. Why not to do the osteotomy in the beginning of the treatment?

Osteotomy should not be performed in "active rickets" (very high ALP and without any sign of radiological healing of ricketic bony lesions) because
1. The deformity tends to remodel with the medical treatment, bracing and age. Hence, the severity of deformity may decrease with time or get self-corrected, and might not require any surgical treatment.
2. An osteotomy performed in active rickets may result in:
   a. Non-healing of osteotomy
   b. Recurrence of corrected deformity

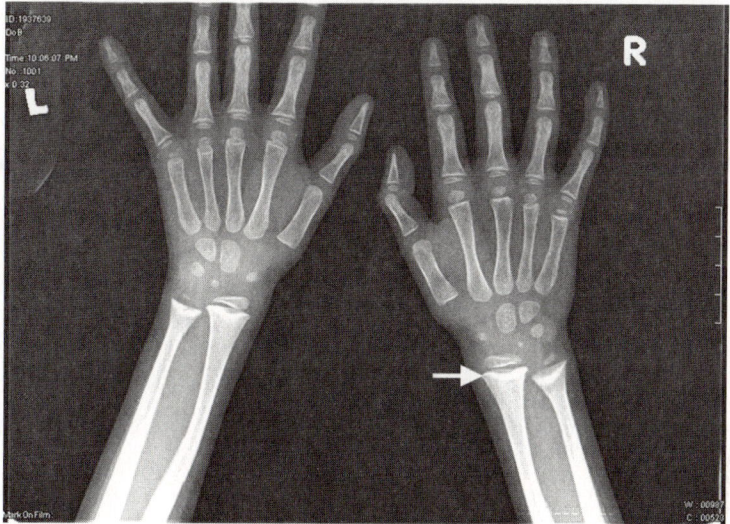

Fig. 6.3: Plain X-ray of wrist shows zone of calcification at the lower end of radius (white arrow) which is a sign of healing in rickets after treatment with vitamin D

Q. What are corrective osteotomies for knee deformities (valgum and varum)?

Genu valgum: Supracondylar femur osteotomy
Genu varum: Proximal tibial osteotomy

Q. Define rickets?

Rickets is defined as *inadequate mineralisation at the growth plate of a long bone in a growing skeleton.*

The inadequate mineralisation of bony matrix or osteoid area (organic collagenous scaffold of bone) results in 'soft bones'. These soft bones are prone for:
• Chronic bending deformity of long bones of lower limb under loading
• Fractures

Q. What is the etiology of rickets?

1. *Hypocalcemic rickets (HCR):* Due to deficiency of calcium or vitamin D (main cause)
2. *Hypophosphatemic rickets (HPR):* Due to phosphate deficiency. For etiology of rickets is given in Table 6.2.

Q. What is pathophysiology of rickets?

Calcium or phosphate mineral deficiency prevents the normal process of bone mineral deposition at the growth plate resulting in rickets.

In HCR, the primary defect results from lack of dietary calcium or vitamin D or vitamin D effect causing decreased calcium absorption from the gut. This reduction in calcium absorption increases parathyroid hormone secretion, which acts to preserve blood calcium levels by:
1. Osteoclast induced bone resorption,

2. Decreasing renal calcium loss,
3. Increasing renal phosphate loss, and
4. Increasing vitamin D activation by upregulating the vitamin D 1-alpha-hydroxylase enzyme in the kidney.

The combination of decreased calcium and phosphate availability results in rickets.

In HPR, there is severe renal phosphate wasting resulting in decreased phosphate availability causing rickets.

Q. What is osteomalacia?

Osteomalacia is defined as poor mineralisation of organic bone matrix bone (osteoid area) following growth plate closure in adults resulting in a greater proportion of unmineralised osteoid.

Note: Rickets occurs at the growth plate in children where osteomalacia can occur in both children and adults as osteoid areas are present in both children and adults.

Q. What are the clinical features of osteomalacia?

- Adult with diet poor in vitamin D, poor exposure to sunlight
- Bone pain
- Proximal muscle weakness
- Fracture

Q. How do you investigate osteomalacia?

The investigations are similar to rickets.

Q. What is the typical radiological finding in osteomalacia?

Typical radiological finding in osteomalacia is **Looser's zone*** (milkman fracture). It lies perpendicular to the cortical margins of the bone. Looser's zone are often bilateral and symmetric, and are seen over

a. Medial border of scapula
b. Pubic and ischial ramus
c. Femoral neck, upper medial part of proximal femur

*Looser's zone indicate insufficiency fracture or unossified matrix.

Other features of osteomalacia are:

1. Osteopenia
2. Long bone end resorption: Distal clavicle, distal femur, distal humerus
3. Cystic areas in bone
4. Rugger jersey spine: Sclerotic bands present at the end plate of the vertebra

Q. What is the treatment of osteomalacia?

Calcium and vitamin D.

Table 6.2: Rickets etiology	
Calcium/vitamin D deficiency	*Phosphate deficiency*

1. **Vitamin D/Ca deficient**
 • Lack of sunlight exposure
 • Lack of Ca/vitamin D_3 in diet
 • Poor absorption 'malabsorption syndrome' celiac disease
 • Drugs preventing absorption: Phenytoin
 • Chronic liver disease
 • Chronic renal disease (renal osteodystrophy)
	1. **Renal phosphate wasting (most common cause)**
	 a. Genetic hypophosphatemic rickets
	   • X linked hypophosphatemic rickets OR familial hypophosphatemic rickets (vitamin D resistant rickets)
	   • Autosomal dominant hypophosphatemic rickets
	   • Autosomal resistant hypophosphatemic rickets
	   • McCune-Albright syndrome
	   • Fanconi's syndrome
	   • Renal tubular acidosis
	 b. **Oncogenic hypophosphatemia:** It is 'tumor induced hypophosphatemia' wherein certain tumors (hemangiopericytoma, mesenchymal tumor) secrete fibroblast growth factor 23 (FGF-23) which is phosphaturic in nature.

2. **Type I vitamin D dependent rickets** • *Autosomal recessive disorder:* Lack of 1-α hydroxylase enzyme in kidney. Hence, no active vitamin D is synthesised in body from 25HCC (calcidiol) to 1,25 DHCC (calcitriol). • Symptoms within 1st year of life • Normal calcidiol level, low calcitriol level • *Treatment* with calcitriol supplements	2. **Poor phosphate intake**
3. **Type II vitamin D dependent rickets** • Autosomal recessive disorder: Receptor resistance to 'calcitriol/ active Vitamin D' • Symptoms of rickets within 2 years of life • *Alopecia* is very characteristics of this type of rickets, and *other ectodermal anomalies* (multiple milia, oligodentia, ectodermal cyst) • *Treatment:* Very high doses of calcitriol and calcium	

Bone Tumors

EWING'S SARCOMA

Common Presentation of Ewing's Sarcoma

Case summary: An 8-year-old boy complained of painful, rapidly growing swelling over middle of the left thigh for last two months. He gave history of minor fall prior to the onset of painful swelling. There is irregular fever, loss of appetite and weight for 4 weeks. There are no similar swellings anywhere else in the body. General examination revealed mild pallor and fever. Local examination of left thigh revealed diffuse swelling over the mid shaft of the femur which was tender and of variable consistency. There were dilated veins over the swelling. Range of movement of knee was 0–120°. Inguinal lymph nodes were palpable. The distal neurovascular examination was normal.

Q. What is the clinical diagnosis?

The clinical diagnosis is malignant lesion of left femur, most likely to be Ewing's sarcoma.

Key point

Age and site of lesion are two most important factors in deciding the diagnosis of bone tumor.

Q. Why do you think that it is Ewing's sarcoma?

It is because of following reasons:

History
1. Painful, rapidly growing bony swelling: Indicates malignancy
2. Loss of appetite, weight and irregular fever
3. Young age: Ewing's occurs between 5 and 15 years

Examination
4. Bony, tender swelling in diaphysis region: Ewing's occurs in diaphysis
5. Variable consistency, dilated veins: Indicates possibility of malignant swelling
6. Enlarged lymph nodes

Students must know the bone tumor classification. It is often asked in viva.

Q. What are the common sites of Ewing's metastasis?

Chest, other bones, and rarely lymph nodes.

Q. How will you investigate this patient?

1. *Complete blood picture:* TLC, DLC may be high and this may raise suspicion of infection as differential diagnosis
2. *ESR, CRP:* Often high
3. *Serum alkaline phosphatase (ALP), and LDH:* Elevated
4. *X-ray of the limb:* AP and lateral view (Fig. 7.1)
   a. Skeletally immature
   b. Diaphyseal lesion
   c. Onion peel appearance
   d. Periosteal elevation
   e. Moth eaten appearance of lesion
5. *MRI scan of thigh:* For soft tissue involvement and intramedullary spread.
6. *Bone scan:* To assess the skeletal metastasis
7. *Biopsy of the lesion:* Confirmatory investigation
8. *Investigation for visceral metastasis:* CT scan of pelvis, abdomen, chest

Note: **Biopsy** is the ***investigation of choice*** to confirm any tumorous lesion

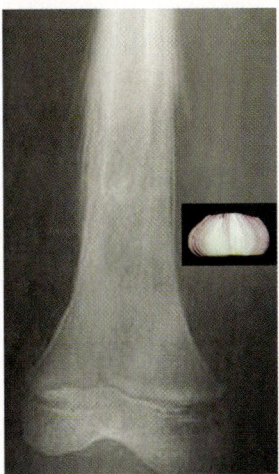

Fig. 7.1: Plain X-ray of femur showing onion peel type periosteal reaction in diaphysis of skeletally immature patient. Inset image shows comparison with onion peel appearance

Once my chief, Prof. Sripathi Rao asked me to come to his chamber and examine a 9-year-old child who presented with a swelling over his proximal thigh for 6 weeks along with fever. Clinically and radiologically, it appeared to be chronic osteomyelitis and that's what I told him. He asked me to admit and investigate. When I was about to leave his chamber; he told me that, keep Ewing's in mind! On exploration of the swelling, it contained pus. But the biopsy turned out to be Ewing's sarcoma! He was treated successfully! Hence, differential diagnosis of Ewing's is chronic osteomyelitis and vice versa.

Investigations for metastasis:
1. CT scan of chest: for pulmonary metastasis
2. USG abdomen
3. *Bone scan:* To look for skeletal metastasis.

Q. What is the classical biopsy finding in Ewing's sarcoma?

Histopathology examination (HPE) shows:
a. Sheets of monotonous, small blue round cells
b. Pseudorosette formation (circle of cells with necrosis in center)

Key point

Bone ALP is produced by osteoblasts. Hence, it is high in all "new bone forming" conditions where osteoblastic activity is high producing more ALP

1. **Fracture healing** after trauma
2. **Osteomyelitis** as there in involucrum formation
3. **New bone forming tumors** like osteosarcoma and Ewing's sarcoma (very high).
4. **Paget's disease**
   Hence, high ALP is a sensitive sign but not specific.

Key point

Bone scan done using Tc99 is actively taken up in high concentration in those areas which have **abnormally high blood supply**. Hence, it is interpreted as hotspot. Abnormal blood supply is present in areas of

1. Fracture healing
2. Infection
3. Inflammation
4. Tumors with new bone formation

So, **bone scan is sensitive** but **not specific** investigation.

Note: Bone scan is negative in multiple myeloma where there is no new bone formation.

Q. How will you treat Ewings sarcoma?

Ewings is treated by chemotherapy followed by surgery.
1. *Neoadjuvant chemotherapy:* 8–12 weeks
   - Vincristine
   - Doxorubicin
   - Cyclophosphamide, isosfamide
   - Etoposide
2. *Surgery:*
   - Wide surgical resection followed by limb salvage
   - Rarely, amputation
3. *Adjuvant chemotherapy:* 6–12 months

Q. Is radiotherapy indicated in Ewing's sarcoma?

Though tumor responds well to the radiotherapy, but it is kept reserved for non-resectable tumors and widespread metastasis.

Q. What is the differential diagnosis of Ewing's sarcoma?

The differential diagnosis of Ewing's sarcoma is chronic osteomyelitis because
- Often there is fever as constitutional symptom
- CBC, ESR and CRP is elevated
- The biopsy of Ewing's tumor could reveal pus like material!
  Similarly, the *differential diagnosis of osteomyelitis is Ewing's sarcoma!*

Q. What is the genetic basic of Ewing's sarcoma?

t(11:22). The characteristic translocation between chromosome 11 and 22 results in a fusion gene EWSR1-FL11 which is present in 90% of cases.

Q. What is role of mild trauma in such cases?

Often children do give a history of minor fall but it remains coincidental, and cannot be implicated in the pathophysiology of the tumor.

OSTEOSARCOMA

Common Presentation of Osteosarcoma

Case summary: A 14-year-old boy complained of painful, rapidly growing swelling over lower end of left thigh for three months with difficulty in walking. He gave history of minor fall prior to onset of these symptoms. There was history of loss of appetite and weight. There are no similar swellings anywhere else in the body. On examination, a diffuse swelling was present at the lower end of femur arising from bone which was tender, diffuse and of variable consistency with dilated veins over the skin. Range of movement was restricted (0–120°). Inguinal lymph nodes are not palpable. There was no limb length discrepancy or distal neurovascular deficit. There are no other systemic symptoms.

Q. What is the clinical diagnosis?

The clinical diagnosis is malignant lesion of left femur, most likely osteosarcoma.

Q. Why do you say so?

It is because of following reasons:

History:

1. Young age, 2nd decade
2. Rapidly growing painful swelling in thigh
3. Loss of appetite and weight (systemic symptom)

Examination

4. Swelling in metaphyseal region (Fig. 7.2)
5. Variable consistency, tender with dilated veins over skin

Q. How will you investigate a patient with suspected osteosarcoma?

1. *Complete blood picture:* TLC, DLC may be high
2. *ESR:* High

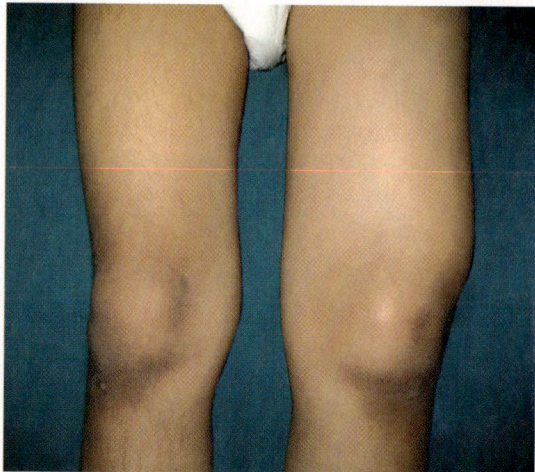

Fig. 7.2: Clinical picture of left thigh showing swelling at the lower end of thigh

Important features of osteosarcoma
- Most common primary malignant bone tumor
- *Age:* Bimodal distribution; 10–20 years, 55–60 years
- Location: Metaphysis of long bone
- Deep boring pain often at rest
- Gradually increasing swelling, variable in consistency

3. Serum Alkaline phosphatase **(ALP)**: Very high
4. *X-ray:* AP and lateral view of the limb (thigh) (Fig. 7.3)
   a. Skeletally immature bone
   b. Metaphyseal lesion
   c. Codman's triangle
   d. Sunburst appearance
   e. Combination of lytic and blastic lesion in metaphysis
5. *MRI scan of thigh:* For soft tissue involvement and intramedullary spread.
6. *Biopsy* of the lesion: Confirmatory investigation
7. Investigation to assess the metastasis:
   a. CT chest, abdomen and pelvis
   b. Tc^{99} bone scan for skeletal metastasis

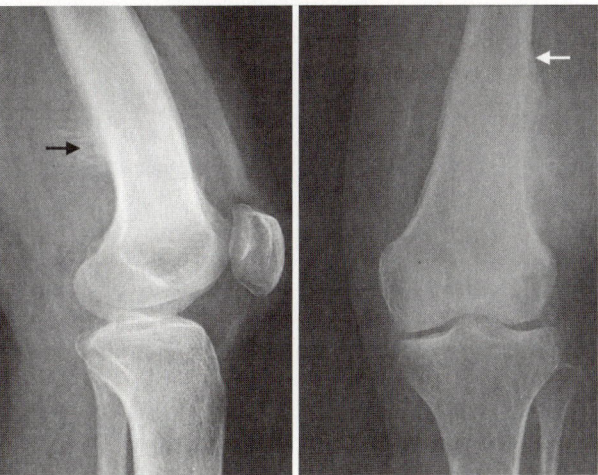

Fig. 7.3: Plain X-ray (AP and lateral views) of left femur shows sunburst appearance in lateral view (black arrow) and Codman's triangle in AP view (white arrow) with periosteal reaction

Q. What is the classical biopsy finding in osteosarcoma?

Histopathology examination shows:
a. Atypical tumor cells with **large areas of "lacey osteoid"**
b. Chondroblastic, osteoblastic or fibroblastic appearance of cells

Q. How will you treat osteosarcoma?

Osteosarcoma is treated by chemotherapy followed by surgery.

1. *Neoadjuvant chemotherapy:* 8–12 weeks
   • Doxorubicin
   • Isosfamide
   • Cisplatin
   • Methotrexate
2. *Surgery:*
   • Wide/radical surgical resection followed by limb salvage surgery (Fig. 7.4)
   • Rarely, amputation
3. *Adjuvant chemotherapy:* 6–12 months

Common side effects of chemotherapy drugs
1. Isosphamide: Hemorrhagic cystitis
2. Methotrexate: Hepatic and renal damage, leucoencephalopathy
3. Doxorubicin: Cardiotoxic
4. Cisplatin: Neuropathy

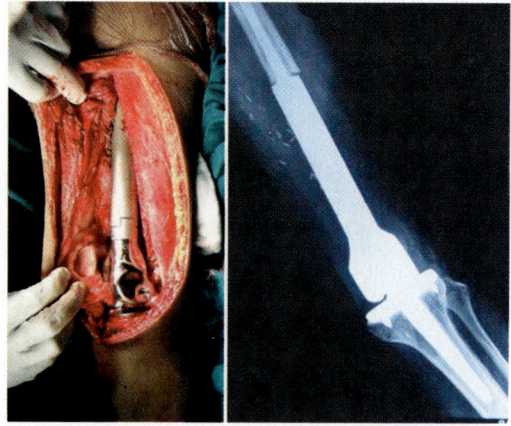

Fig. 7.4: Intraoperative photograph of left femur after radical excision of osteosarcoma of lower end of femur and application of custom made prosthesis (limb salvage surgery). X-ray of same limb shows prosthesis *in situ*. (Photograph of limb salvage surgery. *Courtesy:* Dr. Kishore Reddy, Hyderabad)

Q. What is the rationale of neoadjuvant chemotherapy?

Neo-adjuvant chemotherapy helps in shrinking local tumor size by:
a. Killing rapidly dividing tumor cells almost by 90% and
b. Reducing vascularity of the tumor

Once tumors size and vascularity is reduced, it is easier to resect tumor with tumor clear margins and the chance of perioperative micrometastasis is reduced. It also kills the micrometastatic tumor at the time of primary diagnosis of tumor.

Q. What is limb salvage surgery?

In the past, amputation of limb was primary treatment of choice for most of the malignant bone tumors. However, recently trend is of limb salvage where only tumor is resected (wide or radical), the defect is filled by reconstructive procedure like 'endoprosthesis, allograft, autograft or other reconstructive procedure', and rest of the distal limb is not removed.

The limb salvage helps in preserving the appearance of patient and the limb and provides most optimal function to the limb.

The concept of limb salvage is based on a FACT that the *survival rate of patient with amputated limb and salvaged limb is similar.*

Q. What is the contraindication of limb salvage?

1. Involvement of neurovascular bundle
2. Infection
3. Pathological fracture
   (Remember!: NIP)

Q. What are the problems of limb salvage?

The major problems of limb salvage is associated with 'graft or endoprosthesis'
• Infection
• Prosthesis loosening

Q. When would be amputation performed?

When limb salvage is not possible.

Q. What are the risk factors for development of osteosarcoma?

There are multiple factors which can predispose development of osteosarcoma
a. *Genetic:* Retinoblastoma gene, p53 gene, increased risk in Rothmund-Thomson syndrome
b. *Prior radiotherapy:* Leads to development of secondary osteosarcoma
c. *Patients with Paget's disease*
d. *Watch dial painters with radium* (not seen anymore as not practiced)

Q. What are the various types of osteosarcoma?

There are several types of osteosarcoma.
1. Central (intramedullary type)
   a. Primary osteosarcoma: From normal bone
      i. Classic
      ii. Telangiectatic
      iii. Small cell
      iv. Multicentric
   b. Secondary osteosarcoma (from diseased bone)
Bone infarct, irradiated bone, Paget's disease, pre-existing tumor (fibrous dysplasia, enchondroma) or infection
2. Surface osteosarcoma
   a. Periosteal osteosarcoma
   b. Parosteal osteosarcoma
   c. Dedifferentiated

Q. What are other primary metaphyseal bone tumors?

Other **metaphyseal tumors** are:

a. Chondrosarcoma (malignant)

b. Osteochondroma

c. Adamantinoma (in tibia, mandible)

d. Osteoid osteoma

e. Simple bone cyst

f. Fibrous dysplasia

g. Aneurysmal bone cyst

Epiphyseal tumors

1. Giant cell tumor (osteoclastoma)
2. Chondroblastoma

Q. There are two classical epiphyseal tumors; GCT and chondroblastoma. How will you differentiate between them?

One can differentiate between them by clinical and radiological picture.

Chondroblastoma:

Age: Before skeletal maturity,

X-ray: Single lytic epiphyseal lesion with popcorn calcification

Giant cell tumor:

Age: After skeletal maturity,

X-ray: Epiphyseal, expansile, eccentric lesion (3Es) with soap bubble appearance on X-ray.

Q. Name some diaphyseal tumors?

Yes. These are a few of **diaphyseal tumors**

a. Ewing's sarcoma

b. Multiple myeloma

c. Osteoid osteoma

Q. Classify bone tumors?

a. *Type of tumor:* Benign or malignant

b. *Based upon age of presentation*
   1. 1st decade: Aneurysmal bone cyst, simple bone cyst, neuroblastoma
   2. 2nd decade: Osteosarcoma, Ewing, chondroblastoma
   3. 3rd decade: GCT
   4. 4th decade: Chondrosarcoma
   5. 5th decade: Multiple myeloma
   6. 6th decade: Secondaries

c. *Based upon site of lesion:* Epiphyseal/metaphyseal/diaphyseal

d. *Based upon type of cell of origin:* Read WHO classification and try remembering one tumor of each cell of origin

SOLITARY EXOSTOSIS/OSTEOCHONDROMA

Common Presentation of Solitary Exostosis

Case summary: A 14-year-old boy complained of painless swelling which was growing slowly over inner aspect of the upper end of left calf for two years. However, he complained that off late the swelling is blocking his knee movement, and he cannot bend his left knee completely. There is no history of trauma, fever or any systemic features. There are no similar swellings anywhere else in the body. On examination, nontender, bony hard, a single swelling was arising from upper end of posterior aspect of tibia which was continuous with underlying bone. Range of movement was restricted (ROM: 0–110°). There was no limb length discrepancy or distal neurovascular deficit.

Important features of osteochondroma/solitary exostosis
- *Cell of origin:* Osteoblast/chondroblast or aberrant subperiosteal nest of physeal cartilage
- *Age:* 10–30 years
- *Location:* Metaphysis. It grows away from the joint
- *Common site:* Rapidly growing end of bone around knee, proximal humerus, distal radius
- *Symptoms*
  i. Painless swelling growing away from joint and stops growing once skeletal growth is complete.
  ii. Occasionally blocks the joint movement, becomes painful due to overlying bursa becomes inflamed, compress the adjacent neurovascular bundle or might get fractured

Q. What is the diagnosis?

The clinical diagnosis is solitary exostosis or osteochondroma of left tibia (Fig. 7.5).

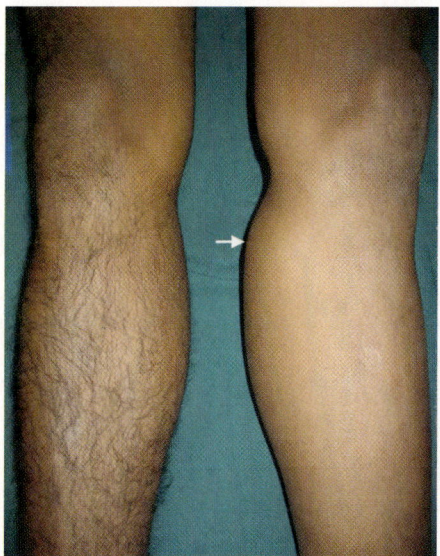

Fig. 7.5: Clinical photograph of left leg showing a swelling at the back of calf (arrow)

Q. Why do you say so?

It is so because of the following reasons:

History

1. Young age
2. Painless, solitary slowly growing bony swelling

Examination

3. Close to metaphysis region, while growing away from the joint
4. Bony hard swelling

Q. Did you look for similar swelling elsewhere in the body? If present, what is the significance?

There are no similar swellings in the body. If there are multiple such swellings over various bones, it is known as multiple hereditary osteochondromatosis (HMO) or multiple hereditary exostosis or diaphyseal aclasis.

Q. What is the other name of multiple hereditary osteochondroma?

It is also known as diaphyseal aclasis (osteochondromatosis) as the end of the long bones in such patients is broad and deformed.

Note: Diaphyseal aclasis an autosomal dominant condition.

Q. What is the other clinical feature which may give clue that the patient might be suffering from diaphyseal aclasis?

• Bilateral multiple osteochondromas all over body
• More common in long bone with angular or rotational deformity of the bone
• Many of these patients are short statured due to associated dyschondroplasia

Q. Patient has reported that the swelling continues to grow slowly? Do you expect it to slowly enlarge in size?

The osteochondroma gradually enlarges till the skeletal maturity, and then it stops growing.

Q. In what all ways, an osteochondroma or solitary exostosis could become symptomatic?

There are various reasons why would an exostosis would become symptomatic such as:

• Mechanical block to joint movement
• Bursitis (over cartilage cap)
• Fracture (of pedunculated exostosis)
• Compression of the neurovascular bundle
• **Sudden change in size of cartilage cap may suggest** malignant change in cartilage cap

Q. What could be the reason if the exostosis suddenly starts increasing in size and becomes painful?

The cause for sudden enlargement in the size of osteochondroma along with pain is possibly malignant change as chondrosarcoma.

Note: The malignant change occurs in the cartilage cap of the osteochondroma.

Q. How will you investigate?

Plain radiograph of affected limb reveals (Fig. 7.6)
a. Lesion at **metaphysis**
b. **Pedunculated or sessile** growth
c. **Growing away from joint**
d. Medullary cavity of lesion is continuous with medullary cavity of bone
e. Cortex of lesion is continuous with cortex of bone
f. On X-ray, lesion appears smaller than actual clinical size as the lesion is covered by a cartilage cap which is radiolucent, and it is not seen on the X-ray.

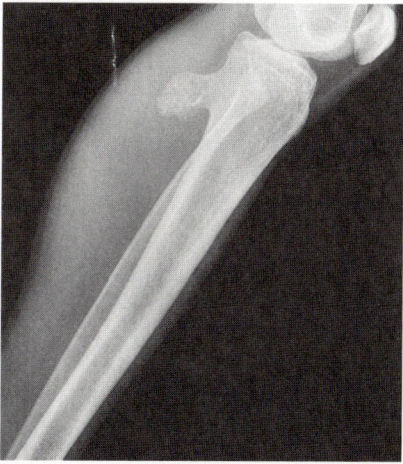

Fig. 7.6: Plain X-ray of tibia lateral view shows pedunculated solitary exostosis (osteochondroma) arising from metaphysis growing away from joint towards diaphysis

Q. How will you confirm the diagnosis?

The diagnosis is confirmed by biopsy.

Q. How will you treat this patient?

Since this swelling is causing blockage in knee flexion, it needs **complete extraperiosteal excision of swelling**. It means that swelling should be completely excised with a rim of surrounding periosteum to prevent its recurrence (Fig. 7.7).

Note:
1. Swelling should be sent for histopathological examination to confirm the diagnosis and rule out any malignant changes.
2. The other swelling which requires extraperiosteal excision is 'Cervical rib'.

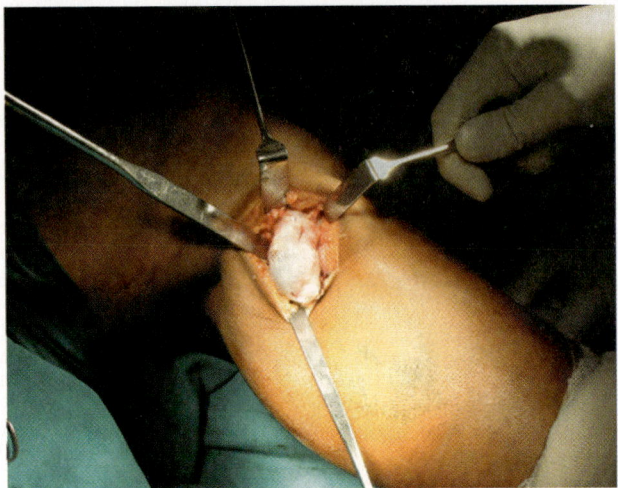

Fig. 7.7: Intraoperative photograph of same swelling shows whitish cartilage cap over the exostosis

Q. Does all patients with solitary exostosis require treatment?

No. Only symptomatic ones are treated.

Q. What are the indications for osteochondroma excision?

a. Mechanical block
b. Compression of neurovascular structures
c. Painful swelling
d. Fracture of the osteochondroma
e. Malignant change

Q. What could be the cause of a painless, solitary benign osteochondroma converting into painful one?

a. Inflammation of bursa over the cartilage cap
b. Neural compression
c. Malignant changes in swelling
d. Fracture of stalk of osteochondroma

Q. Which one, solitary or MHE has more chance of malignant changes?

MHE has higher chance of malignant change (5–25%) whereas solitary exostosis carries 1–5% chance of malignant transformation.

Note: Malignant transformation is more common in flat bone MHEs (pelvis, scapula).

GIANT CELL TUMOR/OSTEOCLASTOMA

Common Presentation of GCT

Case summary: A 26-year-old female presented with a gradually progressive swelling at the upper of left tibia for 6 months, and has become painful for 4 weeks. There are no constitutional symptoms. Local examination revealed a bony swelling with soft to firm areas over upper end of tibia just below the joint line. There was mild tenderness over the swelling with normal skin. Range of movement and neurovascular examination was normal.

Q. What is the clinical diagnosis?

Benign bone tumor of upper end of the tibia; most likely to be a giant cell tumor (GCT) (osteoclastoma) (Fig. 7.8).

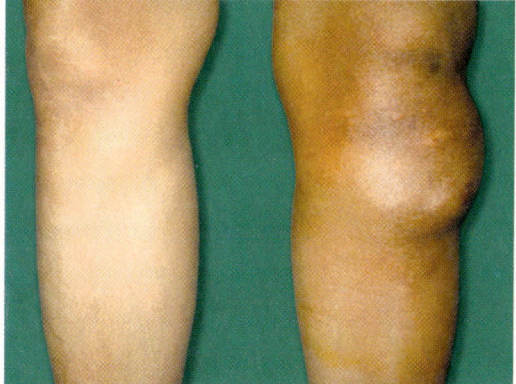

Fig. 7.8: GCT of left tibia

Q. Why do you say so?

History
1. Gradual onset of swelling, minimal pain
2. Female: GCT is more common in females

Examination
Location of bony swelling is upper end of tibia (just below the joint line), i.e. epiphysis, which is the location for GCT.

Q. How will you confirm the diagnosis?

1. *X-ray of the knee:* AP and lateral view

   It will reveal (3Es)
   • Epiphyseal tumor
   • Eccentric in location
   • Expansile (cortical thinning)
2. *MRI:* Shows the bony and soft tissue extension of the tumor.
3. *Biopsy:* Presence of giant cells

Q. What is the treatment of GCT?

GCT is treated in following ways.
1. **Curettage of the cavity:** Helps in removing the gross tumor from cavity
2. **Treat the cavity:** This helps in killing the micro tumor cells in the cavity, and in the tumor wall
   a. *Chemical:* Phenol, hydrogen peroxide
   b. *Thermal:* Liquid nitrogen
   c. *Mechanical:* Burr
3. **Fill the cavity:** Bone grafting, bone cement

Other treatments
4. Resection and arthrodesis
5. Turn-o-plasty in GCT around knee

Q. Is GCT a benign tumor?

Largely. However, rarely it can be locally malignant and very rarely it can metastasize.

Q. Is there any chemotherapy recommended for locally invasive GCT?

Denusumab.

Low Back Pain

LOW BACK PAIN DUE TO IVDP

Common Presentation of Intervertebral Disc Prolapse (IVDP)

Case summary: A 39-year-old male patient complained of low back pain for 3 months, which started after lifting heavy luggage. The pain increases while bending forward, lifting weight, cough, sneeze and turning in the bed. The pain has started radiating to his right lower limb from back of thigh, leg up to the great toe since one week. On examination, there is mild paraspinal spasm and list. He has tenderness over L4, L5 vertebral spinous process. Forward bending is painful and limited. Neurological examination revealed hypoaesthesia over L5 dermatome. The power in extensor hallucis longus (EHL) tendon is grade 4. On affected side, straight leg raising (SLR) is possible up to 50°, and Lasegue sign is positive.

Q. What is the diagnosis?

The diagnosis is low back pain due to intervertebral disc prolapse (IVDP) between L4 and 5 vertebra with radiculopathy on right side.

Q. Why do you think that the back pain is due to IVDP?

History

1. Young age (IVDP is common in younger population)
2. Pain started after lifting heavy weight in forward bending position (common mechanism of IVDP)
3. Radiation of pain to one side (indicates the irritation of a nerve root by a prolapsed disc)
4. Pain increases on bending forward, cough, sneeze and turning in bed (all activities increase intradiscal pressure)

Examination

5. Tenderness present over L4, 5 spinous process
6. SLR limited (50°)
7. Lasegue sign positive
8. L5 root involvement (hypoaesthesia over L5 dermatome and weak EHL)

Q. Why young age is in favor of IVDP?

In the young age, nucleus pulposus remains more hydrated. Hence, there is more chance of prolapse of hydrated nucleus pulposus through the annular tear. As the age advances, the disc **loses its hydration and water content (dessicated)** and hence, disc becomes lesser prone for prolapse (IVDP).

Q. You told that EHL is weak, what does it signify?

EHL weakness signifies involvement of L5 nerve root which is compressed by the prolapsed disc between L4 and L5 vertebra.

Commonly, both at cervical and lumbar level, the nerve root compressed corresponds to lower adjacent vertebra.

Example:
1. When the disc between L3 and L4 vertebrae is prolapsed, root compressed is 'L4'
2. Between L4 and L5 disc, root compressed is 'L5'
3. When the disc between C4 and C5 prolapses, the root compressed is 'C5'
4. When the disc between C5 and C6 prolapses, the root compressed is 'C6Q.

Sensory loss pattern and muscle weakness is a clue for root involvement
1. Weak knee extension (quadriceps): L2,3,4
2. Weak ankle dorsiflexion: L4
3. Weak EHL: L5
4. Weak plantar flexion: S1

Q. What is the most common cause of lumbar IVDP?

'Lifting weight in forward flexion' is the commonest mechanism of injury to the disc of the lumbar spine.

Q. How history of trauma is relevant for IVDP?

Lumbar spine: Fall over the buttocks
Cervical spine: Sudden or chronic load over head

Note: Fall over buttocks leads to sudden rise in axial pressure leading to rise in intradiscal pressure. This can rupture posterolateral aspect of annulus fibrosis which is part of the disc followed by point and consequent prolapse of nucleus pulposus through the rent.

Q. You said that pain started after lifting heavy weight. What relation it has with the prolapse of lumbar intervertebral disc?

When person bends forward without bending his/her knee to lift weight, the lumbar intradiscal pressure raises. This can result in tear of annulus fibrosus, leading to prolapse of soft gelatinous material of nucleus pulposus through the tear in annulus fibrosus.

The prolapsed disc material could result in compression of the thecal sac of spinal cord or nerve roots or both resulting in back pain or radiating pain or both.

Q. Why should lumbar IVDP result in back pain?

Due to rich nerve supply, periphery of annulus fibrosus is pain sensitive. Any stretch of annulus due to prolapsing disc material (nucleus pulposus) results in low back pain. Further, the central prolapse of disc material also presses upon the duramater (thecal sac) causing back pain.

Note: The cervical IVDP would cause neck pain due to similar reasons as above discussed. Also, in the cervical spine, the prolapsed disc could compress the spinal cord along with thecal sac.

Q. Why should IVDP result in radiating pain in the limb?

Any radiating pain in the limb indicates pressure and or irritation (due to inflammation) of the nerve root. The inflammatory reaction occurs as nucleus pulposus is antigenic. When the prolapsed material exits out of annular tear, its paracentral prolapse could press upon the nerve root resulting in radiating pain along the course of nerve in the limb. Usually the nerve indentation is one side, hence the pain is unilateral.

Q. Could IVDP result in bilateral limb pain?

Yes. Large central disc herniation can cause bilateral radiating pain.

Q. What is straight leg raising test (SLRT) and its significance?

The straight leg raise (SLR) is a passive test. Each leg is tested individually with the normal leg being tested first. While performing the SLRT, the patient is positioned in supine without a pillow under the head of the patient. The clinician lifts the patient's leg by the back of the ankle while keeping the knee in a fully extended position. The clinician continues to lift the patient's leg by flexing at the hip until the patient complains of pain in the back of the thigh or leg. The angle between the leg and the horizontal is the angle of SLR. The same is repeated over the affected side.

Note: Positive SLRT above 70° may not have any value. Further mere tightness at the back of thigh, and not pain is attributed to hamstring tightness.

Q. How do you elicit Lasegue sign?

Patient's lower limb is elevated above the examination couch like in SLR test. At a certain angle from horizontal, the patient complains of radiating pain in the affected limb up to the calf, foot or toes. Then, the affected lower limb is slightly lowered till the pain is reduced or relieved. At this point, the ankle is gently dorsiflexed, which again exacerbates the pain. This is known as positive Lasègue sign.

Note: Lasègue's test is sensitive but not specific for IVDP

Q. What is well leg raising test and its significance?

In well-leg raising test, **"well"** or **"normal"** leg is lifted above the examination couch like SLR test. If the patient experiences radiating pain in the affected limb, the well-leg test is considered to be positive.

The well-leg test is quite specific for IVDP of lumbar spine.

Q. How to investigate a case of suspected intervertebral disc prolapse?

1. Plain X-ray of the lumbar spine
   a. Loss of lumbar lordosis
   b. Decrease in disc space especially in chronic disc prolapse
   c. Also, it helps in ruling out several other differential diagnosis such as infection, tumors, fracture, osteoporosis, spondylitis or spondylolisthesis.

2. MRI of the lumbar spine (confirmatory)

MRI of lumbosacral (LS) spine would reveal intervertebral disc prolapse with or without root compression (Fig. 8.1).

MRI helps in identifying the:
- Level of prolapse,
- Degree of prolapse (disc bulge, disc prolapse, extrusion and sequestration)
- Number of disc involved, and
- Type of prolapse (central, paracentral or far lateral).

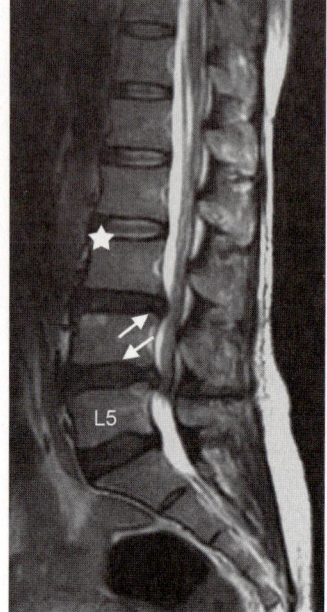

Fig. 8.1: Sagittal section of MRI of lumbosacral spine shows intervertebral disc prolapse at L3–L4 and L4–L5 levels (white arrow). Disc is normal between L2 and L3 (white star) and above

Q. How will you conservatively manage a patient with lumbar IVDP?

1. *General measure*
   a. Bedrest for few days followed by progressive activity.
   b. Patient is advised to avoid lifting heavy weight while bending forward. He is taught to lift weight while keeping his knee flexed and back straight.

2. *Medications*
   i. *Analgesics*
   ii. *Muscle relaxants:* Thiocolchiside, tizanidine
   iii. *To reduce radiating neuralgic pain:* Pregabalin/gabapentin

Many at times in exams (viva/theory), students mention muscle relaxant to be used in back pain as scoline. Scoline is a systemic muscle relaxant used in general anesthesia. It paralyses whole body including respiratory system. Patient will die within a few minutes if used in back pain!

3. *Physiotherapy:* For pain relief and rehabilitation
   a. Intermittent lumbar pelvic traction
   b. Local heat therapy: Moist heat/short wave diathermy/interferential therapy
   c. Spinal extension exercises: Very beneficial
   d. Once patient has considerable pain relief, patient can be advised to wear **lumbosacral corset** for a few weeks and continue **spinal extension exercises.**

4. *Epidural/selective nerve root steroid injection:* If "radiating pain" does not relieve with conservative treatment or the radiating pain recurs later, the steroid injection in lumbar epidural space or around the selective nerve root is quite beneficial in relieving the radiating nerve root pain.

Note: Epidural injection of steroid may not have any major effect in relieving low back pain.

Q. How does advice of avoiding bending forward while lifting weight helps?

The **intradiscal pressure** changes according to various positions
1. **Lowest** in **supine** position
2. **Highest** during **flexed forward** with weights in hand.

Since the intradiscal pressure are highest during flexed forward with weights, this leads to annular rupture and consequently prolapse of nucleus pulposus material through the annular rent.
Hence after IVDP, forward flexion movement especially with weights in hand should be avoided.

Q. By offering conservative trial, patient has to wait for a few days to weeks for some recovery. Why not to offer a surgical treatment for the prolapsed disc especially in your patient who has hypoesthesia and weak great toe extensor?

The **result of conservative treatment is excellent.** Most patients get symptomatic relief in a few weeks and do not require any surgical intervention. Even neurological deficits tend to recover over a few months.

Note: Neurological deficits may not recover completely with either form of treatment, conservative or surgical

Q. What is the indication of surgery in IVDP?

The surgery is indicated in the following situation:
1. **Progressive pain which is not responding** to sincere conservative treatment even after a few weeks to months
2. **Progressive neurological deficit**
3. **Cauda equina syndrome**
4. **Bladder and bowel involvement** due to massive disc prolapse
5. Recurrent root symptoms not responding to conservative treatment

Q. What surgery would you like to do in such cases?

Fenestration and discectomy of the involved intervertebral disc is the treatment of choice.
   Note: The discectomy can be performed as:
1. *Open discectomy:* Discectomy done without the use of visual enhancement
2. *Microdiscectomy:* Entails the use of visual enhancement like a microscope or loupes.
3. *Endoscopic microdiscectomy:* It entails the use of tubular retractors over serial tissue dilators followed by a light source and or microscope.

Q. What is cauda equina syndrome (CES)?

Varying symptoms and signs due to compression of multiple roots in lumbosacral region characterised by:
- Low back pain
- Bilateral radicular pain
- Saddle anesthesia
- Sensorimotor changes in lower limb
- Bladder and bowel involvement

Q. What is the etiology of CES?

- Multiple level lumbar disc prolapse
- Lumbar canal stenosis
- Tumor in LS canal
- Vertebral fracture resulting in 'retropulsion of fragments in canal'
- Postsurgical hematoma

Q. What is conus medullaris syndrome (CMS)?

Sudden and bilateral clinical features due to compression of 'conus medullaris' characterised by:
- Low back pain +/– radiation to lower limb
- Bladder dysfunction
- Impotence

Q. In lumbar IVDP, the pain increases on forward flexion. In which condition of spine, the pain increases on extension or backward bending?

Pain on extension is seen in three conditions:
1. Spondylolysis and spondylolisthesis
2. Lumbar canal stenosis
3. Facet joint arthropathy

Q. What is spondylolysis and spondylolisthesis?

Spondylolysis is characterised by a break in pars interarticularis. Spondylolisthesis is characterised by forward slipping of the upper vertebra over the lower one.

Q. Could this pain be due to spondylolysis/spondylolisthesis?

Unlikely that this is pain is because of spondylolysis or spondylolisthesis as the patients with spondylolysis or spondylolisthesis would present with
1. Patients have more **pain on extension**
2. In case of listhesis, there is a palpable step felt over the spinous process of the slipped vertebra.
3. Attenuated lumbar lordosis

Q. What is pars interarticularis?

Pars interarticularis is the **bony bridge between the two articular facets**, superior and inferior.

Q. What are the causes of spondylolisthesis?

a. *Dysplastic:* Due to congenital anomaly of facets
b. *Isthmic:* Due to defect in pars interarticularis
c. *Degenerative:* Due to facet joint degeneration
d. *Traumatic:* Due to damage to neural arch
e. *Pathological:* Metastatic carcinoma, Pagets
f. Iatrogenic

Q. What is the grading of spondylolisthesis?

Grade 1: <25% slip
Grade 2: 25–50% slip
Grade 3: 50–75% slip
Grade 4: 75–100% slip
Grade 5: >100% slip (spondyloptosis)

Q. How can you confirm the diagnosis of spondylolysis/listhesis?

1. A plain X-ray of lumbosacral spine with oblique views can confirm the diagnosis (Figs 8.2 and 8.3).
2. CT scan can identify the bony anomaly.
3. MRI of lumbosacral spine can detect the compression of neural elements.

Q. What is the typical radiological sign observed in the oblique X-ray of the LS spine with suspected spondylolisthesis/spondylolysis?

Scottish Terrier dog sign is the diagnostic of spondylolysis.

Q. How will you manage spondylolisthesis/lysis?

1. Conservative treatment is same as for IVDP
2. **Spinal flexion exercises** are recommended (instead of spinal extension which are recommended in IVDP).

If conservative treatment fails, then posterior stabilisation of unstable vertebra with instrumentation and lumbar interbody fusion of the involved vertebrae with bone graft is performed.

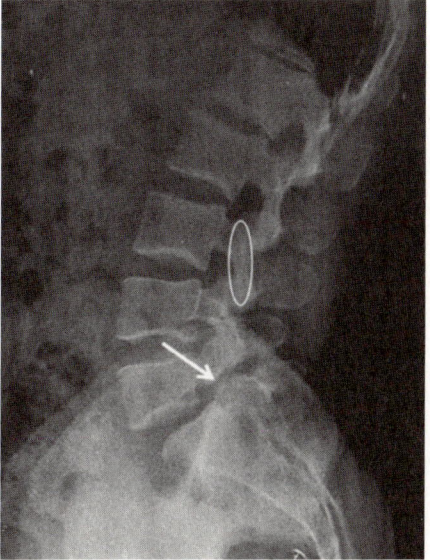

Fig. 8.2: Plain X-ray lateral view of lumbar spine shows spondylolisthesis between L5 and S1 vertebra (white arrow) which is a break in pars interarticularis. It also shows normal pars interarticularis at L3 vertebral level (white oblong area)

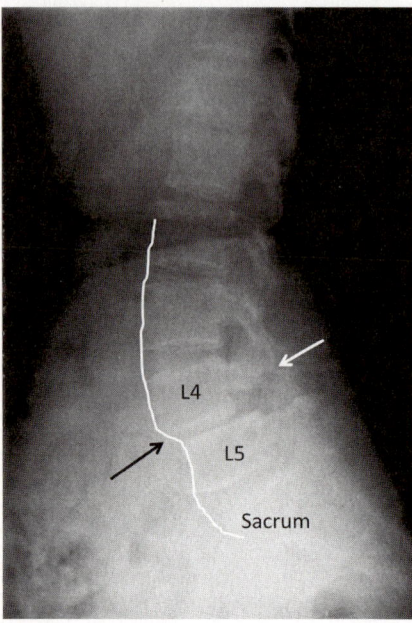

Fig. 8.3: Plain X-ray lateral view of lumbar spine shows a step on the anterior border of body between L4 and L5 (black arrow) indicating spondylolisthesis. There is a break in the pars interarticularis of L4 vertebra (white arrow)

Q. What is lumbar canal stenosis, and its clinical manifestation?

Lumbar canal stenosis is usually observed in older age group after 55–60 years.

Pathologically, the volume/space available for spinal cord and cauda equina (nerve roots) in lumbar portion of spinal canal decreases.

Commonly, stenosis is due to degenerative process resulting in hypertrophy of facet joint and ligamentum flavum, osteophytes encroaching the lumbar canal, and chronic disc prolapses or spondylolisthesis.

Stenosis results in increased pressure over the nerve roots resulting in manifestation of clinical features in three ways.
1. Low back pain with bilateral radiation of pain in lower limbs
2. Neurogenic claudication
3. Painful extension

Note: Typical presentation of lumbar canal stenosis is an **old person** complaining of **low back pain** with **bilateral radiation** to both limbs which increases on walking, climbing downhill or downstairs and prefers sitting with forward bending.

Classical example of **neurogenic claudication** is **lumbar canal stenosis.**
Neurogenic claudication starts immediately after standing and
increases while walking, coming downhill and downstairs; relieves by stair climbing, sitting and bending forward. Peripheral pulses are well felt and associated neurological deficit may be present. **Vascular claudication** is due to atherosclerosis or TAO (thromboangiitis obliterans). Pain increase on walking, going uphill or downhill, stair climbing and pulses are feeble. There is no neurological symptom.

Q. Why does pain in lumbar canal stenosis increases on extension?

The effective diameter or space available for lumbar roots further decreases in extension resulting in low back pain and neurogenic claudication. Hence, pain increases in walking downhill/downstairs as spine is extended in both positions.

Q. How to investigate Lumbar canal stenosis

1. X-ray lumbosacral spine
2. MRI LS spine
   - To assess canal diameter
   - Changes in the disc, longitudinal ligament and ligament flavum, facetal hypertrophy

Q. What is the conservative treatment of lumbar canal stenosis?

The conservative method (mentioned in IVDP) is same but for a few differences.
1. Spinal flexion exercises instead of spinal extension
2. Lumbar traction may not be helpful

   If conservative treatment fails, **laminectomy** is the treatment of choice.

   Removing the lamina and thickened ligamentum flavum increases the space available for lumbar roots which alleviates the pressure over the nerve roots and hence, relieves the radiating pain.

Q. What are other common causes of back pain?

1. Spondylosis or spondylitis
2. Seronegative spondyloarthropathy

Q. What is spondylosis?

- Commonly, it is also known as spondylitis affecting the lumbar and cervical regions. Hence, called lumbar or cervical spondylitis. *It is one of the most common causes of pain in lumbar and cervical region.*
- It is defined as natural degenerative process of vertebral motion segment (vertebra, disc and facet joints).

Q. What is the etiology of the spondylitis?

- Increasing age
- Repetitive strain
- *Occupational hazard:* Repeated lifting, loading, bending, driving, weight lifting on head
- Smoking

TAO is also known as Buerger's disease whereas Buerger's disease is IgA nephropathy!

Q. What are the clinical features of spondylosis?

Lumbar spondylosis
- *Low back pain:* More on activity, relieves on rest
- Difficulty in movements,
- Local vertebral tenderness
- Neurological signs: Rare

Cervical spondylosis
- *Chronic neck pain:* More on activity, relieves on rest
- Difficulty in neck movements
- Local vertebral tenderness
- Neurological signs: Rare

Q. What are the investigations in spondylosis?

1. *X-ray of spine:* Osteophytes, sometimes loss of disc height, facet joint arthropathy
2. *MRI:* Disc disease, osteophytes

Q. How will you treat spondylosis?

Conservative treatment (alike IVDP) is the mainstay.

Q. What is the surgical treatment of spondylosis?

Very rarerly, spondylosis of cervical/lumbar region may require surgical treatment especially when degeneration results in severe root or cord compression or cervical myelopathy.

    Laminectomy and decompression of the canal.

Q. What is seronegative spondyloarthropathy?

Seronegative spondyloarthropathy is another common cause of back pain with key features as:
- Usually male <40 years
- Seronegative (RA factor negative)
- Usually HLA B27 +
- Pathological Hallmark: Enthesitis
- Back pain usually felt more after rest along with morning stiffness
- Cardinal feature is sacroiliac joint involvement as sacroiliitis
- Peripheral joints: Oligoarticular, asymmetric
- Extra-articular manifestation

    The leading cause of seronegative spondyloarthropathy induced sacroiliitis is ankylosing spondylitis.
- Young patients with low back pain and morning stiffness. The stiffness and pain improves after activity, pain increases after inactivity and at night.
- Examination reveals tender sacroiliac joint, restricted spine movement and restricted chest expansion.

 – Often round back kyphotic deformity of the dorsal spine
 – Increased occiput-wall distance

Q. What are the extra-articular manifestation of ankylosing spondylitis?

• Uveitis, iritis
• Cardiac conduction abnormality
• Aortic stenosis
• Pulmonary fibrosis

Q. What is the genetic association of ankylosing spondylitis (AS)?

It is associated with HLA-B27.

Q. What is the basic pathology in ankylosing spondylitis?

The fundamental pathology in AS is 'enthesitis' resulting in bony erosion, ossification and eventual bony ankylosis

Note: The enthesis is connective tissue between tendon or ligament and bone. It is associated with HLA-B27.

Q. What are various tests to confirm the involvement of the sacroiliac joint?

1. Figure of four test
2. Gaenslen test
3. Pelvic compression and distraction test

Q. Which test will confirm the limited lumbar spine motion?

Modified Schober's test

Q. What is Modified Schober's test?

Modified Schober's test is performed to assess the mobility in lumbar spine.

While patient is standing, three points are marked over the midline at lumbar spine. 1st point at the level of PSIS, second point 5 cm below the level of PSIS (A1) and third point 10 cm above it (A2). Now, patient is asked to flex forward.

In a normal patient: The normal distance between highest and lowest mark (A1,A2) must move at least 5 cm apart in forward flexion indicating normal mobility of lumbar spine.

In patient with stiff spine: The distance between the two marks (A1, A2)/points is less than 5 cm.

Q. Why chest expansion is limited in ankylosing spondylitis?

Chest expansion is limited due to involvement of **costovertebral** joints.

Q. What are the investigations in a patient with suspected ankylosing spondylitis?

1. *Serology:* HLA-B27+ (in 90% cases), ESR is high
2. Plain X-ray of dorsolumbar spine and pelvis (Figs 8.4 and 8.5)

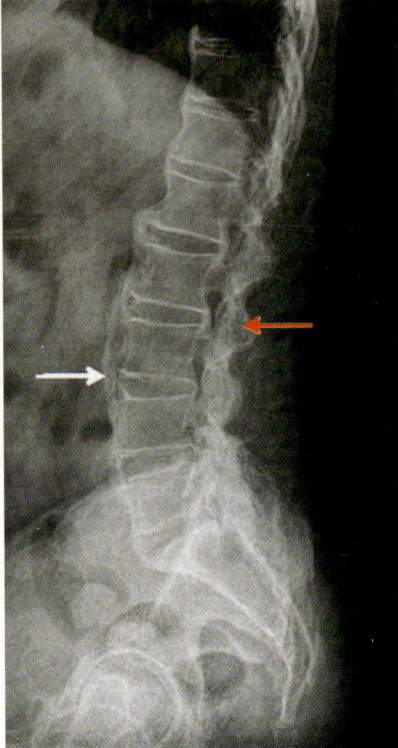

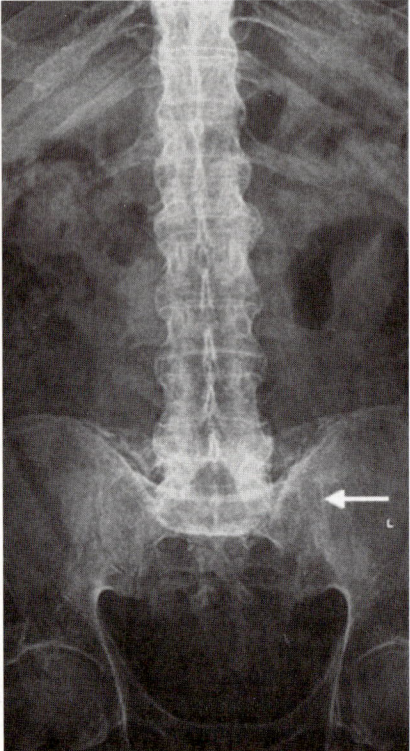

Fig. 8.4: Plain X-ray lateral view of lumbar spine shows ossification of anterior longitudinal ligament (white arrow) and fusion of facet joint (red arrow)

Fig. 8.5: Plain X-ray anteroposterior view of lumbar spine shows fusion of sacroiliac joint of left side (white arrow). Bamboo spine appearance of lumbar vertebra is clearly seen

   i. Pelvis X-ray: Feature of sacroiliitis and joint fusion.
  ii. **Squaring of vertebra:** Anterior vertebral border is straight rather than concave
 iii. **Marginal osteophytes or syndesmophytes:** Thin dense spicules bridging the vertebral bodies
  iv. Bamboo spine
   v. Trolley track sign
  vi. Dagger spine
 vii. Apophyseal and costovertebral ankylosis
viii X-ray hip: Arthritis, protrusio acetabuli, bony ankylosis
  ix. X-ray shoulder: Hatchet sign (defect on anterolateral aspect of head humerus)

Q. How will you manage ankylosing spondylitis?

Conservative treatment is the mainstay which aims in providing pain relief, disease control and maintaining the mobility of the pelvis, spine, and chest.

A. Physiotherapy
  • Physical therapy to maintain joint flexibility, deep breathing exercise for chest
  • *Pain relief:* Moist heat, SWD, IFT

B. Medical treatment
- *Analgesics:* NSAIDs (indomethacin), COX-2 inhibitors
- *Disease modifying agents:* Sulphasalazine
- *Biologic agents:* Infliximab, etanercept

C. Surgical treatment
- *Spinal osteotomy:* To correct severe kyphotic deformity of dorsal spine
- Total joint replacement for ankylosed hip, knee or shoulder joints

Q. What are the other causes of seronegative spondyloarthropathy?
- Ankylosing spondylitis
- Psoriatic arthopathy
- Reactive/Reiter's arthritis
- *Enteropathic arthritis:* Associated with inflammatory bowel disease

Q. What is Reiter's syndrome?

Reiter's syndrome is characterized by:
1. Oligoarticular arthritis
2. Urethritis
3. Conjunctivitis
4. Sacroiliitis

Q. What is psoriatic arthropathy?

It is characterised by:
- Dermatological features of psoriasis
- Sacroiliitis
- Distal interphalangeal joint arthritis is common while PIP and MCP arthropathy is uncommon
- Arthritis mutilans
- Nail changes: Nail pitting, onycholysis.

Pott's Spine

TUBERCULOSIS OF SPINE

Common Presentation of Tuberculosis of Spine

Case summary: A 27-year-old hotel worker presented with insidious onset of mid backache for 2 months. The back pain was localized and progressive. Any attempted movements of back were quite painful. The pain was quite severe in night with painful turning in bed. One month back, he was seen by a physician for chronic cough, low grade fever and weight loss. He was found to have left side pleural effusion which was aspirated and conservative treatment was provided. General examination revealed pallor. Spine examination revealed prominent and tender 7th and 8th thoracic vertebra spinous process with a small swelling in the mid axillary line in the 7th intercostal space on the right side of the chest wall. Dorsal spine movements were painfully restricted. Cervical spine and lumbar spine were found to be normal. Neurological examination was otherwise normal except for exaggerated deep tendon reflexes in lower limb with up-going plantar response. The breath sounds were decreased on the left side of the chest. Per abdomen examination was normal.

Q. What is the clinical diagnosis?

Spinal tuberculosis (D7–8) with early stage of Pott's paraplegia with left side pleural effusion.

Q. Why do you suspect tuberculosis of spine?

It is because

History
- Mid back pain which is severe in night (rest pain in night indicates inflammation, infection or tumor)
- Chronic cough, low grade fever and weight loss with pleural effusion (indicates possible infective etiology likely to be TB in Indian scenario).

Examination
a. Tender D7–8 vertebra spinous process
b. Knuckle deformity over D7 vertebra (indicates vertebral body destruction)

c. Exaggerated deep tendon reflexes in the lower limb with upgoing plantar reflex (indicates that pathology is compressing the cord resulting in UMN sign)

d. Swelling over axillary intercostal region (signifying presence of cold abscess)

Q. What is knuckle deformity?

Knuckle is a type of kyphotic deformity, commonly observed in thoracic spine where the spinous process of the vertebra becomes prominent due to involvement (collapse of body after destruction) of single vertebra.

> **Deformity of spine** (in sagittal plane)
> **K**nuckle: Single level vertebral collapse
> **A**ngular: 2–3 level vertebral collapse
> **R**oundback: 4 or more vertebrae
> **Mnemonic: KAR**

Q. What is the name of deformity when it affects 2 or 3 adjacent levels of vertebra?

Gibbus (also known as angular deformity)

Q. What are the causes of round back deformity?

Young patient: Scheuermann's disease of dorsal spine (common in young females)

Old patient: Osteoporosis with multiple vertebra # (Dowager's hump), ankylosing spondylitis, Paget's disease.

Q. How do you say it has involved D7–8 vertebrae?

By using the surface landmarks and counting the spinous process, the level of vertebra can be localised.

- C7 is the most prominent cervical process.
- Spine of the scapula corresponds to D3 spinous process,
- Inferior angle of scapula corresponds to D7 vertebral spinous process
- Highest point of iliac crest corresponds to disc space between L4 and L5.

Q. Which is the most common region involved in tuberculosis of spine?

Commonest area is involved dorsal spine especially dorsolumbar junction.

- Dorsal spine: 42%
- Lumbar: 26%
- Dorsolumbar and cervical: 12% each
- Lumbosacral: 3%

Q. What are the sites of TB in a vertebra?

1. Paradiscal (90%): The Paradiscal part of two vertebrae (upper and lower) is the commonest site of TB affection in a vertebra.
2. Anterior: Over anterior surface of the vertebral body
3. Central: Over central part of the body
4. Posterior: In neural arches (pedicle, lamina, transverse, and spinous process)

Q. Why TB vertebral infection is common in paradiscal space?

It is common in paradiscal space because of common blood supply to the two adjacent vertebra.

Q. What is the meaning of Pott's paraplegia?

The paralysis of lower limbs (paraplegia) due to compression of the spinal cord and/nerve roots due to tuberculosis of spine is known as Pott's paraplegia.

Q. What are the various causes of Pott's paraplegia?

Extrinsic causes: Caseous material, granulation tissue, sequestrated disc, vertebral bony fragments, kyphotic deformity.

Intrinsic causes: Cord stretching, cord edema, infarction and myelomalacia, spinal artery thrombosis.

Q. What are the different stages of Pott's paraplegia?

There are 4 stages (Kumar and Tuli) in tuberculosis of based predominantly upon motor deficit.

1. *Stage I:* Patient is unaware of neurological deficit but physician detects plantar extensor response and ankle clonus (earliest sign).
2. *Stage II:* Patient finds clumsiness in gait (earliest symptom), aware of deficit but walks with support.
3. *Stage III:* Patient is non-ambulant, paralysis in extension with sensory deficit <50%.
4. *Stage IV:* Patient is non-ambulant, paralysis in flexion with bowel and bladder sphincters involved and sensory deficit > 50%.

Q. What is early onset and late onset Pott's paraplegia?

Early onset paraplegia: Starts within 2 years, in active phase of TB
Late onset paraplegia: Starts after 2 years of disease onset

Q. What are the causes of paraplegia in early phase or active disease?

Spinal cord compression due to:
1. Tubercular granulation tissue,
2. Tubercular cold abscess and inflammatory edema, arterial thrombosis
3. Sequestered disc or bony fragments.

Q. What is the cause of late onset paraplegia?

The late onset paraplegia is due to mechanical pressure over the cord due to stretching of the spinal cord over the internal gibbus in severe kyphosis, ligament ossification and dural fibrosis.

Q. Which spinal region TB is most likely to result in neurological deficit?

Dorsal spine. It is due to less space available for spinal cord in the spinal canal of dorsal spine.

Q. Why neurologic involvement is less common in lumbar spine?

Lumbar spinal canal is wider and spinal cord ends at lower border of L1.

Q. What is clinical surface location of the tubercular cold abscess?

The tubercular cold abscess has a tendency to track along the nerve plexus or musculofascial planes. Hence, it is usually detected far from original site of infection.
1. **Cervical region:** Retropharyngeal abscess, abscess in the posterior triangle of the neck or in the axilla.
2. **Thoracic spine:** Presents as mediastinal mass or as swelling in the intercostal space over lateral or anterior chest wall.
3. **Lumbar spine:** Presents as retroperitoneal mass, iliac fossa swelling, swelling in the groin in the femoral triangle, Petit's triangle (Fig. 9.1) or gluteal region along sciatic nerve.

Q. What is the role of per abdomen examination in TB of dorsolumbar spine?

Abdominal examination helps in ruling out any abdominal mass (cold abscess) in iliac fossa which can cause flexion deformity of hip due to iliopsoas irritation and inflammation.

Other, if any, abdominal organ involvement with TB can also be detected.

Q. How will you investigate a patient with spinal TB?

1. **Serological investigations:**
   a. CBP: Low Hb, lymphocytosis
   b. ESR: Elevated
2. **Investigation for local disease assessment**
   a. X-ray of the spine

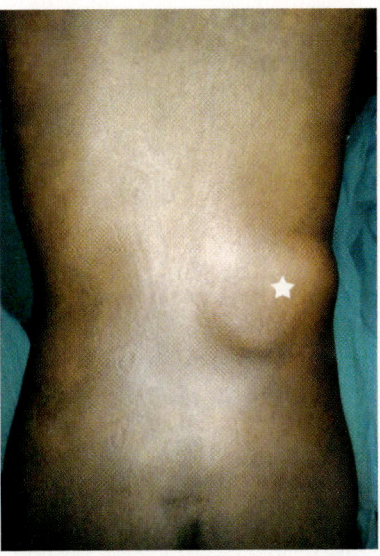

Fig. 9.1: Clinical photograph of patient with Pott's spine with paraspinal abscess (white star)

    b. CT and MRI scan of affected part

    c. Bone scan: To assess multifocal TB

    d. Vertebral biopsy: It is diagnostic. Often done under the guidance of image intensifier or CT. The specimen is sent for AFB stain, cultures, CBNAAT, LPA for MTB

3. Investigations to look for primary foci

    a. Chest X-ray

    b. Sputum for AFB, culture

    c. USG abdomen and pelvis

    d. Mantoux test

    e. Urine: Sterile pyuria may indicate TB of urinary system

> Spinal tuberculosis (or for that matter, musculoskeletal tuberculosis) is always secondary to some primary focus lying in lungs/urogenital system/GIT/lymph nodes. These foci may be covert or overt.

Q. What is the role of ESR?

It is usually elevated in active case of tuberculosis. It is used as a prognostic indicator.

Q. What are the radiological features of spinal tuberculosis on plain X-ray?

There are several features (Fig. 9.2):

a. Localized osteopenia is the **earliest feature**.

b. Reduction in the involved disc space with loss of definition of paradiscal margins is the **most common feature**.

c. There may be collapse of vertebral height (concertina collapse) with paravertebral soft tissue shadow.

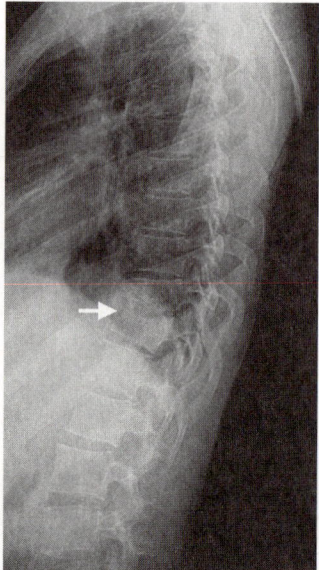

Fig. 9.2: Plain X-ray of dorsolumbar spine lateral view showing decreased intervertebral disc space (white arrow) with collapse of vertebra

In cervical spine

d. There may be increase in the prevertebral soft tissue shadow in case of cervical spinal involvement.

In dorsal spine

e. In thoracic spine, the cold abscess appears as a fusiform swelling in the AP view (bird nest appearance)

f. Varying degree of Kyphosis

In lumbar spine:

f. Tubercular psoas abscess may appear as a bulky psoas shadow in the AP view of lumbar spine.

Q. What are the advantages of MRI scan?

MRI is quite useful to detect

- Number of vertebra involved, cold abscess, vertebral destruction
- Cord compression and condition (edema, myelomalacia) (Fig. 9.3).

Q. What are the principles of treatment of tuberculosis spine?

There are several principles of treatment.

1. Achieve healing of the disease by anti-tubercular drugs
2. Good nutrition
3. To detect, treat and prevent complications like spinal deformities and neurological manifestations by strict bedrest, spinal braces and surgery.

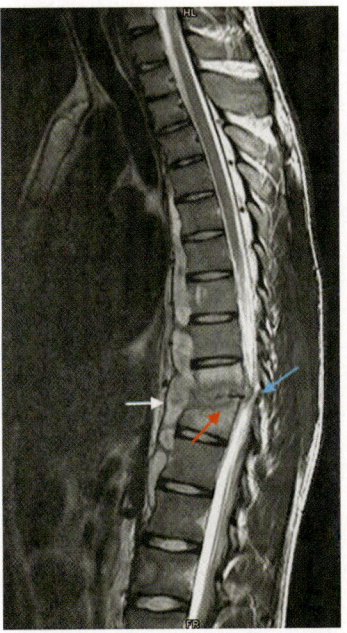

Fig. 9.3: MRI of dorsolumbar spine shows prevertebral abscess (white arrow) in front of affected vertebra. The disc space is between the vertebra is collapsed (red arrow) and abscess is seen extending posteriorly into the spinal canal (blue arrow)

Q. How do you treat spinal TB?

1. General

    a. Rest: Essential for pain relief, prevents further vertebral collapse and possibly reduces the chance of neurological deficit

    b. Nutritional support, correct anemia

    c. Analgesics

2. Medical treatment with ATT and orthotic support (braces)

    a. ATT course: 4 drugs (IREZ) for 2 months **(intensive phase)** followed by 3 drugs for (IRE) next 10–16 months **(maintenance phase)**

    b. Various spinal orthosis to provide support and rest to the spine

3. Surgery: It is indicated when there is

- No response to medical management
- Increasing neurological deficit, unstable spine
- Progressive deformity
- Spastic paraplegia with severe spasm in lower limbs

Principles of surgical management:

a. Debridement of infected bone and debridement of paravertebral abscess

b. Decompression of spinal canal

c. Prevention or correction of spinal deformity with instrumentation, graft and or cage.

Surgical options

1. Anterolateral decompression: Resection of rib, transverse process, pedicle and part of vertebral body

2. Costotransversectomy: Resection of part of rib and transverse process

3. Hong Kong procedure

Q. What is Hong Kong procedure?

Hong Kong procedure comprises several principles.

1. Debridement of infected bone

2. Decompression of spinal canal

3. Correction of kyphotic deformity using structure grafting

4. Instrumentation to support the vertebral column after debridement and grafting.

Q. Which surgical procedure is contraindicated in tuberculosis of spine?

Laminectomy is contraindicated (except in 2 conditions: Spinal tumor syndrome and posterior element involvement).

Q. What is spinal tumor syndrome?

Rarely tubercular granulation tissue proliferates inside the spinal canal resulting in spinal cord compression with no associated radiological changes in the bone.

Q. What are the complication of spinal tuberculosis?

- Early or late onset para- or quadriplegia/paresis
- Bladder and bowel involvement
- Cold abscess
- Deformity

Q. What are the good prognostic signs?

- Early onset with short duration
- Young patient with slow progression
- <60° kyphotic deformity
- Normal spinal cord on MRI.

Painful Shoulder

PAINFUL SHOULDER

Aim of the Shoulder Module

- Understanding a painful and stiff shoulder
- Common presentation of a frozen shoulder
- Differentiation with other common pathologies in shoulder
- Treatment plan

Remember: Age is one of the most important clue in clinical diagnosis of shoulder pathology

1. *15–30 years:* Shoulder dislocation
2. *30–50 years:* Rotator cuff (RC) tendinopathy, impingement syndrome
3. *40–55 years:* Frozen shoulder
4. *55 years onwards:* RC tear, acromioclavicular arthritis
5. *70 years onwards:* Glenohumeral (GH) arthritis

Common Presentation of Patient with
Frozen Shoulder/Adhesive Capsulitis/Periarthritis Shoulder

Case summary: A 48-year-old man case of pain and difficulty in movements in his left shoulder for last 4 months. Pain was insidious in onset and was felt more at night. He had difficulty in elevating his hand above shoulders and reaching at the back There was no history of trauma, fever, loss of weight or appetite. There was no other joint involvement. He was not diabetic or having any thyroid dysfunction. General and systemic examinations were normal. Local examination revealed tenderness over the anterior joint line of shoulder with slight supraspinatus wasting. All movements (active and passive) are grossly restricted especially rotations (external and internal) and abduction. Jobe's supraspinatus test was negative. Other rotator cuff were normal.

Q. What is your clinical diagnosis?

The clinical diagnosis is left side primary frozen shoulder.

Q. Why do you say so?

It is because of following reasons.

Symptoms
1. Middle aged patient (frozen shoulder common in patients in 40–55 years)
2. Insidious onset pain and stiffness of shoulder

Signs
3. All active and passive movements are restricted (this is the single most important feature of frozen shoulder).
4. Tests for rotator cuff integrity are normal.

Q. Which movements are predominantly affected in frozen shoulder?

Abduction and rotations are predominantly affected.

Q. What is the basic pathology in frozen shoulder?

1. Capsular and rotator interval inflammation, capsular thickening and fibrosis
2. Thickening of coracohumeral ligament
   This results in global restriction of both active and passive movements of shoulder.

Q. What are the clinicopathological phases of frozen shoulder?

Classically, there are three phases/stages which may last for 12–18 months
1. *Freezing phase (0–6 months):* In this stage, patient complains of severe pain but has fair range of movements (ROM).
2. *Frozen phase (6–12 months):* In this stage, patient complains of gradually decreasing pain but loss of ROM is severe.
3. *Thawing phase (12–18 months):* This stage is characterized by minimal pain and gradual return of ROM.

Note: The 'stages of frozen shoulder' can be compared like making an ice in fridge wherein one keeps water in freezer. Initially water remain semi-liquid (freezing stage), then gradually becomes ice (frozen stage) and finally once the ice is out of freezer, it melts (thawing stage). The hardness of ice in various stages is comparable to loss of ROM.

Q. What is the natural history of frozen shoulder?

Frozen shoulder gradually resolves over 12–18 months after going through three clinicopathological phases.
   In diabetics/thyroid disorder patients, it may stay for longer duration.

Q. What else did you ask in history?

I asked about the history of diabetes and thyroid dysfunction.

Q. Why it is important to rule out diabetes or thyroid disorder?

Frozen shoulder (adhesive capsulitis) is more common in both disorders.
   However, the cause and effect between these disorders and frozen shoulder is still not well understood!

Remember: Many at times, the diabetes or thyroid dysfunction is first time detected in orthopedic department while evaluating the patient with shoulder pain.

Remember: Night pain in musculoskeletal system pathologies or otherwise is a symptom which indicates sinister problems like inflammatory (rheumatoid, ankylosing spondylitis), infective (tuberculosis) or malignant pathologies. And, that should alert the physician to further investigate the symptoms.

However, patient with "degenerative shoulder pathologies" like frozen shoulder, tendinitis, GH arthritis, calcific tendinitis will always complain of night pain, and that he cannot sleep on the affected side due to pain in night.

Also, patients with cervical spondylitis/ cervical IVDP with root involvement also have night pain when they lie on affected side as neural foramina gets narrowed due to lateral flexion of neck while lying on side.

So, night pain is usually present in the shoulder and neck pathologies even though they are degenerative in nature.

Note: Cervical spine and shoulder degenerative pathologies often co-exist! Both need diagnosis and treatment together for optimal results.

Q. What is the role of cervical spine examination in such cases?

Cervical spine must be examined because

1. Pathologies like cervical spondylitis or IVDP of cervical spine often co-exist with frozen shoulder or other degenerative shoulder pathologies. The radiating pain due to cervical spine pathologies can overlap with shoulder pain.

2. Further, cervical spondylitis or cervical IVDP could initiate frozen shoulder as patient does not move his shoulder much due to radiating pain from neck towards arm and forearm. Less movement at the shoulder joint for a few weeks is enough to precipitate frozen shoulder.

Hence, both conditions require treatment together and missing any one would not give adequate relief to the patient.

Q. What is primary and secondary frozen shoulder?

Primary (idiopathic): No known cause.

Secondary: Any underlying cause can precipitate frozen shoulder like
- Trauma: Fracture around shoulder, soft tissue injury
- Rotator cuff tear
- Nerve injury/affection induced palsy of shoulder muscles
- Calcific tendinits
- Tumors around shoulder

Q. Why it is important to differentiate between primary and secondary frozen shoulder?

It is important to differentiate between the two because

a. Primary frozen shoulder is self-limiting, responds well to conservative treatment with excellent prognosis, and manipulation under general anesthesia (MUGA) can be performed.

b. In secondary frozen shoulder, one must treat the secondary cause along with management of frozen shoulder. Further, secondary frozen shoulder may not respond to routine conservative treatment, prognosis depends upon the pathology and MUGA should not be done. It mostly requires arthroscopic capsular release.

Q. Do you think that this patient is suffering from rotator cuff tendinopathy/tendinitis?

No. It is not rotator cuff tendinopathy/tendinitis because patients with RC tendinitis exhibit near full ROM (active and passive) except terminal restriction of ROM due to pain. However, frozen shoulder results in gross restriction of both active and passive movements.

Q. Clinically, why it cannot be rotator cuff tear?

It is unlikely to be rotator cuff (RC) tear because
1. Patient is young (age 48 years) whereas RC tears are more common in older age (after 55 to 60 years.)
2. In frozen shoulder, there may be subtle wasting of rotator cuff muscle whereas there is gross supra- and/infraspinatus muscle wasting in RC tear.
3. Active range of movement may be limited in RC tear but passive range of movement at joint is usually not restricted in cuff tears unless there is secondary frozen shoulder.
4. Tests for RC tear (Jobe's test, external rotation lag or belly press) are negative whereas it would be positive in patients with cuff tear.

Q. Can it be acute calcific tendinitis?

Unlikely, because acute calcific tendinitis has quite acute (a few days) and a very painful presentation. All movements are severely restricted and very painful, almost giving a pseudoparalytic appearance.

Q. Can it be monoarticular arthritis (inflammatory/tubercular) of shoulder?

It is less likely because in case of:

In inflammatory arthritis, usually there is
1. Morning stiffness
2. Oligo- or polyarticular involvement
3. There may be systemic feature: Malaise, anemia

In infective arthritis
1. Systemic features (fever/loss of weight/loss of appetite)
2. Possible history of TB in past (musculoskeletal TB is always secondary to primary elsewhere)

Q. Can it be primary osteoarthritis of glenohumeral joint?

Unlikely because
1. Patient is young (48 years). Primary GH arthritis usually occur after the age of 65–70 years.
2. In frozen shoulder, history is usually short and shows symptoms and signs of recovery over period of 12–24 months. In GH arthritis, history is long (few months

to years) and patient's symptoms of pain and stiffness worsen over months and years.

3. In GH arthritis, the joint line will be tender with crepitus and restricted range of motion.

Q. How will you investigate your patient?

First, I would like to investigate my patient.

1. *X-ray of shoulder:* AP and axillary view. It is done to rule out any secondary causes (arthritis, tumor, calcification, infection) (Fig. 10.1). Also, it can assess the amount of osteoporosis in the head humerus

2. *Ultrasound of shoulder:*
   a. In frozen shoulder: Capsular and coracohumeral ligament thickness, rotator interval inflammation
   b. To rule out RC tendinitis or rotator cuff tear

3. *MRI of shoulder:* To rule out other pathologies in rotator cuff and labrum which can cause secondary frozen shoulder.

4. **Blood sugar levels**—to rule out diabetes (MUST)

5. **T3, T4 and TSH** levels to rule out thyroid disorder

Q. What is the role of X-ray in frozen shoulder?

Though the plain radiograph is normal in frozen shoulder, it is important for certain reasons

1. It helps in **ruling out secondary causes of frozen shoulder** like chronic calcific tendinitis, post-traumatic, infections or other inflammatory causes

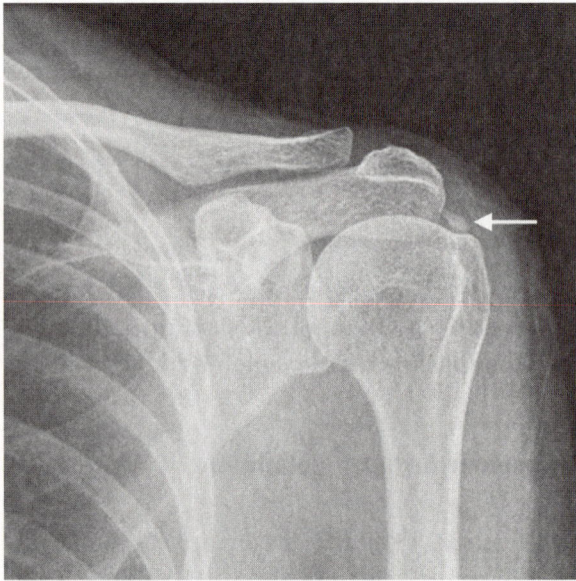

Fig. 10.1: Plain radiograph of left shoulder shows calcific deposit (white arrow) in the site for supraspinatus tendon

2. If there is **osteoporosis of upper end of humerus,** then MUGA is contraindicated as there is chance of fracture of upper end of humerus while manipulating the shoulder.

Q. How will you treat your patient with frozen shoulder?

A. In the freezing or early frozen stage

1. **Medications**
   a. NSAIDs
   b. Local diclofenac gel application
2. **Physiotherapy**
   a. Moist heat
   b. Short wave diathermy/local ultrasound therapy
   c. Gentle active shoulder mobilization exercises (pendular and wall climbing exercises)
3. **Intra-articular injection of steroid (methyl prednisolone/triamcinolone)**

B. Late stage of frozen shoulder (frozen) or Thawing stage:

- Continue mobilisation, and rehabilitation
- Analgesics sos (as and when required)
- Rarely, may require MUGA or arthroscopic capsular release

Aim of conservative treatment

1. Minimize pain by medication, physiotherapy and steroid injection
2. **Retain** the remaining movement and **regain** further movement by physiotherapy

---

Q. What if patient gets no relief; pain remains same and movements do not improve especially in late frozen stage?

1. **Manipulation under general anesthesia** (MUGA) followed by intra-articular injection of steroid. Manipulation causes in 'tearing of the fibrosed capsule' resulting in improved movements.

   Caution: MUGA should be done only after 6 months of onset of frozen shoulder while ROM remains grossly restricted and shows no improvement on prolonged physiotherapy.

   However, currently MUGA is not preferred due to possible complications of fracture of humerus, tears of labrum and cuff.

2. **Arthroscopic release of fibrosed capsule** should **performed** in case there osteoporosis of upper end of humerus or in cases of secondary frozen shoulder.

Q. What are the advantages and disadvantages of manipulation under anesthesia (MUGA)?

Advantages

1. Non-invasive procedure (no scar/infection), less costly

Disadvantage
1. Overzealously done MUGA can cause fracture of proximal humerus, especially in osteoporotic bone. So, MUGA to be avoided in osteoporotic bones
2. MUGA could result in labral tear or rotator cuff tear.

Q. What are the advantages and disadvantages of arthroscopic capsular release?

Advantages
1. The complete all-round capsular release is performed under arthroscopic vision in a very controlled fashion.
2. No risk of any structural damage (bone/cuff/labrum)
3. Best suited for secondary frozen shoulder wherein the primary pathology can also be tackled in same setting.

Disadvantages
1. Invasive procedure, costly, skin scars
2. Very rare risk of infection

Q. When is arthroscopic capsular release is recommended?

1. Osteoporotic upper end of humerus
2. Associated cuff, labral tear
3. Secondary frozen shoulder.

Q. What is done after MUGA or arthroscopic release?

Patient is started on extensive shoulder mobilization physiotherapy to retain all movements which have been regained during procedure.

Q. What is the prognosis of adhesive capsulitis?

Generally, the prognosis is excellent. Once completely treated or resolved, it does not recur and leaves joint nearly pain free and patient attains near full range of movement.

Q. What is the natural history of adhesive capsulitis (frozen shoulder)?

This condition tends to naturally resolve over 12–24 months (even if no medical or surgical management is taken!). However, since it is very painful, some intervention is usually required in form of medications, physiotherapy, intra-articular injections or MUGA/arthroscopic capsular release.

> Once, we saw a patient on consultation (who was admitted in some other department) that had frozen shoulder. We decided to manage him with medication and physiotherapy and so, wall climbing exercise was mentioned in consultation sheet. After a few hours, we got a frantic call from ward resident. He said that he himself and patient is quite upset that orthopedic doctors have not mentioned "which wall to climb and how to climb"?

Q. What is rotator cuff tendinopathy/rotator cuff tendinitis?

It is a condition wherein the rotator cuff tendon undergoes internal degeneration resulting in pain, decreased strength and performance of the shoulder. It occurs due to imbalance between damage and repair process of the tendon.

Q. What is the etiology of the rotator cuff tendinopathy?

It is seen in overuse and abuse of the shoulder which could be occupation related (overhead athletes, carpenters, painters, electricians, etc.) coupled with ageing.

Q. What are the clinical features of rotator cuff tendinitis/tendinopathy?

- Usually seen in patients aged >40–45 years
- Pain with overhead abduction
- ROM is nearly normal except terminal restriction of ROM due to pain
- Neer's and Hawkin's sign is positive.

Note: Usually, the symptomatology of the condition is self limiting and subsides in 6–9 months after the onset. However, mild degeneration of tendon may persist without any symptom.

Q. How will you manage rotator cuff tendinitis?

Since most cases of RC tendinopathy resolve over 6–8 months, it is largely managed conservatively by:

Minimise pain by
1. Avoid or minimize those activities which hurts shoulder
2. Analgesics sos, local diclofenac gel,
3. Physiotherapy: Local moist heat, short wave diathermy (SWD), interferential therapy (IFT) and local ultrasound therapy.
4. Subacromial steroid injection

Rehabilitation of shoulder
1. Rotator cuff strengthening and scapular stabilization exercises
   I will do only conservative management in form of NSAIDs and physiotherapy. If patient still experiences pain, I will give subacromial steroid injection.

Q. What is the etiology of the rotator cuff tear?

- Traumatic
- Degenerative

Q. What are the clinical features of rotator cuff tear?

- Usually seen in patients aged >55–60 years
- History of trauma (fall) in traumatic tears
- Pain with overhead abduction
- Passive ROM is nearly normal except terminal restriction of ROM due to pain.

However, active ROM is limited due to loss of power

- Neer's and Hawkin's sign is positive.
- Tests for cuff tear (Jobe's, External rotation lag sign, Belly press test, Hornblower sign) may be positive depending upon which tendon is torn.

Q. Which investigation is performed to confirm the diagnosis of rotator cuff tear?

- MRI: Investigation of choice
- USG

Q. What is the treatment of rotator cuff tear?

1. *Traumatic rotator cuff tear:* Surgical repair (open or arthroscopic)
2. Degenerative Rotator cuff tear:
   a. *Conservative:* Analgesics (sos), physiotherapy. However, if conservative treatment fails to improve pain, movements and strength
   b. Surgical repair can be done

Q. What is the treatment of glenohumeral joint arthritis?

Initially, a painful arthritic shoulder joint should be managed conservatively (analgesics sos and physiotherapy).

Surgical options must be given if pain and disability is not manageable in conservative ways.

1. *Total shoulder replacement:* If rotator cuff is normal
2. *Reverse shoulder replacement:* If there is complete irreparable rotator cuff tear.

Q. What is painful arc syndrome?

In painful arc syndrome, both active and passive abduction between 60 and 120° remain painful whereas rest of ROM is relatively painless.

Note: Unlike adhesive capsulitis, ROM is not restricted in painful arc syndrome.

Note: Painful arc syndrome (PAS) is a syndrome representing any of the following etiology:
1. Calcific tendinitis
2. Malunited greater tuberosity fracture
3. Subacromial bursitis.
The diagnosis and treatment of PAS depends upon the etiology.

Q. What is impingement syndrome?

Normally, the rotator cuff with subacromial bursa moves freely in flexion and abduction of shoulder between the spaces occupied by acromion (A, superiorly) coracoacromial ligament (CAL, anteriorly) and greater tuberosity (GT, inferiorly) without getting impinged between them.

However, in certain pathologies, the space available for free movement of subacromial (SA) space for rotator cuff and/subacromial bursa during the flexion-abduction is reduced, and the cuff-bursa complex gets 'impinged' between these static structures resulting in pain while movement. It is known as impingement syndrome (impingement of rotator cuff and/bursa).

There are several causes for impingement syndrome

a. Subacromial bursitis (a thick bursa gets impinged between A–CAL–GT)
b. Rotator cuff tendinopathy (thick inflamed tendon occupy more SA space and gets impinged between GT–A–CAL)
c. Thickened coracoacromial ligament (reduce SA space for cuff)
d. Spur at the anterior tip of acromion or type III acromion (reduce SA space for cuff during flexion).

Q. What are the clinical features of impingement syndrome?

Symptoms: It is seen in patients in middle age who present with activity related pain and difficulty in moving the shoulder. They also complain of night pain.

Signs
1. *Neer's impingement sign:* Patient experiences pain with forward flexion of shoulder especially flexion between 70 and 90°. However, ROM is nearly full and rotations are not restricted.
2. *Neer's test:* The pain of impingement is relieved following the subacromial injection of xylocaine.
3. *Hawkins sign:* With shoulder in forward flexion of 90°, it is internally rotated resulting in pain. The appearance of pain with this maneuver indicates subacromial bursitis.

Q. What is the management of impingement syndrome?

Conservative treatment in form of:
• Physiotherapy
• Analgesics
• Subacromial steroid injection

Rarely, arthroscopic surgery which comprises of:
• Arthroscopic debridement of inflamed, thickened bursa and frayed tendon.
• Excision of acromial spur, release of CAL

Q. What is the typical sign associated with impingement syndrome?

It is called Neer's impingement sign. Patient experiences pain with forward flexion of shoulder. But the ROM is nearly full and rotations are not restricted. It is relieved when subacromial injection of xylocaine is injected in subacromial space. The latter is known as Neer's test.

Remember: All painful shoulders are not frozen shoulder. There is much more in shoulder than frozen shoulder!

Spine Injury its Complications and Rehabilitation

INJURY TO THE SPINE

Common Presentation of a Patient with Dorsal Spine Injury

Case summary: A 36-year-old man sustained RTA two months back while driving a motorbike. He sustained injury to his lower back. Following the injury; he had severe back pain, inability to move his both lower limbs, loss of sensations over his legs and loss of control over bladder and bowel. His clinical examination revealed tender L1 vertebra with mild kyphotic deformity. He had no sensation below T12 dermatome with no power in both lower limbs. Lower limb muscle tone was increased and reflexes were exaggerated with Babinski's positive. He had no control over his bladder and bowel.

Q. What is the diagnosis?

The diagnosis is 2-month-old traumatic paraplegia complete below L1 with bladder and bowel involvement.

Q. Why do you say so?

History

a. History of trauma with loss of sensation and power in lower limbs along with loss of bladder-bowel control

Examination

b. Tenderness and deformity at the lumbar region (L1 vertebra)
c. Loss of sensation from L1 dermatome
d. Loss of motor power in the lower limb
e. Exaggerated reflexes
f. Loss of control over bladder and bowel

Q. What are various clinical scores to classify the spinal cord injury (SCI)?

1. Frankel's grading
   Frankel A: No motor or sensory function; complete SCI
   Frankel B: Sensory normal, motor deficit

Frankel C: Sensory normal, motor power <3/5 (useless)
Frankel D: Sensory normal, motor deficit >3/5 (useful)
Frankel E: Sensory normal, motor normal; No SCI
2. **ASIA (American Spinal Injury Association) scoring**

Q. What is the meaning of unstable spine fracture?

1. Associated with deformity of spine
2. Associated neurological deficit
3. Asymmetric gap between spinous process of spine or rotational malalignement
4. Injury to two or more columns of Denis
5. All spinal cord injuries/spine injuries are considered unstable unless the neurological status and spine completely is assessed.

Q. How will you investigate a patient with spine and/spinal cord injury?

1. **X-ray of spine:** Reveals fracture and/dislocation of vertebra
2. **CT scan:** Confirms extent of bony injury and fracture fragment displacement especially in the spinal canal
3. **MRI scan:** Detects extent and type of injury (contusion, laceration, transection) to the spinal cord.

Q. What is the principle of spine injury management?

1. Initial management of SCI and spine fracture with as per ATLS protocol.
2. Early protection of spine with immobilisation
3. Definitive management of fracture of spine
4. Care of paraplegic
5. Rehabilitation

Conservative and operative management of the fracture of spine
Braces for various spine #
1. Cervical spine: Hard cervical collar, Philadelphia collar, four post collar, halo ring immobilisation
2. Dorsal spine: Taylor's brace, modified Jewett brace, ASHE (anterior spinal hyperextension) brace
3. Lumbar spine: Knight spinal brace

Operative fixation for spine fracture:
Open reduction and internal fixation with pedicle screw system is performed for unstable fractures of spine.

Note: The operative fixation of spine does not guarantee early return of functions of spinal cord. It merely facilitates an easier rehabilitation of a patient with SCI and helps in avoiding the complications of recumbent position (UTI, RTI, bedsores, DVT, etc.)

Q. What are the complications anticipated in this patient?

Note: Every system in body is prone for complication after paraplegia or quadriplegia.

1. *Central Nervous System*

a. Post-traumatic stress disorder
b. Depression, anxiety

2. *Cardiovascular System*

a. ***Deep vein thrombosis:*** Due to no or poor muscle contraction in paralytic limb, prolonged immobilisation and dehydration results in venous stasis.
b. ***Hypotension:*** Especially seen after high cervical injury due to poor sympathetic outflow.
c. ***AV conduction block:*** Due to vagal overtone at heart in quadriplegics with lesions higher than C5–6.

3. *Respiratory System*

a. ***Hypostatic pneumonia:*** It is more common in quadriplegics due to their inability to clear secretions as a result of poor or absent cough reflex with added palsy of diaphragm and intercostal muscles while dehydration results in thick alveolar secretions which are difficult to cough out.
b. ***Aspiration pneumonia:*** Prone for aspiration due to poor cough reflex.

4. *Gastrointestinal System*

a. ***Constipation:*** Bowel denervation leading to poor motility of bowel, coupled with dehydration and less food intake or loss of appetite.
b. ***Incontinence:*** Due to bowel denervation and loss of anal sphincteric tone.

5. *Hepatobiliary System*

a. ***Cholecystitis and cholelithiasis:*** Due to stasis in biliary system

6. *Urinary System*

a. ***Urinary tract infection:*** Due to repeated catheterisation or indwelling urinary catheter.
b. Urolithiasis, diverticulosis
c. Vesicoureteric reflux, renal failure

7. *Skin*

Bedsores

8. *Musculoskeletal System*

a. Joint stiffness: Due to paralysis
b. Muscle wasting: Due to disuse
c. Osteoporosis: Due to disuse
d. Myositis ossificans: Especially if vigorous massage is performed over affected joints

Q. How will you prevent and/or treat these complications?

Undermentioned table outlines the various systems of body and their complication.

System	Complication	Prevention	Treatment
CNS	Depression/post-traumatic stress disorder	Counseling	Psychiatry and psychological treatment
CVS	DVT	Regular mobilization of joint	Anticoagulants
CVS	Sinus bradycardia, orthostatic hypotension, conduction disorder/heart block due to vagal overtone (seen in cervical spine injuries) this entire table need horizontal lines after each 1st side heading too to divide it	Atropine, pacemaker if life-threatening conduction defect	Pacemaker for heart blocks
RS	Hypostatic pneumonia	Deep breathing exercise Proper hydration (keeps secretion fluidic) Steam inhalation, respiratory	• Antibiotics • Respiratory therapy • Deep breathing exercise • Maintain hydration (keeps secretion fluidic)
Skin	Bedsore	• 2 hourly side—side turning • Keep skin dry • Keep bed sheet clean and without crease • 6 pillow techniques over bony prominences • Spirit can be applied over skin to keep it hard • Adequate hydration • Water bed	Treatment of bedsore as per grade of bedsore
Urinary system	UTI	• Proper hydration • Regular change of catheter • CIC should be performed with proper antisepsis	Treatment of UTI
GIT	Constipation	• Proper hydration • Bulk laxative • High fiber diet	• Enema • Suppository • Maintain hydration
Musculo-skeletal system	Joint stiffness Disuse osteoporosis	• Regular passive mobilization of joint • Splintage of joints in functional position • Baclofen to reduce spasticity in muscle • Regular mobilization of patient over wheel chair • Mobilization of joints • Active mobilization of joints which are uninvolved	• Physiotherapy • Contracture release • Tendon lengthening

Q. What can be done for the fracture of spine?

Fracture can be managed by braces or internal fixation.

Q. Which brace is suitable for vertebral fracture?

1. *Cervical vertebra fracture:* Hard collar, Philadelphia collar, sterno-occipital mandibular immobilizer (SOMI) brace, four post-collar brace.
2. *Dorsal vertebra fracture:* Modified Jewett brace, anterior spinal hyperextension (ASH) brace and Taylor's brace for multiple level # in dorsal spine.
3. *Lumbar vertebra fracture:* Knight spinal brace.

Q. What are the skeletal tractions used to immobilise the cervical spine fracture?

Patient can be kept on Crutchfield tong/Gardener well tong skeletal traction applied over the skull for 6–8 weeks followed by 4–6 months of hard cervical collar.

Note: Skeletal traction through outer table of skull is a highly specialized job as hole is made only in outer table of skull to place the traction pin.

Q. What is the advantage of surgical fixation of fractured vertebra?

The **most significant advantage** of surgical stabilization of vertebra is **early mobilization and prevention** of complication arising due to recumbence.

Q. Does surgical fixation ensures early spinal recovery?

No. It does not ensure early recovery as spinal cord recovery is guided by extent and type of injury to cord. Therefore, even after surgical fixation, patients may not achieve any neurological recovery.

Q. What is the prognosis of spinal cord injury leading to para- or quadriplegia?

It depends upon extent of injury to the spinal cord. Mild cases of SCI may recover gradually whereas extensive lesion may recover partially or not at all resulting in a forever paralytic patient.

Q. How will you ambulate a paraplegic?

A paraplegic can be ambulated with the help of wheelchair. Paraplegic patient can be taught to transfer themselves onto the wheelchair. Those who have some power around hip can be made to walk with crutches and orthosis.

Once, a patient was admitted with cervical spine injury. Gardener well tong traction was applied. Immediate X-ray showed satisfactory placement of traction pin onto the outer table only. A few days later, patient developed features S/O meningitis. Skull X-ray revealed that the traction pins were too much inside the skull poking onto the brain matter. Everyone was surprised, how did it happen? When further probed, patient told that he thought that everyday the side nuts have to be tightened, so kept on doing so. However, removal of traction and pins led to complete recovery without residual neurological deficit.
So, moral of the story is
"Some screws and nuts of brain need to tightened regularly (pun intended) but not of Gardener well tongs".

Q. How will you ambulate a quadriplegic?

Once a quadriplegic is transferred on wheelchair, they can mobilize themselves if they have enough power in upper limbs. **A motorized electric wheelchair** may be more convenient especially in those who do not have enough power in upper limb.

Q. What are main problems of spine injury patients?

Main problems are:
1. **Bedsore**
2. **Urinary tract infection,** and
3. **Respiratory tract infection**
4. Deep vein thrombosis (DVT)
5. Joint contractures
6. Depression, anxiety

Q. How will you rehabilitate spine injury patients?

Once these patients can be mobilized onto wheel chair
1. Appropriate vocational training to self-sustain them.
2. Self-care training and transfer onto wheel chair techniques
3. Appropriate tendon transfer to restore some power in upper limbs.
4. Psychological counselling

Q. What is spinal shock?

Spinal shock is defined as complete loss of all neurological activity below the level of lesion including sensory, motor, reflex and autonomic function.

It is a short-term temporary phenomena of spinal cord. Spinal shock may persist till 6 weeks.

Q. What is the meaning of incomplete spinal cord injury?

Incomplete injury is characterized by: Sparing of residual sensory or motor function below the level of lesion.

Complete spinal cord injury is characterized by:
No sensory or motor function below the level of injury.

Q. What are the superficial reflexes to be elicited after spinal cord injury?

1. Abdominal (D7–12)
2. Cremasteric (L1–2)
3. Bulbocavernosus (S2–4)
4. Anal (S2–4)
5. Plantar (S1–2)

Q. What is the importance of bulbocavernosus (BC) reflex?

The **return** of bulbocavernosus reflex **marks the "end of spinal shock"**. It also indicates the **incomplete nature of spinal cord injury**.

BC reflex returns within 24–48 hours in 99% patients.

(BC reflex is elicited by tugging the indwelling Foley's catheter or squeezing the tip of glans penis and anal wink is watched for)

Q. Which are the deep tendon reflexes to be elicited after spinal cord injury?

1. Biceps (C5–6)
2. Supinator (C5–6)
3. Triceps (C7)
4. Knee (L3–4)
5. Ankle (S1–2)

Q. What is the difference between superficial and deep reflex?

Both are reflex arcs where deep reflex is predominantly a typical **monosynaptic** spinal reflex whereas superficial reflex is **polysynaptic** with a **cerebral or supraspinal component.** Hence, superficial reflex is not elicitable in complete spinal cord injury due to the absence of supraspinal component whereas the deep reflex returns once the spinal shock is over whether there is complete or incomplete type of SCI as deep reflex does not depends upon any supraspinal component.

Q. What does presence of clonus suggest?

Presence of **clonus** suggests **upper motor neuron lesion**.

Q. With spinal cord injury (SCI), there is cessation of sensory and motor activities. But what is the characteristic of autonomic nervous system (ANS) dysfunction?

This **depends upon the level of injury**. The sympathetic component of ANS arises from D1–L2 spinal cord segment (**thoracolumbar outflow**). This is responsible for heart rate and blood pressure. Once the sympathetic outflow is cutoff, it leads to **bradycardia** (vagal overtone at heart) and **hypotension** (due to loss of tone at the level of arterioles).

The effect is **more prominent** when the spinal cord **lesion is in cervical region** as whole sympathetic supply is disrupted. However, spinal cord lesions below D6 have much less affect as by that level most of the sympathetic supply is already given to heart and blood vessels.

However, later the tone of ANS recovers and patient's cardiovascular system does stabilize.

Q. What is the origin of parasympathetic nervous system?

Parasympathetic nervous system arises from craniosacral outflow. Cranio through vagus nerve and sacral through the S2, 3, 4 spinal segment.

Q. What are the types of bladder dysfunction you know of in SCI?

There are two types of neurogenic bladder in SCI.
1. *Atonic type (LMN type):* When SCI is below D12
2. *Automatic type (UMN type):* When SCI is above D12.

Q. What is atonic bladder?

In atonic or LMN type of bladder; the reflex arc itself is disrupted either at afferent, bladder sacral center in the spinal cord or efferent. In such a case, urine gradually fills up in the bladder resulting in incremental rise in the intravesical pressure. Once intravesical pressure exceeds the urethral sphincteric pressure, some urine dribbles out. This lowers the intravesical pressure and once, intravesical pressure is lower than spincteric pressure, the dribbling of urine stops. So, in atonic bladder, large volumes of residual urine (post dribbling) is left predisposing the bladder for recurrent UTI, bladder stones, renal failure and diverticulosis.

Q. What is automatic bladder?

Automatic bladder or UMN bladder results after an injury to the SC above the level of sacral center of spinal cord but below the level of pontine bladder center. There is no supraspinal bladder inhibitory control but the local reflex arc is maintained. Here, once the bladder fills up, it stretches the detrusor muscle resulting in afferent signal to the sacral center. The efferent directs the signals back to detrusor which results in contraction of detrusor and simultaneous relaxation of sphincter resulting in evacuation of a large volume of urine and hence lesser residual volume of urine retained in bladder.

Hence, the complications of residual urine (UTI, bladder calculus, etc) are less in UMN than LMN type of bladder.

However, sometimes there can be detrusor-sphincter dyssynergia resulting in lesser volume exiting through the sphincter.

Understanding the urinary bladder innervation and its normal function (Fig. 11.1)

Urinary bladder has three source of nerve supply
1. Sympathetic supply (T10–L2)—relaxing effect on detrusor and contracting effect on sphincters
2. Parasympathetic supply (S2–4)—contracting effect on detrusor and relaxing effect on sphincters
3. Somatic: Pudendal nerves S2–4—voluntary control on external urethral sphincter.

Centers for bladder action!
1. Local sacral center in spinal cord
2. Relay center in pons, and
3. Cerebral center at paracentral lobule on medial surface of brain.

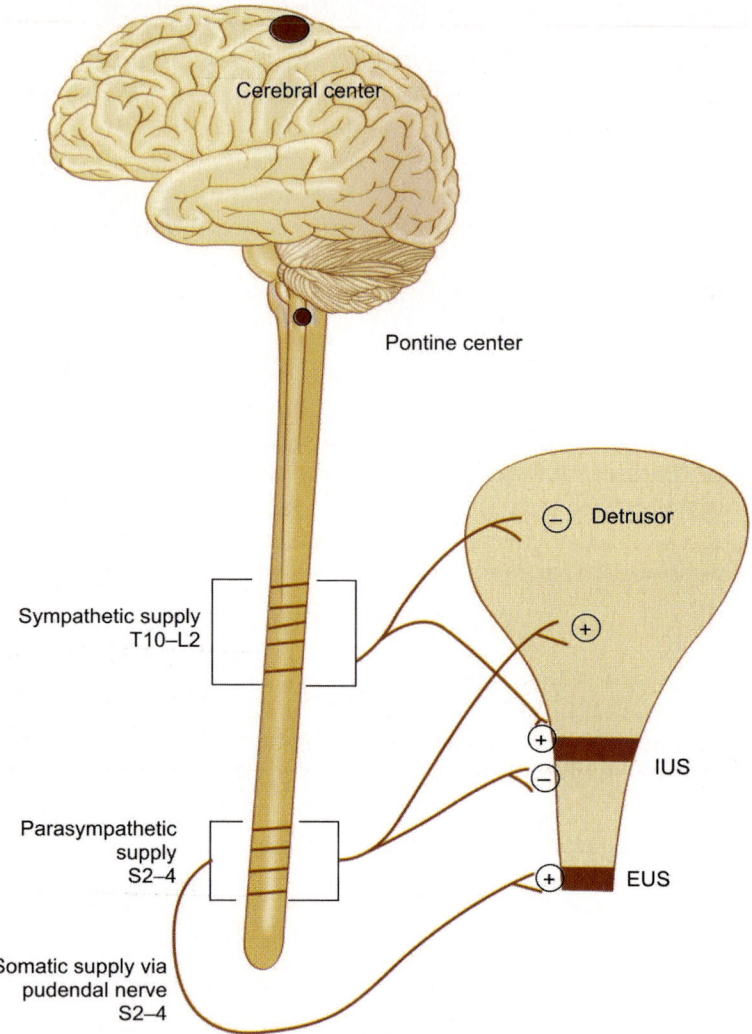

Fig. 11.1: Diagrammatic representation for urinary bladder neurological innervation (*see* Box)

Unstable Knee
(Ligament Injury of the Knee)

A 19-year-old boy complained of repeated buckling of the right knee while playing football since four months. Four months back, he sustained a twisting injury while playing football. He developed immediate pain and swelling of the right knee and inability to bear weight over the knee. He was taken to a hospital where he was given analgesics, knee brace, and advised physiotherapy. A few days later, he started walking normally. However, he continued to experience a weak knee, which occasionally gave way while running, jumping, turning or playing football. Examination revealed tenderness over the medial joint line, positive Lachman, anterior drawer, pivot shift, and McMurray test. The valgus and varus stress test were normal. The neurovascular examination was normal.

Q. What is your clinical diagnosis?

The clinical diagnosis is right knee anterior cruciate ligament (ACL) tear with a medial meniscus tear.

Q. Why do you say so?

It is because
1. History of twisting trauma to the knee followed by immediate painful swelling of knee and inability to weight bear (*observed in fractures, ligament injury*)
2. Repeated episodes of instability (*suggestive of a ligament injury*)
3. Tender medial joint line and positive McMurray test (*for medial meniscus*)
4. Positive Lachman, anterior drawer and Pivot shift test (*for anterior cruciate tear*)

Q. How to investigate the patient?

1. **Plain X-ray of the knee:** AP, lateral view
   - Usually normal. However, it is always done to rule out any fractures or bony avulsion injury of the ligaments
   - *Segond's sign:* In AP view of the knee, a small bony flake is observed adjacent to the anterolateral aspect of the lateral tibial plateau. It is quite specific for an ACL tear.
2. **MRI of the knee:** *Diagnostic investigation*
   Apart from cruciate ligament tear; it can detect meniscal and collateral ligament tear, injury to muscles, tendons and cartilage, and bone contusions.

Q. How will you treat the patient?

Since this patient has meniscal and ACL tear, we need to manage both.

A. **Meniscal tear:** The management would depend upon the location of a meniscal tear
   1. *Peripheral tear (red-red and red-white zone):* Repair the meniscus
   2. *Inner (white-white) zone:* Resect the meniscus (partial meniscectomy)

B. **ACL tear:** Since the patient is experiencing repeated instability, he should undergo arthroscopic ACL reconstruction.

Q. Which test is performed to rule out collateral ligament injury?

Varus stress test: To evaluate the integrity of lateral collateral ligament (LCL) injury.
Valgus stress test: To evaluate the integrity of medial collateral ligament (MCL) injury.

Q. Which other ligament injuries could result in instability of the knee?

1. Posterior cruciate ligament (PCL) tear
2. Medial patellofemoral ligament injury: It results in patellar instability.
3. A complete tear of collateral ligament: Very rarely, it occurs in isolation. Most of the time, it is injured in combination with cruciate ligaments.

NOTEWORTHY POINTS ABOUT MENISCUS, ITS INJURY, AND ITS MANAGEMENT

Q. What is the function of meniscus?

1. It acts as a load-bearing, shock absorber and helps in distributing stress to the tibia bypassing tibial articular cartilage
2. Joint stabilizer: By deepening the tibial articular surface
3. Helps in lubrication and nutrition of the joint cartilage

Q. What is the peculiarity of meniscal blood supply, and what is the meniscal zone system?

- The periphery of the meniscus has an excellent blood supply. Therefore, it is known as **red-red zone**.
- The middle part of the meniscus has a lesser blood supply, and consequently known as **red-white zone**.
- The inner third is quite avascular, and therefore known as **white-white zone** (Fig. 12.1).

Q. What is surgical importance of meniscal zone system?

The healing potential of a zone is directly proportional to the vascularity of the zone. The meniscal zone with good vascularity *(red-red and possibly red-white zone) has good healing potential* while the inner third *(white-white zone) is nearly avascular with poor healing potential.*

Therefore, peripheral meniscal tears and the middle third must be repaired (due to better vascularity) while zone with minimal vascularity (inner third; white-white zone) must be excised.

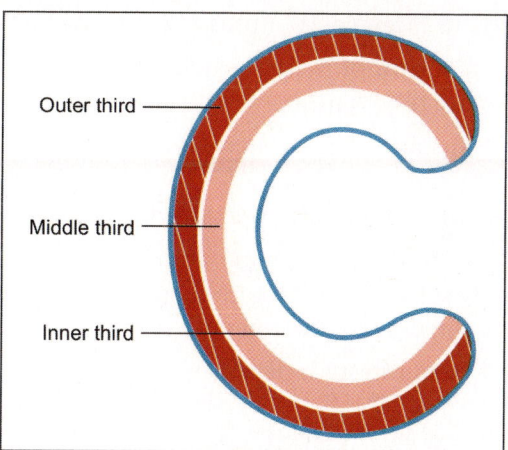

Fig. 12.1: The zones of a meniscus

Q. What are the common mechanism of injury to the meniscus?

1. Meniscus is commonly injured while twisting injury to the knee joint during sporting activity wherein twisting and jumping is common (football, basketball, volleyball)
2. Road traffic accident
3. Degenerative injury to the meniscus in osteoarthritis of the knee

Q. What are various morphological types of meniscal tears?

1. Longitudinal
2. Bucket handle
3. Radial
4. Parrot beak
5. Horizontal

Q. What are the common symptoms of the meniscal injury?

1. Mechanical pain: Pain while walking, running, jumping, squatting, or sitting cross-leg.
2. Locking: Quite typical of bucket handle tear of the meniscus
3. Clicks

Q. What are the standard tests performed to diagnose a meniscal tear?

1. **Joint line tenderness:** Sensitive test
2. **McMurray test:** Specific test
3. **Apley's distraction-compression test:** To differentiate between collateral and meniscal tear
4. **Thessaly test:** 'Most sensitive and specific test for meniscus.'

Q. Which is the diagnostic investigation to detect meniscal injury?

MRI

Q. What are the options to manage meniscus tear?

1. *Partial meniscectomy:* If it cannot be repaired
2. *Meniscus repair:* If repair is possible
3. *Meniscus replacement:* In case of total meniscectomy

Q. What would happen when meniscus is excised, partially or totally?

Whenever meniscus is excised, the load and contact stress over the articular cartilage dramatically increases resulting in cartilage degeneration and damage. Therefore, knee joint could develop arthritis after several years.

Note: Rate of cartilage degeneration depends upon the amount of meniscal resection (the more meniscus removed, the faster is cartilage degeneration)!

Hence, in most cases, surgeons prefer to repair the meniscus, if possible, to prevent arthritis.

Q. Which meniscus is more prone for injury, and why?

The medial meniscus is more prone for injury because it is more firmly fixed to the tibia, joint capsule, and medial collateral ligament.

The lateral meniscus is more mobile, and therefore, lesser prone for injury.

NOTEWORTHY POINTS ABOUT ACL ANATOMY, ITS INJURY AND ITS MANAGEMENT

Q. How many bundles are present in ACL and their function?

Anatomy: Two bundles—anteromedial and posterolateral

Function: Principle function of ACL is to prevent excessive anterior translation of tibia over the femur. However, each bundle performs different function.

Anteromedial bundle: Resists anterior translation

Posterolateral bundle: Provides rotational stability

Q. What are the common mechanism of injury to the ACL?

1. Twisting injury while playing sports (semiflexed knee with rotational stress over the knee)
2. Direct contact injury

Q. What is the clinical presentation of an ACL tear?

History: Immediately after the injury, the patient develops swelling of the knee joint (due to hemarthrosis) and difficulty to bear weight. Over the next few weeks, the patient regains the confidence to walk but continues to experience instability during 'pivoting activities', landing, running, and jumping. However, normal walking remains smooth.

Examination
- Mild quadriceps wasting
- Anterior drawer, Lachman test and Pivot shift test are positive

Q. Which is the most sensitive and specific test for an ACL tear?

Most sensitive: Lachman test
Most specific: Pivot shift test

Q. Is it possible to have an ACL tear but negative anterior drawer test?

Yes. It could happen due to the *door stopper effect* of the intact posterior third and horn of the medial meniscus.

In a patient with torn ACL but with an intact medial meniscus, the medial meniscus abuts against 90° flexed femoral condyle and acts as a 'door stopper' for femoral condyle. Therefore an intact medial meniscus may prevent anterior translation of tibia and preclude a 'positive anterior drawer sign.'

Q. What are the investigations to confirm ACL tear?

1. *MRI of the knee:* It is the confirmatory investigation for an ACL tear. Besides ACL tear, it can detect meniscal tears, cartilage injury, and other ligament injuries.

Q. What is the appropriate management of ACL tear?

1. **Acute ACL tear:** Traditionally, an acute ACL tear is managed conservatively.
   a. Analgesics for few days, brace
   b. Gradual knee mobilization and weight-bearing
   c. Muscle-strengthening exercise: Quadriceps, hamstrings
   Once the knee achieves painless ROM, *ACL reconstruction* is planned, especially if the patient is young or an athlete/sportsperson.
2. **Chronic ACL tear:** If the patient is experiencing recurrent instability, *ACL reconstruction* must be performed.
3. **Bony Avulsion of ACL:** Usually, ACL avulsion occurs on the tibia side. The bony avulsion should be fixed onto the bone bed with screws/anchors/sutures.

Q. Why ACL is commonly reconstructed rather than repair?

The results of acute ACL repair are not as consistent as compared to ACL reconstruction. Therefore, the reconstruction is preferred over repair.

Q. What are the graft option for ACL reconstruction?

1. Quadrupled hamstring tendons (semitendinosus and or gracilis)
2. Bone-patellar-bone tendon graft
3. Quadriceps tendon graft

NOTEWORTHY POINTS ABOUT PCL ANATOMY, ITS INJURY AND ITS MANAGEMENT

Q. How many bundles are present in PCL and their function?

Anatomy: Two bundles; anterolateral (larger) and posteromedial (smaller).
   PCL is attached 1 cm below the tibial articular surface.
Function:
1. The principal function of PCL is to prevent excessive posterior translation of tibia over the femur especially in a flexed knee.

2. It also helps in screw home mechanism and locking of the knee wherein the knee is enabled to stay stable in complete extension. However, separate bundles of PCL perform different function.
   Anterolateral bundle: Stability predominantly in flexion
   Posteromedial bundle: Stability predominantly in extension

Q. What are the common mechanism of injury to the PCL?

1. Direct injury: Dashboard injury, direct hit over the knee/tibia
2. Hyperextended knee

Q. What is the clinical presentation of PCL tear?

History: Immediately after the injury, the patient develops swelling of the knee joint (due to hemarthrosis) and difficulty to bear weight. Over the next few weeks, the patient regains the confidence to walk.

However, many patients report instability while 'coming down the stairs or ramp' or lifting substantial weight overhead (weight-lifters, manual laborers lifting the weight over the head). Some patient report pain in the knee. Nevertheless, walking on the flat ground may remain smooth.

Examination
- Mild quadriceps wasting
- Posterior drawer, quadriceps active, and sag test are positive

Note: Why some patients complain of instability while descending stairs or downstairs/walking down the ramp/lifting heavy weight overhead?
It is because of:
1. PCL is essential to provide posterior knee stability in a flexed knee (on stairs or lifting weight from ground)
2. Loss of accurate screw home mechanism which requires an intact cruciate ligament.

Q. Why patients with chronic PCL tear develop knee pain?

There are two reasons why a patient with chronic PCL tear develop knee pain. The pain is felt in the medial compartment of the knee and patellofemoral joint due to gradually developing arthritis in these two compartments because

1. Due to posterior sag, the medial meniscus has lesser contact with the condyles resulting in higher stress and contact pressure over the cartilage in the medial compartment resulting in an accelerated degenerative change in the cartilage of the medial compartment.
   Therefore, the patient experiences pain while walking. The local examination may reveal medial joint line tenderness.
2. Chronic PCL tear results in posterior sagging of tibia, which consequently drags the patellar tendon backward. Therefore, the patella moves closer to the trochlea resulting in higher contact pressure in the patellofemoral (PF) joint.
   The increased pressure in PF compartment results in pain while squatting, sitting cross-legged, climbing or coming downstairs as all these activities further increase patellofemoral contact pressures.

Q. What are the investigations to confirm PCL tear?

MRI of the knee: It is the confirmatory investigation. It can confirm the PCL tear. Besides, it can detect meniscal tear and cartilage injury.

Q. What is the appropriate management of PCL tear?

1. **Acute PCL tear:** Traditionally, acute PCL tear is managed conservatively.
   a. Analgesics, knee immobiliser for few days
   b. Gradual knee mobilization and weight-bearing
   c. Muscle-strengthening exercise: Quadriceps, hamstring strengthening exercise
   Once the knee achieves painless ROM, *PCL reconstruction* is planned, especially if the patient is young or an athlete/sportsperson.
2. **Chronic PCL tear:** In case the patient is experiencing instability or pain, *PCL reconstruction* should be planned.
3. **Bony Avulsion of PCL:** Usually, PCL bony avulsion occurs on tibia side. The bony avulsion must be fixed onto the bone bed with screws/anchors/sutures.

Q. Why PCL is commonly reconstructed rather than repair?

The results of PCL repair are not as consistent as compared to ACL reconstruction. Therefore, the reconstruction is preferred over repair.

Q. What are the graft option for PCL reconstruction?

1. Quadrupled hamstring tendons (Semitendinosus and or Gracilis)
2. Bone-patellar-bone tendon graft
3. Quadriceps tendon graft

NOTEWORTHY POINTS ABOUT PATELLA ANATOMY, ITS DISLOCATION, AND MANAGEMENT

Lateral Patella dislocation is another common cause of knee instability.

Q. Which ligament stabilizes patella in the trochlear groove or which soft tissue is predominantly responsible for patellar stability?

Medial patellofemoral ligament (MPFL)

Anatomy: Medially, MPFL is attached between medial femoral epicondyle and adductor tubercle and laterally over the upper 2/3rd lateral border of the patella.

Function: MPFL prevents lateral patella subluxation, especially in 0–30° of knee flexion.

Q. What are the bony factors responsible for patellar stability?

1. *Trochlear groove anatomy:* An appropriately deep trochlea is must for patellar stability. A shallow trochlea predisposes for lateral patellar dislocation.
2. *Q angle:* Larger the Q angle, higher is the chance of patellar dislocation. With larger Q-angle, the lateral displacing forces over the patella increase.
3. Femoral intorsion/anteversion, external tibial torsion, patellar facet anatomy.

Q. What is the clinical presentation of recurrent patella dislocation?

History: Immediately after the injury, the patient develops swelling of the knee joint (due to hemarthrosis) and difficulty to bear weight. Over the next few weeks, the patient regains the confidence to walk.

However, few of them continue to feel instability during their routine activities, especially while performing sports, running, dance, etc. Nevertheless, walking on a flat ground remains normal.

Examination
- Mild quadriceps wasting
- Apprehension test is positive

Q. How limb alignment could change Q angle?

Increasing genu valgum increases Q angle. Thus, predisposes towards 'patella dislocation.'

Q. What are the investigations to confirm patella dislocation?

MRI of the knee: It is the confirmatory investigation which detects
- MPFL tear
- Trochlear anatomy/dysplasia
- Meniscal tear, cartilage injury
- Patella alta

Q. What is the appropriate management of recurrent patella dislocation?

1. **Acute patella dislocation:** Traditionally, acute primary dislocation of the patella is managed conservatively.
   a. Analgesics, bracing for few days
   b. Gradual knee mobilisation and weight-bearing
   c. Muscle-strengthening exercise: Quadriceps, hamstrings
2. **Recurrent patella dislocation:**
   - MPFL reconstruction using Gracilis or any other soft tissue graft.
   - Trochleoplasty (in case of trochlear dysplasia)
   - Femoral osteotomy to correct higher Q angle.

Q. What is patella Alta?

Patella Alta means high riding patella.

Q. How do you measure patella alta?

Patella alta is measured on lateral knee X-ray, CT or MRI with several indices such as:
- Insall-Salvati index
- Caton-Deschamps index

Miscellaneous Conditions

CARPAL TUNNEL SYNDROME

Case summary: A 45-year-old female complained of insidious onset pain around right wrist and tingling over radial 3 fingers since 6 months. Pain and tingling is more at night waking her up. She also gives history of weakness of her right grip. She also gives history of cold intolerance and weight gain. On examination, there is no deformity but tenderness is present over the volar aspect of the wrist. Range of movement at wrist and fingers is full and painless. There is hypoaesthesia in median nerve distribution area. Thenar muscle test reveals weakness of abductor pollicis brevis. Phalen's and Durkan's test are positive.

Q. What is the diagnosis?

The diagnosis is right side carpal tunnel syndrome with suspected hypothyroidism.

Q. Why do you say so?

It is because of following reasons:

History
1. Common in females
2. Pain around wrist and hand
3. Clinical evidence (cold intolerance and weight gain) possibly indicating hypothyroidism

Examination
4. Tingling over the radial side three fingers
5. Phalen's and Durkan's test are positive
6. Weakness in thenar muscles and hypoaesthesia in median nerve distribution area

Q. What is carpal tunnel syndrome (CTS)?

Carpal tunnel syndrome is a median nerve compressive neuropathy due to compression of median nerve in the carpal tunnel causing pain, tingling, numbness and weakness in the area of median nerve distribution.

Q. What is a carpal tunnel?

Carpal tunnel is an osseofibrous tunnel located on the volar aspect of the wrist through which **9 flexor tendons and median nerve** pass. The floor of carpal tunnel is formed by carpal bones and roof is bounded by flexor retinaculum.

Q. What are the common causes of CTS?

Common causes are:

1. Acute or malunited fractures around wrist (Smith's, Colles')
2. Hypothyroidism
3. Acromegaly
4. Rheumatoid arthritis
5. Diabetes mellitus
6. Pregnancy
7. Repeated occupational stress injury (e.g. while prolong working on computer)
8. Idiopathic

Q. Why does median nerve get compressed in the carpal tunnel (CT)?

Any cause which leads to decrease in volume of carpal tunnel space/increase in size of current structures/extra fluid in the space leads to decrease in space available for median nerve resulting in carpal tunnel syndrome.

> **Decrease in volume of CT:** Acute or chronic malunited fracture of distal radius can cause decrease in volume of CT—Smiths #, Colles'#
>
> **Increase in current size of structures:** Synovial sheath of flexor tendons of carpal tunnel gets inflamed and hypertrophied in rheumatoid arthritis. Acromegaly causes increased growth hormone secretion leading to soft tissue growth in the tunnel.
>
> **Extra-substance/fluid in CT:** Fluid retention in pregnancy, Cushing syndrome, hypothyroidism.

Q. What are the signs elicited in CT syndrome?

There are several signs for CTS.

Phalen's sign: Both wrist are gently palmar flexed as far as possible, then holding the position for symptoms to appear. A positive test is one that results in tingling and/numbness in the median nerve distribution while holding the wrist in acute palmar flexion within sixty seconds. The quicker the numbness starts, the more advanced the condition (Fig. 13.1).

Reverse Phalen's sign: Both wrist are gently dorsiflexed as far as possible, then holding the position for symptoms to appear. A positive test is one that results in tingling and/numbness in the median nerve distribution while holding the wrist in acute dorsiflexion within sixty seconds. The quicker the numbness starts, the more advanced the condition (Fig. 13.2).

Durkan's sign: Direct pressure is applied over median nerve over wrist for 30 seconds. This results in tingling and numbness along the median nerve distribution area in hand (Fig. 13.3).

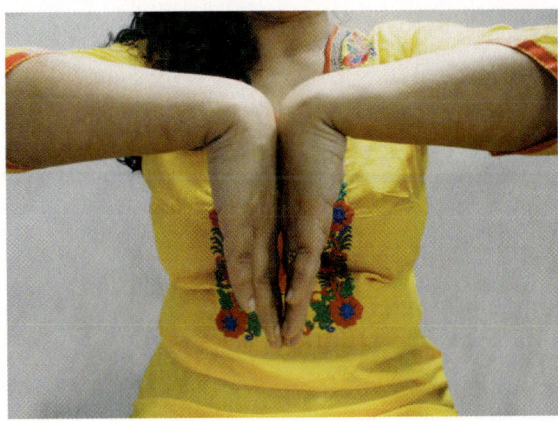

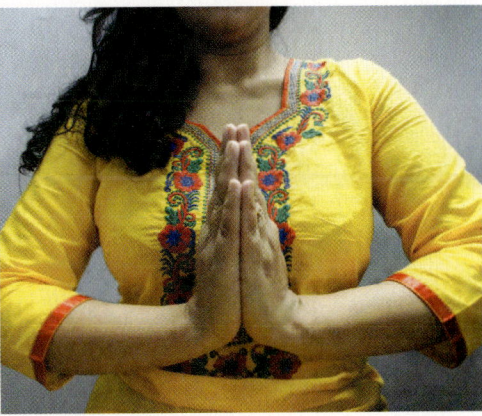

Fig. 13.1: Clinical picture of Phalen's test   **Fig. 13.2:** Clinical picture of reverse Phalen's test

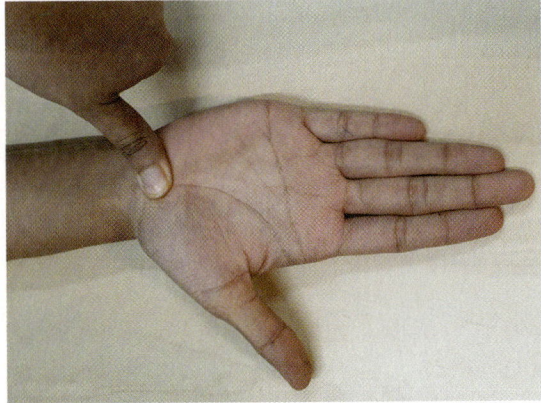

Fig. 13.3: Clinical picture of Durkan's test where in pressure is applied over median nerve above carpal tunnel

Q. How will you confirm the diagnosis?

Diagnosis is confirmed by:
1. Nerve conduction velocity test of nerves of upper limb (of both sides for comparison)
2. USG of carpal tunnel to look for median nerve compression and volume of carpal tunnel.

Q. What is the treatment of CTS?

Treatment of CTS involves:
a. **Treatment of underlying cause:** Hypothyroidism/diabetes/others
b. **Conservative treatment**
   • Carpal tunnel splint, pregabalin, analgesics for symptomatic relief
c. **Surgical release of flexor retinaculum, if conservative treatment fails.**

Q. What can be the other common causes of radiating neuralgic pain from neck on radial side of hand?

Other common cause of radial side neuralgic pain is:

a. Cervical spondylitis or cervical intervertebral disc prolapse with C5, 6 or 7 root involvement. However, such patients may complain of pain in the neck which radiates towards arm, forearm and hand.

b. Local cause of radial side thumb pain could be due to De Quervain's tenosynovitis.

Q. What is common cause of radiating ulnar side pain from neck?

It could be due to:

a. Ulnar nerve neuropathy or entrapment behind medial epicondyle

b. Thoracic outlet syndrome affecting C8, T1 nerve root.

Q. What is the common cause of thoracic outlet syndrome (TOS)?

Cervical rib is common cause of TOS.

TENDO ACHILLIS RUPTURE

Common Presentation of Patient with Tendo Achillis Rupture

Case summary: A 45-year-old male walks into the consultation room of an orthopedic surgeon with complaints of pain at the lower end of the left calf since 6 months with increasing pain and difficulty in walking since 6 weeks. Insidious onset, non-traumatic pain at the back of heel and lower calf has bothered him especially while walking. Pain used to be more with first few steps and then used to decreases a bit while walking. He took analgesic and applied gel to relieve his pain, but to no avail. Then, his doctor gave a local injection at the back of the heel. Pain got relieved for a few days till one day he heard a snap at the back of heel. Pain has increased since then and he finds difficulty in walking more than before. O/E, swelling and tenderness is present along the course of tendo Achillis. 2 cm above the calcaneus tuberosity, there is a 4 cm defect palpable over the lower end of tendo Achillis. Tip toe standing on affected side is not possible. The movements at the ankle are nearly full but painful. Ankle dorsiflexion is slightly more on index side as compared to normal side. Thompson test is positive. Neurovascular examination is normal. Calf wasting is noted.

Q. What is your diagnosis?

The diagnosis is tendo Achillis (TA) rupture of left side.

Q. Why do you say so?

It is because of:

a. Pain around the tendo Achillis (heel) since 6 months
b. History of injection around tendo Achillis (a steroid injection near TA can result in rupture of TA)
c. Palpable defect over tendo Achillis (Fig. 13.4)
d. Increased dorsiflexion on affected side
e. Cannot stand or walk on tip toe
f. Thompson sign is positive.

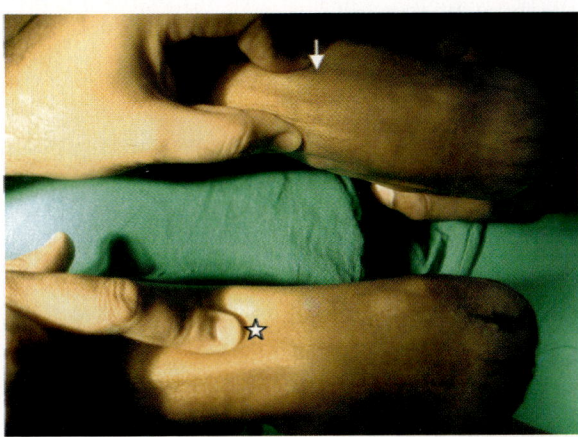

Fig. 13.4: Clinical picture of patient with TA rupture in prone position. Palpation of right side shows intact TA (white arrow) whereas left side shows defect over TA (white star)

Q. What is the relevance of injection around tendo Achillis?

He must have received steroid in/around his tendo Achillis which lead to the rupture of tendon.

Q. Why should steroid injection cause tendon rupture?

Patient was having pain in the region of back of the heel, i.e. around TA since 6 months possibly indicative of TA tendinitis or retrocalcaneal bursitis. Chronic Inflammation and subsequent reparative fibrosis of TA might have weakened the collagen fibres of TA.

Steroid injection into the substance or around the already weakened TA causes further weakening of the TA fibres as steroid are known to damage the collagen framework of tendons by inhibiting tendon repair mechanisms*. So, an already weakened TA tendon is prone for rupture when steroid is injected locally. Also, steroid is a potent anti-inflammatory agent causing pain relief. So, patient may tend to overuse already weakened tendon which may also contribute towards tendon rupture.

*Smith AG, Kosygan K, Williams H, et al. Common extensor tendon rupture following corticosteroid injection for lateral tendinosis of the elbow. Br J Sports Med 1999;33:423–5.

Q. What is the function of TA, and why a person cannot stand over tip toe or cannot walk over tip toe?

TA inserts over the back of calcaneum causing plantar flexion of ankle joint. Standing or walking over tip toe/forefoot or a push off during gait cycle is an antigravity act requiring great strength of plantar flexion which is derived from intact TA. Since TA is ruptured, patient would be unable to perform such an action.

Q. What is Thompson sign?

Patient is made to lie prone with knee flexed. Normally; on gentle active squeezing of calf by the examiner, ankle goes in plantar flexion against the gravity (calf squeeze leads to force transmission along TA to the ankle and hence ankle moves plantar wards). However, on the affected side, no such ankle movement happens because of TA rupture. This is k/a Thompson sign (Fig. 13.5).

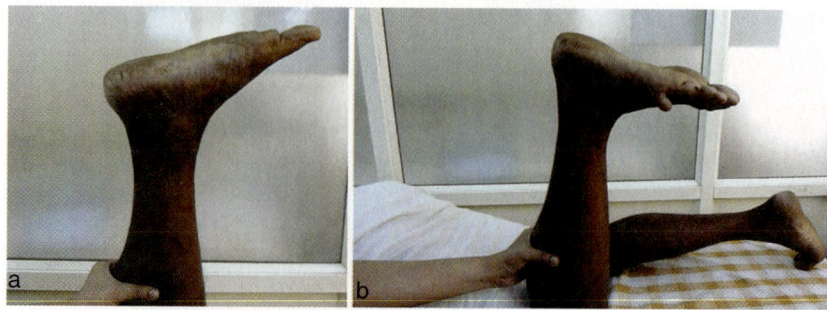

Fig. 13.5: Demonstration of Thompson sign in patient with TA rupture in prone position. (a) Plantar flexion of ankle and foot against gravity when the calf is squeezed on intact TA side whereas (b) shows ankle and foot remains dorsiflexed when calf is squeezed on ruptured TA side

Q. What are the other clinical signs of TA rupture?

1. *Matles test:* Patient lies prone and both knees are passively or actively flexed up to 90° by the examiner or patient, respectively. The foot of intact TA side would remain in slight plantar flexion while the ruptured side would remain neutral.

2. *O'Briens needle test:* A 25 gauge needle is inserted perpendicularly through the skin of calf muscle just medial to midline at a point 10 cm proximal to the superior border of calcaneum. The needle tip should be just within substance of the tendo calcaneus.

   When the ankle is passively dorsi- or plantar flexed, the motion of the hub of the needle is in an opposite direction to that of the tendon during passive dorsiflexion and plantar flexion of the ankle confirms an intact tendon distal to the level of needle insertion.

   However, if needle remains still, it confirms the diagnosis of TA rupture.

Q. Do you think that only local steroid injection cause tendon rupture?

No. Even high dose inhalational steroid can also cause tendon rupture.

Ref: Dilsher singh, Darshan Pandit, Martin Doherty. High dose inhaled corticosteroid can cause Achilles tendonitis. Case report. Respiratory medicine CME 2009;2(1):15–17.

Q. What are the other non-traumatic causes of TA rupture or spontaneous other tendon ruptures?

1. Inflammatory diseases: Rheumatoid arthritis, SLE
2. Metabolic diseases: Gout, pseudogout
3. Chronic renal failure
4. Local steroid injection
5. Prolonged antibiotic intake: Fluoroquinolones
6. Episodic athletes, weekend warriors
7. Chronic Haglunds

Q. How will you confirm the diagnosis?

The diagnosis is confirmed by:

1. *MRI:* Investigation of choice. It can detect
   - Partial or complete rupture
   - Retraction of tendon
   - Degenerative changes in the tendon
   - Cheap, dynamic

Once, a patient presented before my colleague Dr Kiran, with tendo Achillis tendinitis. He prescribed her conservative treatment. After a few days, patient called Dr. Kiran and told that she does not feel much improvement and a physician has advised her to take a local injection near the tendon. Dr. Kiran advised her not to take such injection. Patient called him again after a few weeks and said that she suddenly developed pain and inability to walk properly after hearing a snap at the back of heel. She informed him that despite his advice, she went ahead and took injection at the back of the heel. *So, injections into/ close to TA can lead to tendon rupture with disastrous consequence.*

2. *USG*
  - Operator dependent
  - Hematoma, presence of intact plantaris tendon may give erroneous diagnosis of partial rupture.
3. *X-ray:* To look for any Haglund's bump

Q. How to treat Tendo Achillis rupture?

a. *Acute rupture:* Both conservative and operative methods are acceptable treatment options with contentious arguments for either options.
  1. *Conservative:* Functional brace or below knee cast in resting equinus.
     - Injury is within 1 week and a non-retracted rupture TA
     - Patients with low demand, elderly, medically unfit
  2. *Surgical repair:*
     - Young, athletes, high demand patients
     - Injuries older than 1 week with retracted tendon edges
b. *Chronic rupture:* Usually surgical repair of TA is performed unless there is an indication to conserve (mentioned below)
   Conservative:
   - If medically unfit, elderly patient with low demand
   - Poor vascularity in lower limbs, neuropathies, poor skin condition around heel
   - Major systemic illnesses

Q. What is the advantages and disadvantages of conservative treatment?

Advantage: No scars or wound issues.

Disadvantage
- Higher rate of re-rupture of TA (remains contentious)
- Prolonged rehabilitation
- Difficult repair if there is re-rupture
- Slightly lower power and endurance of heel as healing may happen with elongated tendon.

Q. How acute TA rupture is repaired?

Acute rupture: Acute end to end repair of TA is possible within 6 weeks of rupture.

Q. How chronic TA rupture is repaired?

The TA rupture site is opened, the fibrosed ends are freshened and repair of tendon to the calcaneus is performed using non-absorbable suture material (ethibond, fibrewire) passed through the transosseous tunnels from calcaneum. One can also use anchors in calcaneum to repair the tendon.

  Chronic retracted tears might require:
- V-Y plasty of tendo Achillis
- Supplemental tendon grafting using plantaris tendon.

LATERAL EPICONDYLITIS (TENNIS ELBOW)

Case summary: A 45-year-old male presents with complains of pain in his right elbow for three months. It aggravated on lifting weights and on driving two-wheeler. There was no history of trauma. Pain was localized to outer aspect of the right elbow joint. He does not have any medical illness. There was no neck pain, tingling or numbness in the right forearm. On examination, there was tenderness over the lateral epicondyle. Movements of the elbow were normal and pain-free. Distal neurovascular examination was found to be normal. Cozen's test was positive.

Q. What is the Diagnosis?

The diagnosis is most likely to be right lateral epicondylitis (tennis elbow).

Q. Why do you say so?

It is because of the following reasons:

History
- Non-traumatic pain over the outer aspect of elbow joint (most common cause is tennis elbow)
- Chronic duration (3 months)
- Pain aggravating on activities (especially lifting weights, twisting/squeezing/wringing movements

Examination
- Tenderness over the lateral aspect of the elbow
- Cozen's test positive
- Normal range of movements of the elbow joint

Q. What is lateral epicondylitis (tennis elbow)?

It is the tendinopathy of the common extensors' origin (*typically involving the origin of extensor carpi radialis brevis muscle*).

Q. What are the causes of tennis elbow?

Cumulative trauma disorder: Wear and tear of tendons and muscles due to repetitive movements or excessive use/repetitive microtrauma.

Q. What is the association with tennis?

Although initially discovered among tennis players (forced wrist extension that occurs during backhand stroke), other Racquet sports can also be risk factors for developing this condition. It can happen in person not involved in any sporting activities as well.

Q. Other than sports, what are the risk factors for developing Tennis Elbow?

Manual laborers, construction workers (repetitive hammering, using a wrench), two-wheel driving (accelerator), cooking (squeezing/twisting movements) and not surprisingly orthopedic surgeons (using manual screwdrivers). Working population between 20 and 50 are at risk of developing the disorder.

Q. What are the differential diagnoses for this condition?

- Radial tunnel syndrome (entrapment neuropathy of the posterior interosseous nerve)
- Ligament injuries on the lateral side of the joint
- Intra-articular pathology like loose bodies
- Referred pain from cervical pathology (cervical spondylosis)
- Elbow synovitis or arthritis
- Fractures of the radial head or lateral condyle/epicondyle

Q. What is the special test described for this condition?

Cozen's test

Position: Patient seated; elbow extended and pronated; make a fist.

Test: Active wrist extension against resistance.

Positive result: pain experienced at the lateral aspect of the elbow/inability to perform active wrist extension due to pain.

Q. How will you confirm the diagnosis?

The diagnosis of this condition is primarily *clinical*.

1. *X-rays:* Antero posterior and lateral views of the elbow joint (tennis elbow: Mostly normal; calcifications along the common extensor origin can be infrequently seen). It is helpful to rule out any other bony/intra-articular pathology.
2. *USG:* Degenerative tendinopathy or tendon tears (partial or complete) can be visualized.
3. *MRI:* Can also detect changes in the tendon.

Q. What are the non-operative treatment options for this condition?

Roughly, in one-third of the cases, it is a self-limiting disorder. In acute phase or any primary presentation, it is desirable to give a trial of conservative management for at least 3–6 months.

Conservative Measures

- Activity modification
- Home-based stretching and strengthening exercise program
- Analgesics, topical gels
- Extracorporeal shock wave therapy/ultrasound massage/laser stimulation
- Local injections (steroids, platelet rich plasma, botulinum toxin A)
- Orthotics (counterforce brace): Tennis elbow brace/band

Q. What are the operative treatment options for this condition?

Only a minority of cases are categorized as "resistant" types (who have tried some conservative treatment for a 'considerable' amount of time and failed to respond) which might require surgery.

Options include:
- Radiofrequency micro-debridement
- Arthroscopic (keyhole surgery) debridement of the tendon
- Percutaneous/mini open release of the common extensor origin tendon
- *Open procedure (Nirschl procedure):* Excision/debridement of the tendinopathic tissue at the extensor carpiradialis brevis origin.

MEDIAL EPICONDYLITIS (GOLFER'S ELBOW/PITCHER'S ELBOW)

Case summary: A 29-year-old software professional presents with complains of pain in her left elbow for two months. It aggravated on activities such as typing on computer. There was some relief on stopping the activity but recurred. There was no history of trauma. Pain was localized to inner aspect of the left elbow joint and radiated distally along the forearm. There was no neck or shoulder pain. On examination, tenderness was noted 1cm distal to the medial epicondyle. Elbow movements were unaffected. Distal neuro-vascular examination was found to be normal. Resisted wrist flexion test was found to be positive.

Q. What is the diagnosis?

The diagnosis is most likely to be left medial epicondylitis (Golfer's elbow).

Q. Why do you say so?

It is because of the following reasons:

History
- Non-traumatic pain over the inner aspect of elbow joint
- Chronic duration (two months)
- Pain aggravating on activities

Examination
- Tenderness over the medial aspect of the elbow
- Resisted wrist flexion test positive

Q. What is medial epicondylitis (Golfer's elbow)?

It is the tendinopathy of the medial common flexor origin as a result of overuse.

Q. What are the causes of Golfer's elbow?

Cumulative trauma disorder (wear and tear of tendons and muscles due to repetitive movements or excessive use/repetitive microtrauma) as seen in other tendinopathies.

Q. What is the association with golf?

Wrist goes into flexion during golf swing (this repetitive action is probably the culprit for the development of this condition). This phenomenon can also be seen in other sporting activities such as racquet sports (including tennis!), javelin throw, rowing, baseball. It can happen (more frequently) with construction workers such as carpenters, plumbers, manual laborers, etc.

Q. What are the differential diagnoses for this condition?

- Cubital tunnel syndrome (entrapment neuropathy of the ulnar nerve at the elbow)
- Tardy ulnar nerve palsy
- Entrapment neuropathy of the median nerve/anterior interosseous nerve
- Ligament injuries on the medial side of the joint
- Intra-articular pathology like loose bodies

- Referred pain from cervical pathology (cervical spondylosis)
- Elbow synovitis or arthritis
- Avulsion fractures of the medial condyle/epicondyle

Q. What are the special tests described for this condition?

Resisted wrist flexion test

Position: Patient seated; elbow extended and supinated; wrist neutral
Test: Examiner resists wrist flexion of the patient
Positive result: Pain at the medial epicondyle or 2–4 cm distal to it

Q. How will you confirm the diagnosis?

The diagnosis of this condition is primarily *clinical.*
1. *X-rays*: Anteroposterior and lateral views of the elbow joint (tennis elbow: Mostly normal; calcifications along the common flexor origin can be infrequently seen). It is helpful to rule out any other bony/intra-articular pathology.
2. *USG*
3. *MRI*

Q. What are the non-operative treatment options for this condition?

In majority, it is a self-limiting disorder. In acute phase or any primary presentation, it is desirable to give a trial of conservative management for at least 3–6 months.

Conservative measures
- Activity modification
- Home-based stretching and strengthening exercise program
- Analgesics, topical gels
- Extracorporeal shock wave therapy/ultrasound massage/LASER stimulation
- Local injections (steroids, platelet rich plasma, botulinum toxin A)
- Orthotics (counterforce brace) or a cock-up splint at night-time

Q. What are the operative treatment options for this condition?

Only a minority of cases are categorized as "resistant" types (who have tried some conservative treatment for a 'considerable' amount of time and failed to respond) and warrants surgery.

Options include
- Arthroscopic (keyhole surgery) debridement of the tendon
- Percutaneous (small stab incision) release of the common flexor origin
- Mini-open (1.5–3 cm incision) technique
- *Open procedure:* Excision/debridement of the tendinopathic tissue at the flexor carpi radialis origin

DE QUERVAIN'S TENOSYNOVITIS

Case summary: A 39-year-old female with right hand dominance presents with complains of pain in her right wrist for 2 months. It is associated with difficulty gripping objects and performing the daily activities. There was no history of trauma. Pain was localized to the base of thumb. There was no neck or shoulder pain. On examination, tenderness was noted in the anatomical snuff box. Wrist movements were unaffected. Distal neurovascular examination was found to be normal. Finkelstein test was found to be positive.

Q. What is the Diagnosis?

The diagnosis is most likely to be right de Quervain's tenosynovitis.

Q. Why do you say so?

It is because of the following reasons:

History
- Age of the patient (generally seen between 20 and 50 years)
- Non-traumatic pain over base of right thumb
- Duration of illness (two months)
- Pain aggravating on activities and weak grip strength
- Absence of neck or shoulder pain

Examination
- Tenderness over the anatomical snuff box
- Finkelstein test positive
- Normal range of movements of the wrist joint
- Normal distal neurovascular examination findings.

Q. What is de Quervain's tenosynovitis?

It is the inflammation of the tendons and their sheaths of the first dorsal (extensor) compartment (**abductor pollicis longus** and **extensor pollicis brevis**) as a result of overuse.

It is also called *radial styloid tenosynovitis/de Quervain's disease/stenosing tenovaginitis/ new mother's tenosynovitis.*

Q. What are the causes of de Quervain's tenosynovitis?

- *Cumulative trauma disorder* (wear and tear of tendons and muscles due to repetitive movements or excessive use/repetitive microtrauma) as seen in other tendinopathies.
- **Racquet sports, frequent texting using phones/tablets (texting thumb syndrome), postpartum (unknown reason).**

Q. What are the differential diagnoses for this condition?

Thumb carpometacarpal arthritis, intersection syndrome (inflammation at the crossing point between first (APL and EPB) and second (ECRL and ECRB) dorsal compartment tendons.

Q. Which is the special test described for this condition?

Finkelstein's test:

Position: Patient seated; elbow extended and in mid-prone.
Test: Examiner pulls (traction) the patient's thumb into ulnar deviation *(OPEN FIST)* other hand of the examiner supporting the forearm.
Positive result: Pain at the base of the thumb.

Q. How will you confirm the diagnosis?

The diagnosis of this condition is primarily *clinical*. Others are:
1. *X-rays:* Posteroanterior and lateral views of the wrist joint. It is helpful to exclude any other bony/intra-articular pathology.
2. *USG*
3. *MRI*

Q. What are the non-operative treatment options for this condition?

In acute phase or any primary presentation, it is desirable to give a trial of conservative management for at least 3–6 months.

Conservative measures
1. Activity modification
2. Analgesics/anti-inflammatory
3. Local injections (steroids—USG guided)
4. Orthotics: Thumb spica splint

Q. What are the operative treatment options for this condition?

Only "resistant" types (who have tried some conservative treatment for a 'considerable' amount of time and failed to respond) warrants surgery.

Surgery: Open release of the first dorsal compartment.

Case Taking Format

Case Format and Tips for a Orthopedics Short Case Presentation

Orthopedic cases are presented as short case in examination. The candidate is given brief time of 10–20 minutes to evaluate the patient. Hence, it is important that he/she must know art of quick evaluation and crisp presentation.

General Format for Presentation

Name   *Age*   *Sex*   *Occupation*   *Address*

Handedness
(especially in upper limb case)

Chief Complaint (in chronological order)

> Initial demographic data can be said as "Mr AB, 28-year-old male from Bangalore, health worker by occupation is a right-handed person presents with chief complaints…"

1. AA
2. BB
3. CC

History of Present Illness (HOPI)

- Description of each chief complaint separately
- Important positive history
- Important negative history

Past History

Personal History

Treatment History

Family History

Menstrual History

At the end of the complete history taking, the candidate must be able to arrive at some conclusion about broad category of the diagnosis. The disease could be:

1. Congenital: Present from birth/late presentation
2. Traumatic: History of trauma
3. Inflammatory: For example, many joints involved, malaise, multi-system affection
4. Infective: History of fever
5. Neoplastic: History of rapidly growing swelling, loss of weight, appetite
6. Metabolic: Osteoporosis, gout with relevant history
7. Degenerative: Mostly age related—osteoarthritis, tendinitis
8. Others

So, while taking history, student must take relevant positive and negative history from each category to rule out diseases.

A very common mistake during case presentation is mixing **treatment history** with HOPI. It should always be avoided. It takes away the focus from HOPI. Only case where one can mix present history with treatment history is a case of trauma whereas in all other cases, treatment history should be mentioned separately.

Examination

- General examination
- Systemic examination
- Local examination
  1. Gait
  2. Attitude
  3. Inspection
  4. Palpation
  5. Movements
  6. Measurement
  7. Neurovascular examination
  8. Special tests for individual pathology
  9. Joint above and below

Final Diagnosis

Final diagnosis should have following components:
1. Duration
2. Anatomical site
3. Side
4. Pathology
5. Etiology
6. Complication, if any

Example of a complete diagnosis: One-year-old, right side tibial shaft non-union due to road traffic accident with shortening.

Description: **One-year-old** (duration) **right side** (side) **tibial shaft** (anatomical site) **non-union** (pathology) due to **road traffic accident** (etiology) with **shortening** (complication).

1. Diagnosis should be based upon positive points favoring the diagnosis from history and examination.
2. Student must not give the diagnosis based upon negative points
3. It is not always essential to give a differential diagnosis. For example, there will not be any differential diagnosis for tibial non-union. However, there can be differential diagnosis in patients with rheumatoid arthritis of knee.

Certain Tips while Performing Examination

1. General and systemic examination should *always* be done. However,
   a. If general examination is normal, it can be said as "general examination normal". If there is a significant abnormality, it should be informed, e.g. "pallor present".
   b. If systemic examination is normal, it can be said as "systemic examination normal". In case of a disorder which has a systemic effect or it is a part of systemic illness like rheumatoid arthritis/tuberculosis, it would be worth to do quick systemic examination and report the relevant information alone. For example, "a case of tubercular ankle synovitis", One should do the systemic examination sincerely to look for focus of infection in chest, GIT, etc. It can be reported as right upper lung zone shows clinical evidence of fibrocavitation due to tuberculosis. Rest of the systemic examination is normal.

During regular case presentation/exam viva, it is wrong to say that "I have not done the general or systemic examination". It should always be done even in short cases. If both are normal, it can be summarized as "general and systemic examination normal" and candidate should focus upon the local examination as orthopedic cases are given as short case.

2. In the category of palpation, the point or area of tenderness must be specified as specifying area of tenderness helps in localizing pathology. For example, in the knee examination, one should say that there is tenderness present over tibial tuberosity rather than saying, knee is tender. The latter way of presentation is common and it may suggest that whole knee is tender which may be the case of septic arthritis.
3. In the **category of movement**, candidate should mention range of movement, e.g. knee movement: 0–100°. 0–90° is painless whereas rest 10° is painful. Further is not possible. Both active and passive are same.

Avoid adjective like "knee movement is full/ very good"! Examination is an objective assessment and no adjective should be added during examination.

4. In the **category of measurement**, one can straight away tell the discrepancy/ normalcy of limb length rather than narrating the individual measurements of limb and not calculating the final discrepancy. The objective of limb length measurement is to analyze the discrepancy in the limb length, if any and to assess the area of discrepancy (femur/tibia/both, etc.).

Usual, but wrong way of answer: "The right femur is 52 cm long and right tibia is 35 cm long. The left femur is 52 cm long and left tibia is 33 cm long". After this statement, many students think that the job is over. After the individual measurements of bones, **goal** is to measure the **"limb length discrepancy"** which is 2 cm short tibia in this case.

So, simple way is to calculate the discrepancy, if any and answer accordingly.

Simple and right way of answer: "The right lower limb is 2 cm short as compared to the left, and the shortening is in tibia".

If the limbs are equal in length, then saying that "there is no limb length discrepancy" is enough.

During the presentation of short case, examiner is not interested in the individual measurement of bone length.

5. In the **category of neurovascular (NV)** examination:
   - If the **NV examination is normal**, it can be said as "**neurovascular examination is normal**"
   - If the **NV examination is abnormal**, then **individual finding should be told**. For example, if pulse is absent but neurological examination is normal, then it is appropriate to say that "neurological examination is normal. However, dorsalis pedis artery is not felt on right side."
6. **Joint above and below** should be examined. So, in case of a knee pathology, if they are normal, it can be again summarized as joint above (hip) and ankle (below) is normal.

However, if there is an abnormal finding, it should be informed.

While presenting finding of the case, two things to be avoided unless asked for
1. Methodology of examination
2. Etiology of finding.
Classic example is limb length. How the student examines and what is the cause of short limb is not to be presented while presenting the finding that the tibia is short in measurement section?
- If examiner asks that, how did you measure the limb length; only then examinee should inform the methodology?
- Also, why the tibia is short should be kept reserved for discussion and not to be told during finding presentation? Example; tibia is short because of bone loss during accident.
A structured, crisp presentation is an art inculcated over three and half years in clinics wherein student learns this scientific art by presenting several cases and actively participating in the discussion. It cannot be learnt overnight by reading this manual or any other clinical book. Hence, one must spend as much time as possible in clinics. Medicine is a subject which cannot be learnt by correspondence courses or by staying in the room!

II

Radiological Diagnosis

Trauma Radiographs

1. CERVICAL SPINE FRACTURE AND DISLOCATION

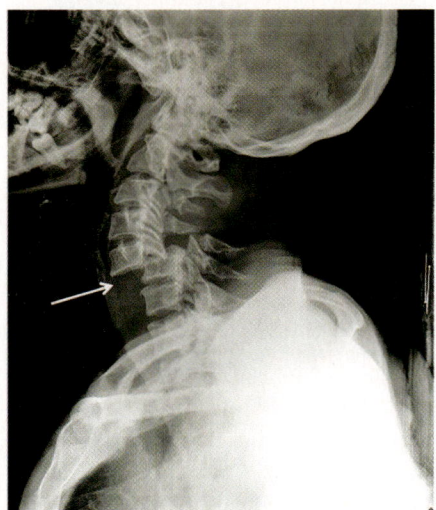

Plain lateral radiograph of cervical spine of skeletally mature patient shows:
- Dislocation of C5 over C6 vertebra
- At the level of C6 vertebra, the size of prevertebral soft tissue is increased (white arrow). Normally, prevertebral soft tissue space is <1/3rd the width of the vertebral body.

Diagnosis. C5–C6 dislocation with fracture of C5 spinous process

Few salient features of cervical spine injury

1. Cervical spine injury occurs in road traffic accidents/fall from height.
2. The injury to cervical spine may result in injury to the spinal cord injury followed by quadriplegia/quadriparesis.
3. It is managed by closed/open reduction of dislocation and then maintain reduction on skull traction (Crutchfield/Gardner-Wells tongs) or internal fixation by cervical plate.

2. FRACTURE CLAVICLE

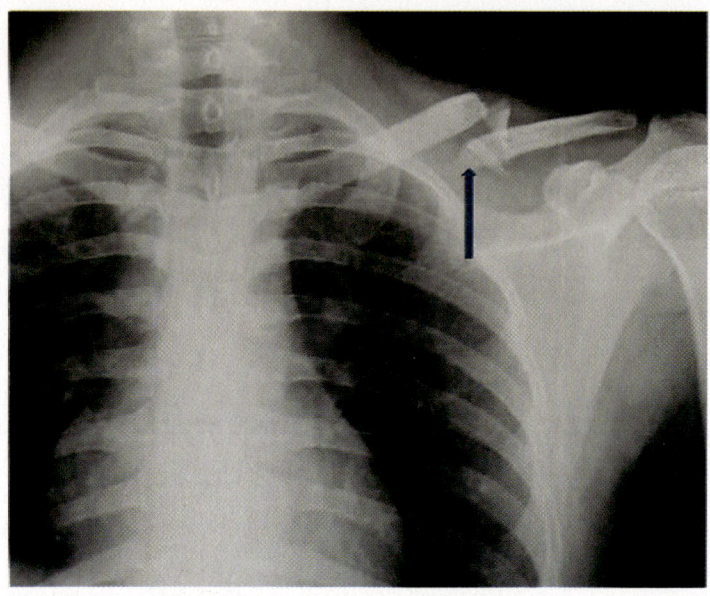

Plain AP radiograph of the chest of a skeletally mature patient shows:
- Comminuted fracture of middle third of the clavicle (left side, black arrow)
- Stenoclavicular joint, acromioclavicular joint and shoulder joints normal

Diagnosis. Left side clavicle middle third fracture

Few salient features of fracture clavicle
1. **Mechanism of injury:** Fall over the affected shoulder, fall on outstretched hand.
2. Commonest complication is malunion. Others; non-union, shoulder stiffness.
3. **Management:** Commonly, it is managed by figure of eight bandage/clavicle brace and arm sling. Sometimes, it requires ORIF with plates and screws.

3. ANTERIOR DISLOCATION OF THE SHOULDER

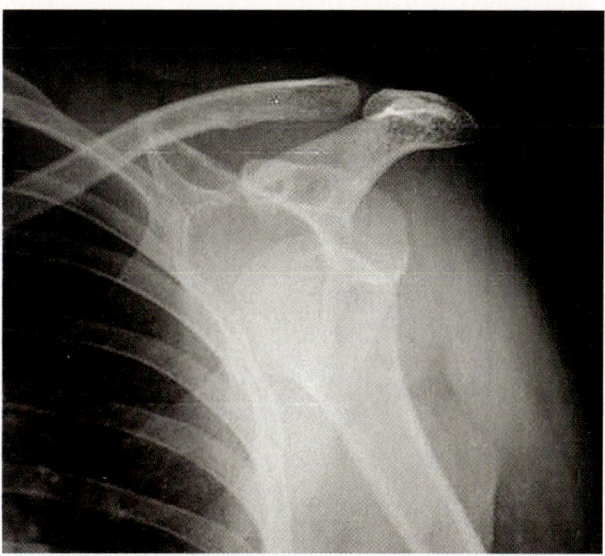

Plain AP radiograph of left shoulder of a skeletally mature patient shows:
- Head of the humerus is out of the glenoid cavity
- The humeral head is lying below the coracoid process
- The long axis of humerus is abducted
- Scapula, humerus and acromioclavicular joints are normal

Diagnosis. Anterior dislocation of the shoulder left

Note: Axillary view is required to ascertain anterior or posterior dislocation of the shoulder. However, sub-coracoid position and abduction of arm is enough to suggest anterior dislocation.

Few salient features of anterior dislocation of shoulder
1. **Mechanism of injury:** Direct or indirect trauma.
2. **Pathological lesion:** Bankart's lesion (anteroinferior labral tear) and Hill-Sachs lesion (posterolateral head impaction fracture).
3. **Common complication:**
   Acute: Axillary nerve injury, rarely; brachial plexus injury, axillary artery injury.
   Chronic: Recurrent dislocation
4. **Treatment:** Reduction is achieved by Milch maneuver. Kocher's maneuver is less practiced.

4. FRACTURE SHAFT HUMERUS

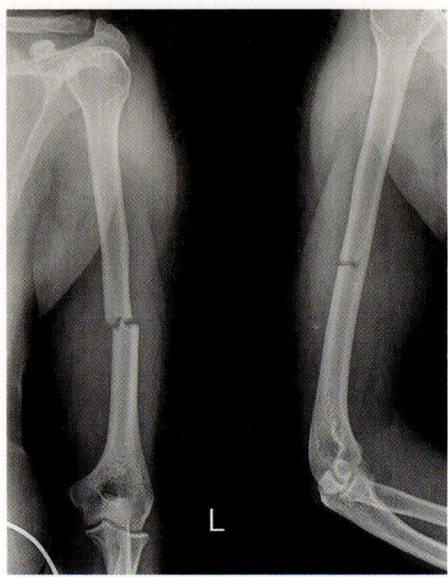

Plain AP and lateral radiographs of left side humerus of skeletally mature patient show:
- Transverse fracture of middle third–lower third shaft of the humerus
- Normal shoulder and elbow joint

Diagnosis. Fracture shaft of humerus left

Few salient features of fracture shaft humerus
1. Radial nerve injury is common in midshaft fractures
2. Managed by hanging cast/U cast method or open reduction and internal fixation by plate or nail

5. FRACTURE SUPRACONDYLAR HUMERUS

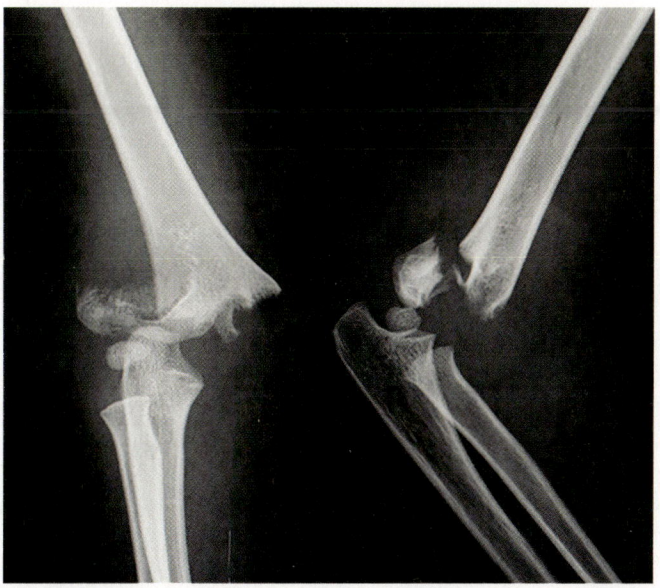

Plain AP and lateral radiographs of elbow joint of skeletally immature patient show:
- Displaced supracondylar fracture of the humerus
- Extension type
- Elbow joint and superior radioulnar joints are normal

Diagnosis. Supracondylar fracture of the humerus

Note: The fracture line in supracondylar fracture runs just above the cornoid and radial fossa.

Few salient features of supracondylar fracture
1. **Mechanism of injury:** Due to fall on outstretched hand
2. **Radiological classification (Gartland):** Extension (95%) and flexion (5%) type
3. **Treatment:** Closed reduction and cast application/closed reduction and K-wire fixation.
4. **Common complications:**
   Acute: Compartment syndrome/Volkmann ischemia, anterior interosseous nerve injury followed by radial and ulnar nerve injury
   Chronic: Malunion resulting in cubitus varus deformity.

6. FRACTURE OLECRANON PROCESS

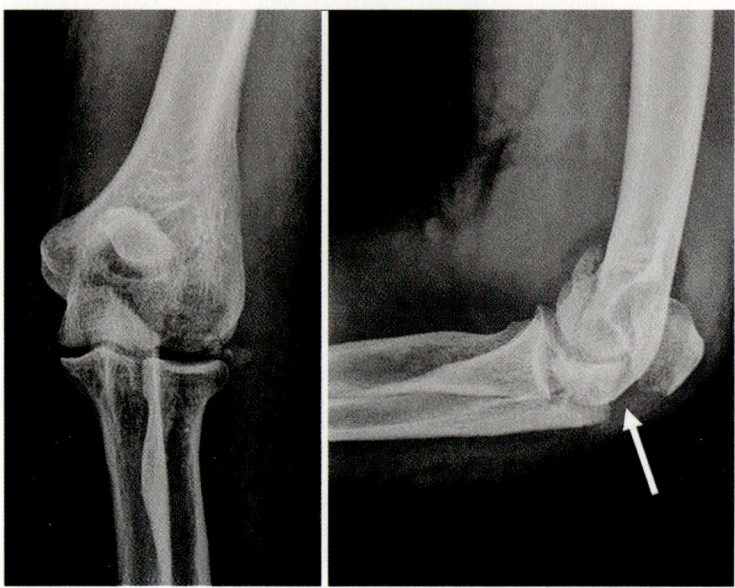

Plain AP and lateral radiographs of left elbow joint of skeletally mature patient show:
- Displaced, transverse fracture (white arrow) of the olecranon process
- Distal humerus, radius and proximal radioulnar joint are normal

Diagnosis. Displaced olecranon fracture

Few salient features of fracture olecranon
1. Triceps is inserted over the tip of olecranon
2. It is managed by open reduction and internal fixation by tension band wiring.

Note:
- **Principle of tension band wiring (TBW):** The distractive forces at the fracture site is converted into the compressive forces resulting in fracture union.
- **Common sites of TBW:** Transverse fracture of olecranon, patella and medial malleolus.

7. POSTERIOR DISLOCATION OF THE ELBOW

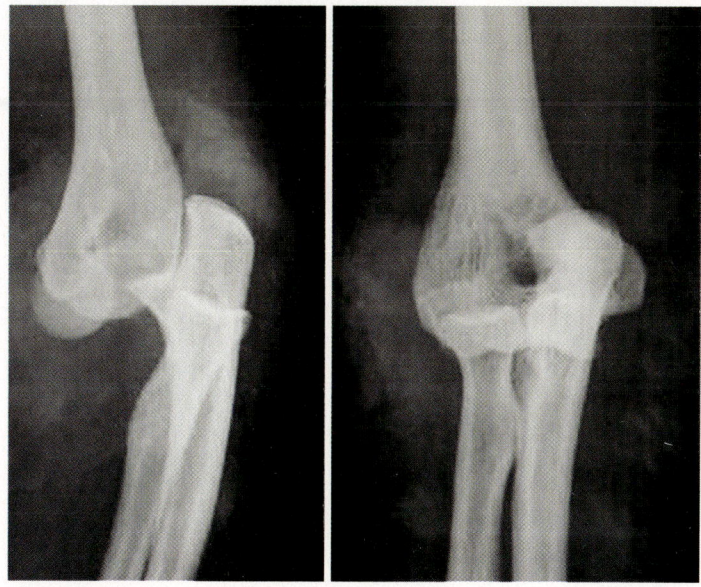

Plain AP and lateral radiographs of left elbow joint of skeletally mature patient show:

- Dislocation of the elbow joint with empty olecranon fossa (normally, the long axis of the radial through radial head must pass through the capitellum. In this case, the axis is not passing through the capitellum in both AP and lateral view.)
- Posterior displacement of radius and ulna
- Distal humerus, proximal radius and ulna normal

Diagnosis. Posterior dislocation of the elbow joint

Few salient features of posterior elbow dislocation
1. **Common complications:**
   Acute: Compartment syndrome, median nerve injury
   Chronic: Stiffness of the elbow joint, myositis ossificans
2. **Treatment:** Closed reduction and above elbow slab application for 2–3 weeks

8. MONTEGGIA FRACTURE DISLOCATION

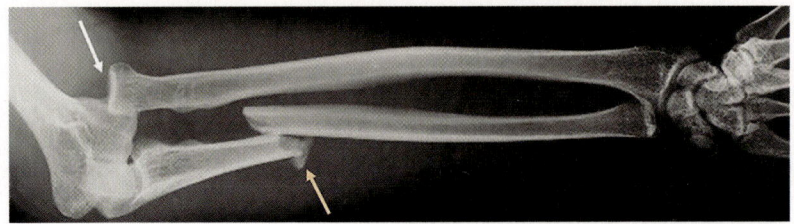

Plain lateral radiograph of forearm of skeletally mature patient shows:
- Comminuted fracture of upper third of ulna (yellow arrow)
- Anterior angulation of the ulna
- Anterior dislocation of the radial head (white arrow)

Diagnosis. Monteggia fracture dislocation (MFD)

Few salient features of Monteggia fracture dislocation

1. MFD is often associated with posterior interosseous nerve (PIN) palsy as PIN winds around the neck of radius resulting in finger and thumb drop due to extensor digitorum and extensor pollicis palsy.

   Note: Wrist extensors (extensor carpi radialis longus and brevis) escapse the palsy as both are supplied by radial nerve.

2. **Treatment:** In adults, MFD is managed by OR and IF by plate and screws.

9. FRACTURE BOTH BONES FOREARM

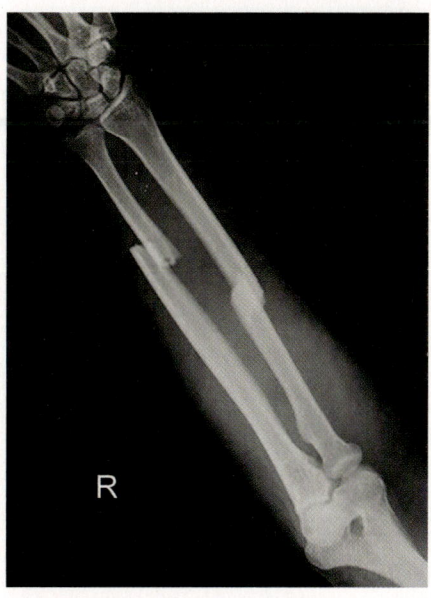

Plain AP radiograph of right radius and ulna of skeletally mature patient shows:
- Transverse, displaced fracture shaft of both bone forearm (radius and ulna)
- Normal elbow and wrist joint

Diagnosis. Fracture shaft of radius and ulna right side

Few salient features of fracture both bones forearm

1. **Acute complication:** Compartment syndrome
2. **Chronic complication:** Malunion (affects pronation-supination), nonunion
3. **Treatment:** Closed reduction and above elbow cast application or OR and IF by plate.

10. GALEAZZI FRACTURE DISLOCATION

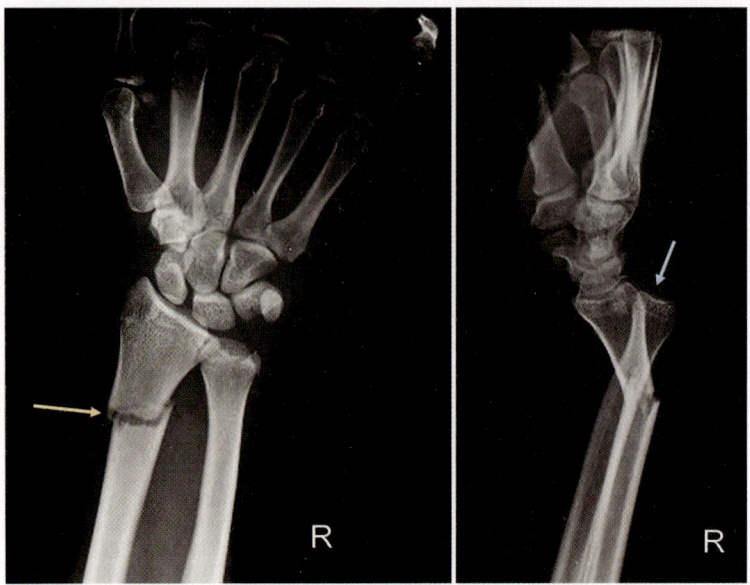

Plain AP and lateral radiographs of right side forearm of skeletally mature patient show:
- Fracture of lower third shaft of the radius (yellow arrow)
- Disruption of distal radioulnar joint (blue arrow)

Diagnosis. Galeazzi fracture dislocation right side

Few salient features of Galeazzi fracture dislocation
1. It is managed by OR and IF by plate.
2. It is prone for malunion which affects pronation–supination.

11. COLLES' FRACTURE

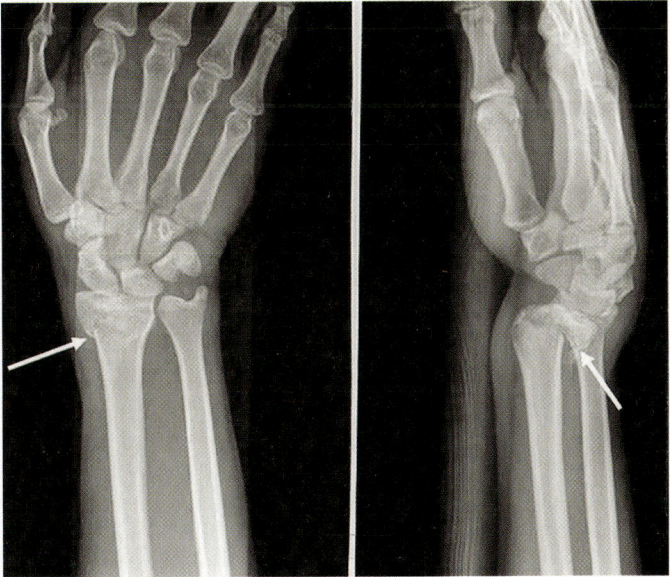

Plain AP and lateral radiographs of the distal radius with wrist of skeletally mature patient show:
- Displaced fracture of distal third of radius right (white arrow)
- Dorsal tilt (on lateral X-ray, white arrow)
- Dorsal displacement
- Lateral displacement
- Lateral tilt
- Impaction (radial styloid process lower than ulnar styloid process)

Diagnosis. Colles' fracture

Few salient features of Colles' fracture

1. **Mechanism of injury:** Fall on outstretched hand.
2. Often associated with osteoporosis especially in elderly.
3. **Treatment:** Closed reduction and below elbow cast application or/ORIF with plate and screws.
4. **Complications:** Malunion, stiffness of wrist, Sudeck's dystrophy, carpal tunnel syndrome, rupture of extensor pollicis longus tendon, osteoarthritis of wrist joint.

12. SMITH'S FRACTURE

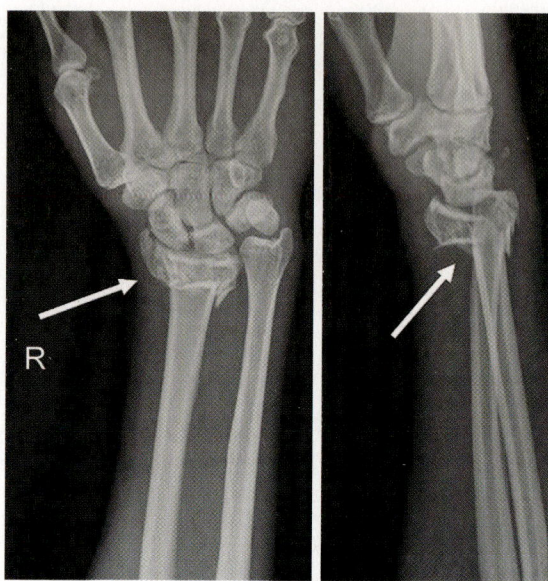

Plain AP and lateral radiographs of the right distal radius with wrist of skeletally mature patient show
- Displaced fracture of distal third of radius right (white arrow)
- Impaction with radial styloid process at the lower level than ulnar styloid.
- **Volar angulation** (on lateral X-ray, white arrow)
- **Volar displacement**
- Radial displacement
- Radial angulation

Diagnosis. Smith's fracture right side

Few salient features of Smith's fracture

1. Injury to the median nerve is common as the fracture fragment displaces volarwards compressing onto the median nerve.
2. Treatment: CR and below elbow cast/ OR and IF by plate.

13. FRACTURE SCAPHOID

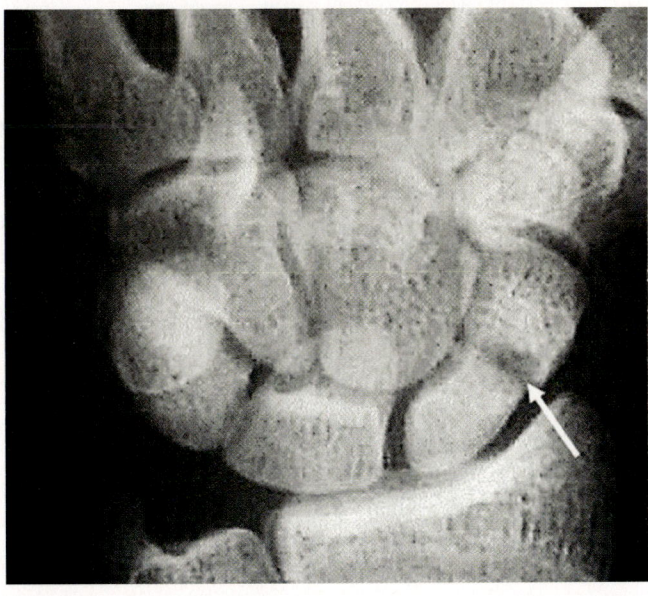

Plain AP radiograph of wrist of skeletally mature patient shows
- Displaced fracture waist of scaphoid

Diagnosis. Scaphoid fracture

Few salient features of fracture scaphoid
1. **Mechanism of injury:** Fall on outstretched hand.
2. **Clinical features:** Tenderness in the **anatomical snuff box**
3. **Treatment:** Below elbow cast application/OR and IF by Herbert screw.
4. **Common complication:** Nonunion, avascular necrosis, later radiocarpal arthritis

14. FRACTURE OF LUMBAR SPINE

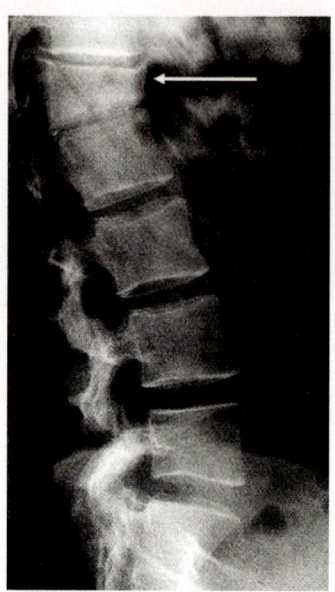

Plain lateral radiograph of lumbar spine of skeletally mature patient shows
• Wedging of L1 vertebral body (white arrow)

Diagnosis. L1 vertebral body wedge fracture

Few salient features of lumbar spine fracture
1. **Mechanism of injury:** Fall from height, RTA
2. **Treatment:** Brace/internal fixation by pedicle screws.
3. **Complication:** Spinal cord injury leading to paraplegia/paraparesis, deformity and chronic low back pain.

15. FRACTURE PELVIS

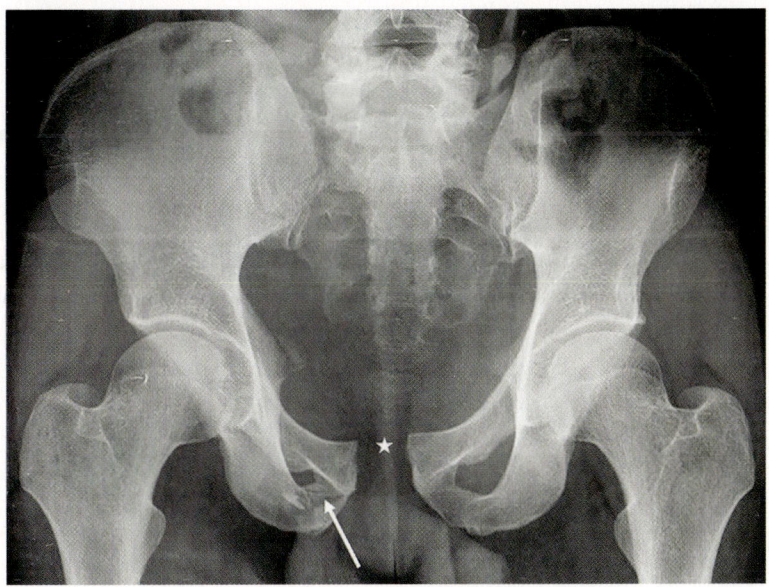

Plain AP radiograph of pelvis with both hips of skeletally mature patient shows
- Fracture of inferior pubic rami right side (white arrow)
- Disruption of pubic symphysis (pubic diastasis) [white star]

Diagnosis. Pubic symphysis diastasis with inferior pubic rami fracture

Normal gap at pubis symphysis is 4–5 mm

Few salient features of fracture pelvis
1. **Mechanism of injury:** RTA, fall from height.
2. **Complications**
   Acute: Hemorrhagic shock, injury to pelvic organs like urinary bladder, urethra, rectum
   Chronic: Malunion, limb length discrepancy.

16. POSTERIOR DISLOCATION OF THE HIP

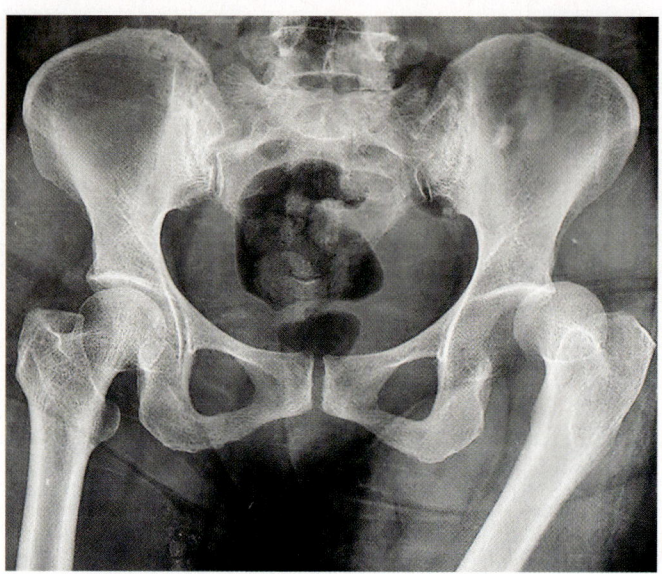

Plain AP radiograph of pelvis with both hips of skeletally mature patient shows:
- Femoral head is out of the acetabular cavity on left side
- Broken shenton line
- Left side hip joint is in flexion, adduction and internal rotation attitude.

Diagnosis. Posterior dislocation of the hip joint left

Few salient features of posterior dislocation of hip
1. **Mechanism of injury:** RTA
2. **Treatment:** Closed reduction
3. **Complication**
   Acute: Sciatic nerve injury leading to footdrop; fracture acetabulum
   Chronic: Avascular necrosis of head of femur, myositis ossificans

17. FRACTURE NECK FEMUR

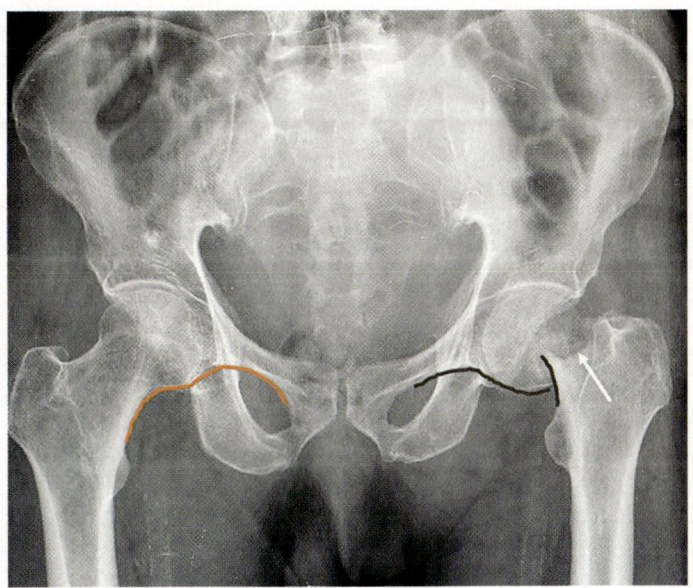

Plain AP radiographs of pelvis with both hips of skeletally mature patient show:
- Displaced fracture neck of femur left side
- Broken Shenton's line (black line)
- Proximal migration of greater trochanter
- More prominent lesser trochanter (signifies external rotation)

Diagnosis. Fracture neck of femur left

Normal shenton line on right side (orange line)

Few salient features of fracture neck femur
1. Usually in old age due to fall.
2. Associated with **osteoporosis**.
3. Usually, **treatment** is dictated by the age of patient
   - *Age < 60 years:* OR and IF by DHS/cannulated cancellous screw
   - *Age > 60 years:* Hemireplacement by Austin Moore prosthesis/Thomson prosthesis. In case of acetabular arthritis, total hip replacement is performed.
4. *Complications:* **Nonunion, avascular necrosis** of head of femur and hip arthritis.

18. FRACTURE INTERTROCHANTERIC FEMUR

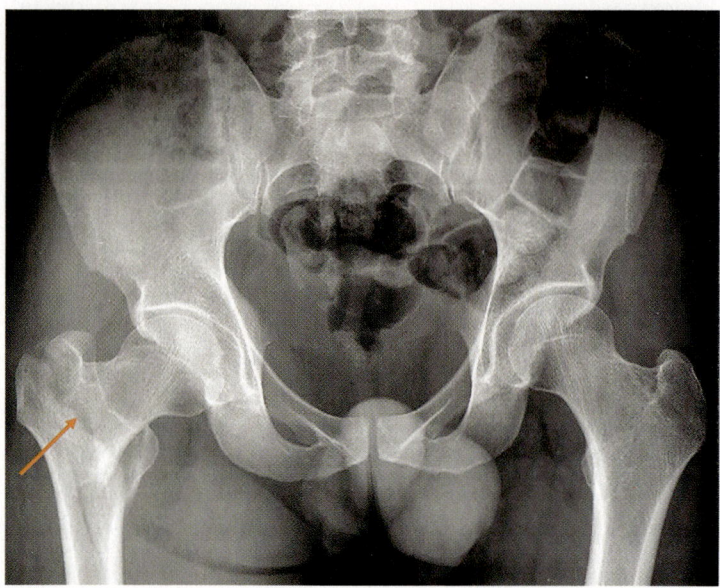

Plain AP radiograph of pelvis with both hips of skeletally mature patient shows:
- Displaced fracture intertrochanteric right side (orange arrow)
- Coxa vara (decreased neck-shaft angle)
- Both hip and sacroiliac joints are normal

Diagnosis. Fracture intertrochanteric right

Note. Normal neck shaft angle—126°

Few salient features of intertrochanteric fracture
1. Seen in elderly population, associated osteoporosis
2. Untreated fractures lead to **malunion** and **coxa vara** deformity.
3. **Treatment:**
   - OR and IF by DHS/proximal femoral nail
   - Rarely by traction and Thomas knee splint application

19. FRACTURE SHAFT FEMUR

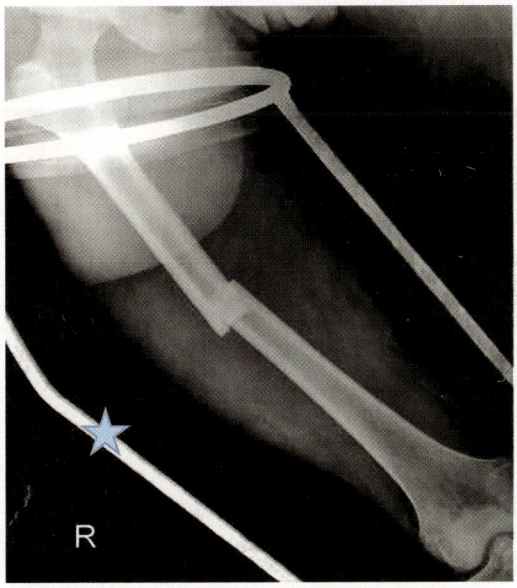

Plain AP radiographs of right femur of skeletally mature patient show:
- Fracture of middle third of shaft femur
- Displaced and transverse fracture
- The metallic shadow all around (blue star) is of Thomas knee splint

Diagnosis. Fracture shaft of right femur

Few salient features of fracture shaft femur
1. **Complications**
   - Within 2 hours: Hemorrhagic shock
   - Within 2 days: Fat embolism
2. Temporary immobilization of fracture by Thomas knee splint
3. **Current preferred method of treatment:** CR and IF by intramedullary interlocking nail; sometimes ORIF by plates

20. FRACTURE PATELLA

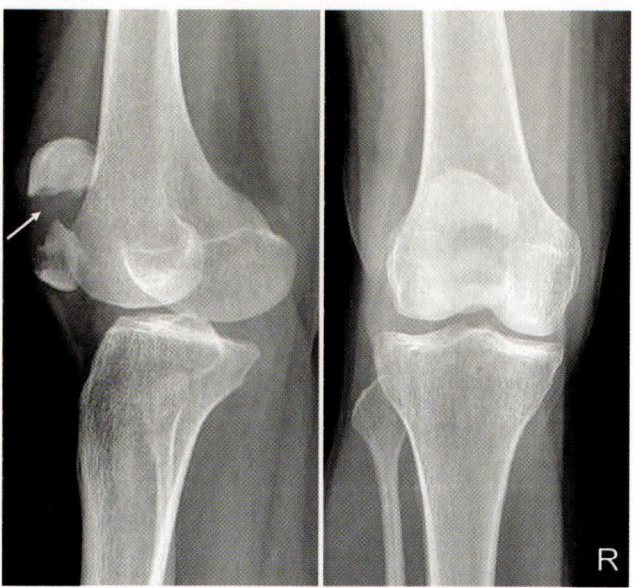

Plain AP and lateral radiograph of right side knee joint of skeletally mature patient shows:

- Fracture of middle third of patella
- Transverse fracture
- Distal femur and proximal tibia normal

Diagnosis. Fracture of patella right

Note. Principal function of patella is to increase lever arm of quadriceps muscle enabling smooth knee extension.

Few salient features of fracture patella

1. *Treatment:*
   - Displaced fracture: Tension band wiring.
   - Undisplaced fracture: Above knee cylindrical cast
2. *Chronic complication:* Malunion, nonunion, patellofemoral arthritis

21. FRACTURE TIBIA—FIBULA

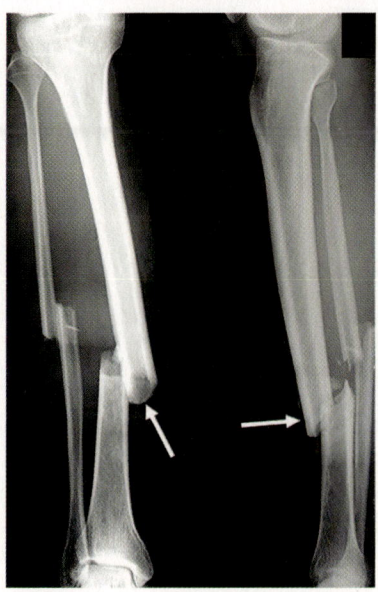

Plain AP and lateral radiographs of right tibia of skeletally mature patient show:
- Fractures of middle third–lower third tibia and middle third–lower third fibula (white arrow)
- Displaced (valgus and hyper extended)
- Oblique fracture
- Normal knee and ankle joint

Diagnosis. Fracture shaft of right tibia and fibula

Few salient features of tibia fibula fracture
1. Acute complication: Compartment syndrome
2. Treated by
   - CR and above knee cast application or
   - CR/OR and IF by intramedullary interlocking nail.
3. *Chronic complication:* Malunion, nonunion

22. BIMALLEOLAR FRACTURE

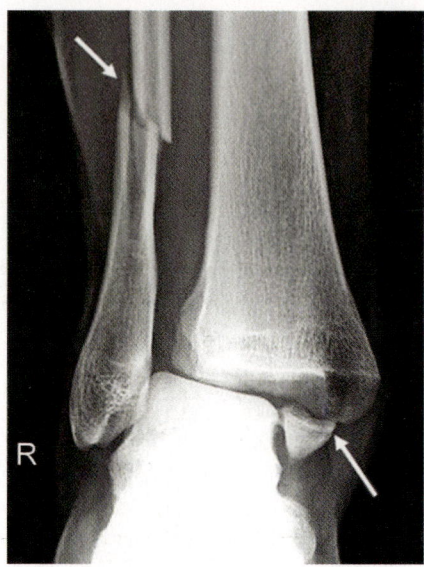

Plain AP radiographs of right side ankle with distal tibia of skeletally mature patient show:
- Transverse fracture of medial malleolus (white arrow)
- Lateral displacement of ankle mortise
- Lower third oblique fracture of fibula (white arrow)
- Disruption of distal tibiofibular joint

Diagnosis. Bimalleolar fracture right side

Few salient features of bimalleolar fracture
1. **Commonest mode of trauma:** Fall from height/twisting injury to ankle.
2. **Treatment:**
   - CR and below knee cast application, or
   - OR and IF by tension band wiring for medial malleolus and plate fixation of fibula
3. **Complications:**
   Acute: Compartment syndrome of foot, fracture blisters
   Chronic: Malunion, nonunion, ankle arthritis

23. FRACTURE CALCANEUM

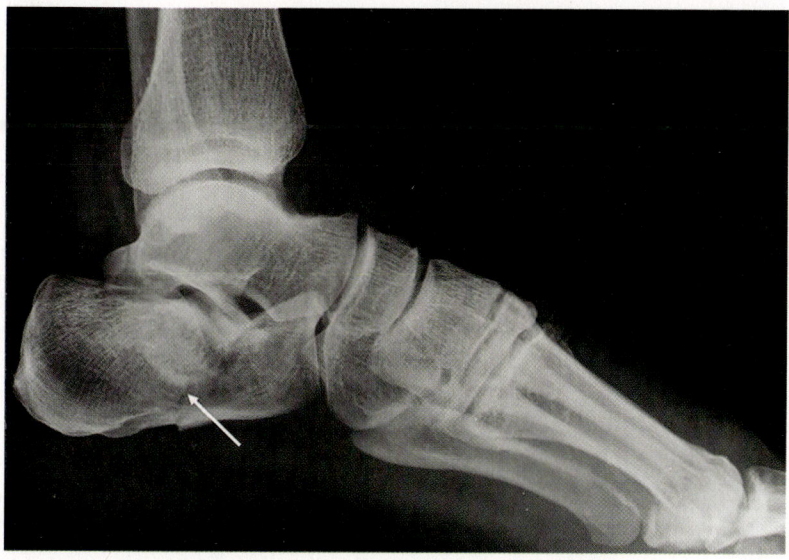

Plain lateral radiograph of left ankle of skeletally mature patient shows:
- Fracture of body of calcaneum (white arrow)
- Depression of the subtalar joint
- Talus, distal tibia and fibula, rest of tarsal bones is normal

Diagnosis. Fracture body of calcaneum left

Few salient features of fracture calcaneum
1. **Mechanism of injury:** Fall from height
2. **Treatment**
    - CR and above knee cast application, or
    - OR and IF by plates
3. **Complications**
    Acute: Compartment syndrome of foot, fracture blisters
    Chronic: Malunion, subtalar arthritis

24. FRACTURE TALUS

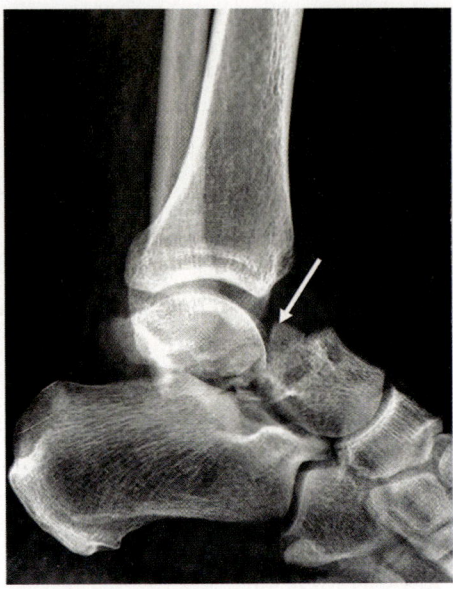

Plain lateral radiograph of left ankle of skeletally mature patient shows:
* Fracture of neck of the talus (white arrow)
* Displaced fracture
* Distal tibia and fibula normal

Diagnosis. Fracture neck of the talus left

Few salient features of fracture talus

1. Also known as Aviator's astragalus
2. **Treated by**
   * CR and below knee cast **or**
   * OR and IF by screws
3. **Chronic complication: Nonunion, avascular necrosis of body of talus**
4. Revascularisation of head is associated with radiological "**Hawkin's sign**"

25. ATROPHIC NONUNION

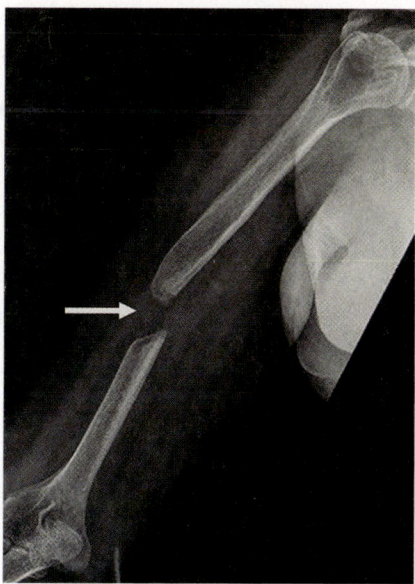

Plain AP radiograph of right humerus of skeletally mature patient shows:
- Fracture of middle third of shaft of humerus
- **No callus at fracture site (atrophic nonunion)**
- Closed medullary canal
- Sclerosed margins of fracture ends

Diagnosis. Atrophic nonunion of the humerus

Few salient features of nonunion
1. Clinical feature: Painless abnormal mobility
2. Atrophic nonunion is characterized by **lack of biological activity at the fracture site**. (Hence bone grafting is required to stimulate union.)
3. **Treatment**
   a. Open reduction
   b. Freshening of sclerosed ends
   c. Opening of medullary canal
   d. Internal fixation
   e. Bone grafting in atrophic nonunion

26. HYPERTROPHIC NONUNION

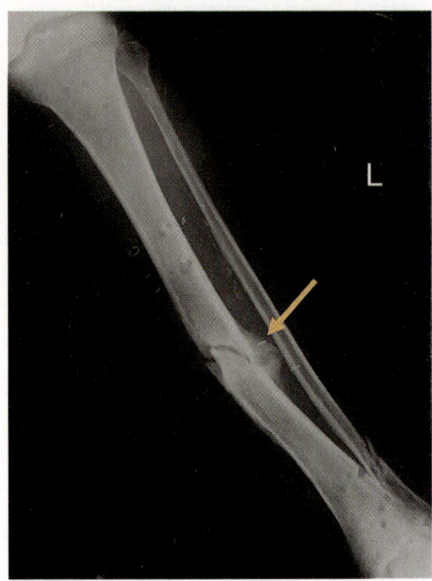

Plain AP radiograph of tibia of skeletally mature patient shows:
- Fracture of middle third of shaft of tibia
- Gap present between proximal and distal fracture fragments with closed medullary canal
- Hypertrophic callus present (orange arrow)

Diagnosis. Hypertrophic nonunion of left tibia

Few salient features of hypertrophic nonunion
1. Hypertrophic nonunion is characterized by presence of callus and visible fracture line. It is due to **lack of mechanical stability at the fracture site**.
2. Treatment is directed at increasing stability by using thicker nail/plate. Bone grafting is usually not required unlike atrophic nonunion.

27. NONUNION LATERAL CONDYLE

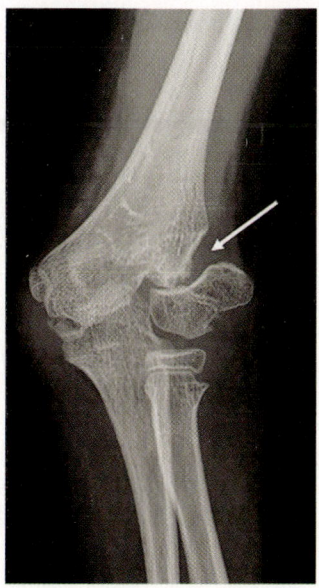

Plain AP radiograph of left elbow of skeletally immature patient shows:
- Fracture of lateral condyle (white arrow)
- Sclerosis of the margin of both fragments with closed medullary cavity
- Cubitus valgus

Diagnosis. Nonunion lateral condyle left side in child

Note: Lateral condyle of humerus comprised of lateral epicondyle, capitellum and lateral half of trochlea.

Few salient features of nonunion lateral condyle fracture humerus
1. It is often associated with tardy ulnar nerve palsy and progressive cubitus valgus
2. Tardy ulnar nerve palsy is treated by anterior transposition of ulnar nerve.
3. Nonunion of lateral condyle is treated by open reduction, internal fixation and bone grafting.

28. MALUNION

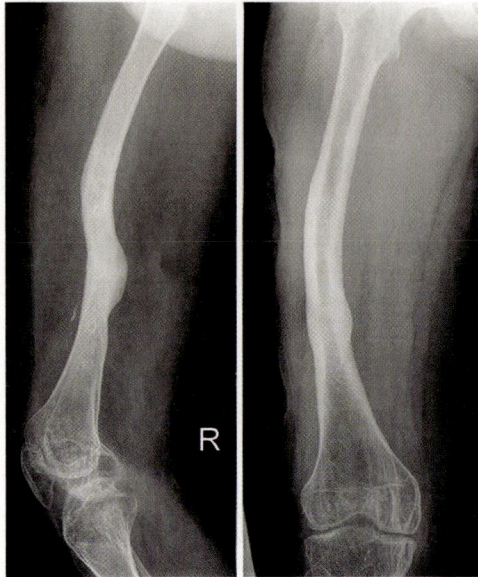

Plain AP and lateral radiographs of right femur of skeletally mature patient show:
- Old healed fracture of middle third shaft of the femur
- Varus angulation at fracture side (AP view)
- Extension angulation at fracture side (lateral view)

Diagnosis. Malunion of shaft of the femur

Few salient features of malunion

1. Malunion causes deformity and may result in functional loss.
2. If symptomatic, malunion is treated by corrective osteotomy.

Non-traumatic Condition Radiographs

1. PEDIATRIC

Developmental Dysplasia of the Hip Joint

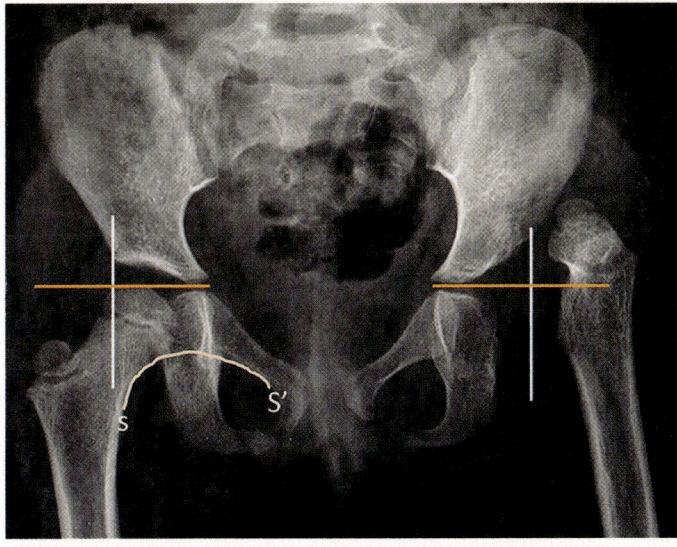

Pelvis with both hips—AP radiograph of skeletally immature patient shows:

- Left side femoral head is out of socket of acetabulum
- Femoral head is in upper and outer quadrant of the hip joint. The four quadrants around hip are divided by *Hilgenreiner's line* (horizontal line connecting the triradiate cartilages) and *Perkin's line* (vertical line from outer margin of acetabulum)

- Left side Shenton line (line along the lower border of the superior pubic ramus which should pass along lower border of neck of the femur [SS']) is broken
- Left side acetabular dysplasia is present

Diagnosis. Developmental dysplasia of the hip left side

Few salient features of DDH

1. Common in first born, left side, female, post-term, breech delivery
2. Barlow and Ortolani tests are performed to detect DDH at birth
3. Managed with Pavlik harness, closed reduction, open reduction, varus derotation osteotomy, pelvic osteotomy.

Perthes' Disease

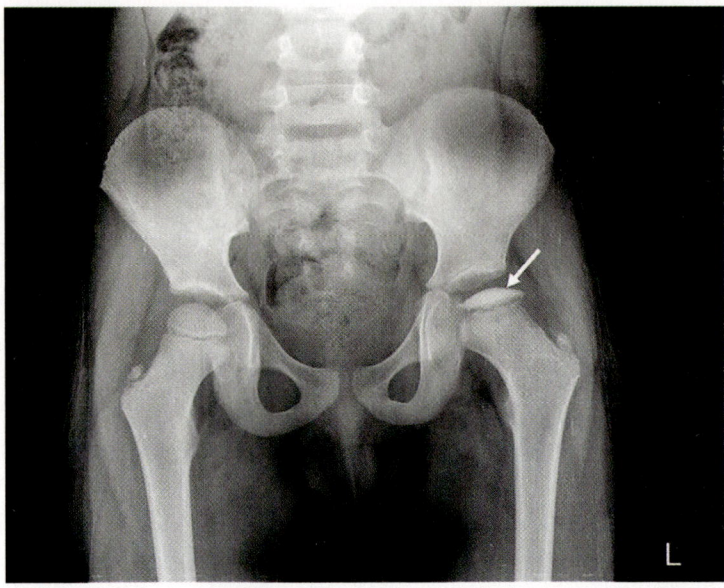

Pelvis with both hips: AP radiograph of skeletally immature patient shows:

- Left side capital femoral epiphysis is sclerosis [radiodense (white arrow)]
- Collapse of capital femoral epiphysis
- Extrusion of the femoral head

Diagnosis. Perthes' disease left side.

Other sign (not present in this radiograph): Fragmentation of the capital femoral epiphysis.

Few salient features of Perthes' disease
1. **Self-limiting avascular necrosis** of the capital femoral epiphysis.
2. Main aim of the treatment to maintain normal spherical shape of the femoral head.

Slipped Capital Femoral Epiphysis

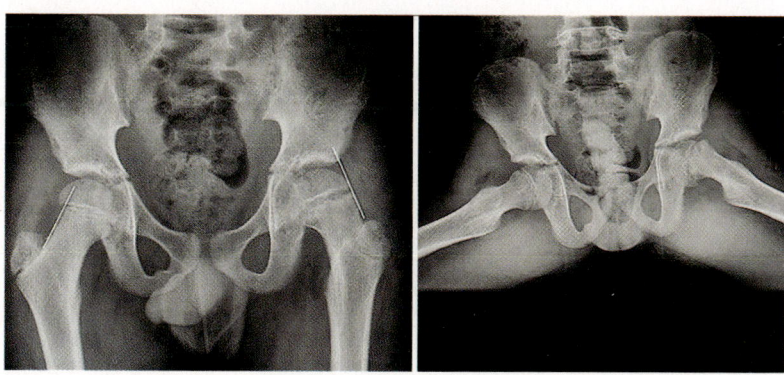

Pelvis with both hips: AP and frog lateral radiograph of skeletally immature patient shows:

- Widening of capital femoral physis left side
- Displacement of metaphysis
- Coxa vara
- *Positive Trethowan sign:* Normally, line drawn through superior border of neck passes through superior part of head. In SCFE, the line along the superior surface of the neck remains superior to the head of the femur.

Diagnosis. Slipped capital femoral epiphysis (SCFE) left side.

Few salient features of slipped capital femoral epiphysis
1. Common in adolescent, obese children. Often associated endocrinal disorders.
2. Prevention of further slip is prime goal of the treatment.
3. *In situ* fixation is standard treatment for SCFE.

2. INFECTION

Osteomyelitis

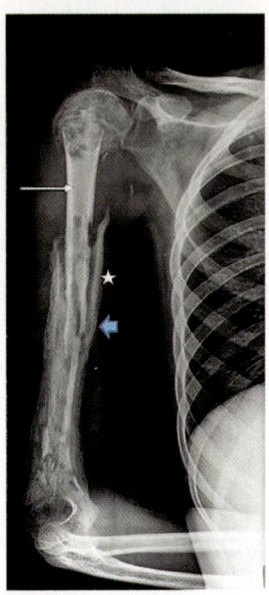

AP radiograph of right humerus of a skeletally immature patient shows:

- Large sequestrum (white arrow)
- Periosteal reaction on medial aspect of humerus forming involucrum (star)
- Cortical (diaphyseal) thickening and irregularity
- Pathological fracture between involucrum and sequestrum (blue arrow)
- Deformed humeral head

Diagnosis. Chronic osteomyelitis of the humerus

Few salient features of osteomyelitis

1. **Commonest organism:** *Staphylococcus aureus.*
2. **Principle of treatment of chronic osteomyelitis is always surgical.** It includes sinus tract excision, sequestrectomy, saucerization and curretage.
3. **Complication of chronic osteomyelitis:** Pathological fracture, deformity, limb length discrepancy, septic arthritis, sinus tract malignancy, amyloidosis.

Sequelae of Septic Arthritis of the Hip (sequelae of Tom-Smith arthritis)

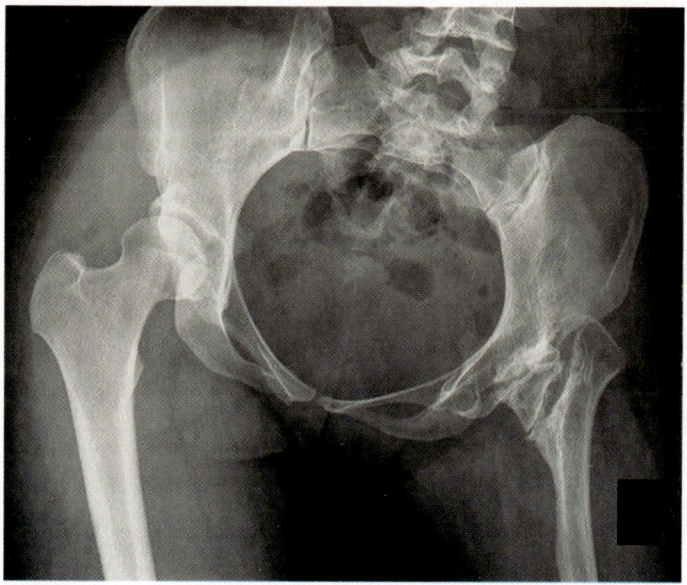

Pelvis with both hips: AP radiograph of skeletally mature patient shows:
- Tilt of the pelvis
- Left side distortion of the shape of the femoral head
- Resorbed femoral neck
- High riding trochanter
- Dysplastic acetabulum

Diagnosis. Sequelae of Tom-Smith arthritis left side.

Other radiological features
- Absence of the femoral head
- Absence of the femoral neck

Few salient features of septic arthritis
1. **Commonest organism:** *Staphylococcus aureus*
2. **Treatment:** Open arthrotomy/arthroscopic debridement of the joint, rest and antibiotics (6–8 weeks)
3. **Common complications:** Septicemia, stiffness, deformity, instability, secondary degenerative arthritis, bony ankylosis, chronic osteomyelitis.

Tuberculosis of Spine

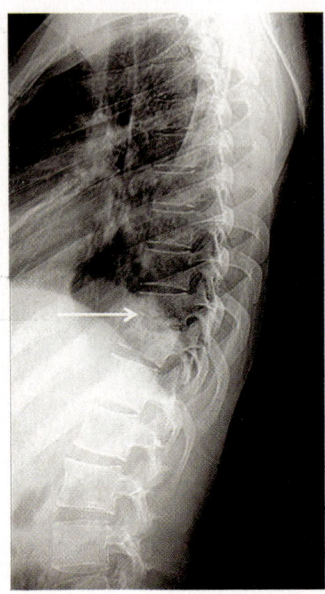

Lateral radiograph of the dorsolumbar spine of skeletally mature patient shows:
- Decreased intervertebral disc space
- Destruction of adjacent vertebral bodies of D10–D11
- Posterior elements are normal

Diagnosis. Potts' spine D10–D11

Few salient features of tuberculosis of spine
1. Spine is the commonest area involved in osteoarticular tuberculosis with thoraco-lumbar junction is the commonest site
2. Paradiscal site is the commonest radiological diagnostic feature
3. Treatment—anti-tuberculosis drugs, rest with/without surgical debridement

3. BONE TUMORS

Osteosarcoma

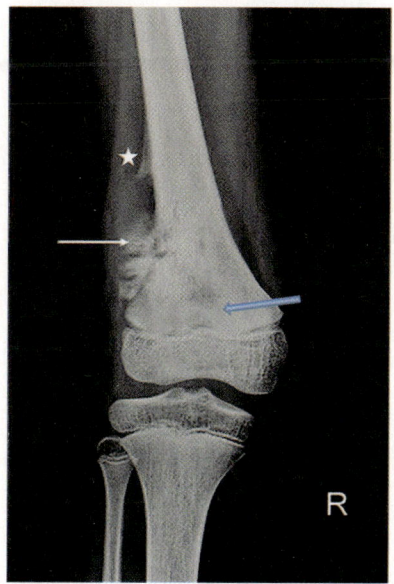

AP radiograph of right side femur of skeletally immature patient shows:
- Ill-defined osteolytic and osteosclerotic lesion in distal metaphysis of femur (blue arrow)
- Permeative lesion
- Poorly defined margin
- Sunray appearance (white arrow)
- Codman's triangle (white star)

Diagnosis. Osteosarcoma of distal femur

Few salient features of osteosarcoma
1. Common in second decade, metaphysis of ***long bones.***
2. **Treatment:** Neoadjuvant chemotherapy, wide excision of the tumor and limb salvage or amputation followed by adjuvant chemotherapy. *Chemotherapy drugs are cisplatin, ifosfamide, methotrexate, adriamycin, gemcitabine.*

Ewing's Sarcoma

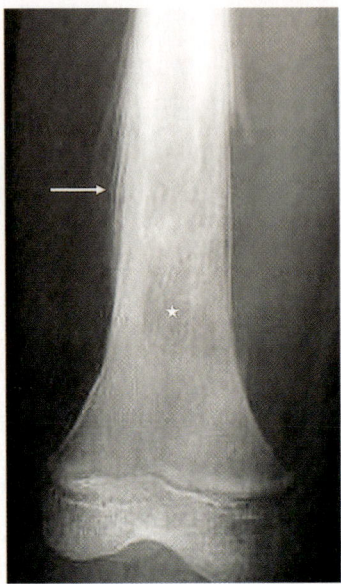

AP radiograph of left side femur of skeletally immature patient shows:
- Ill-defined osteolytic lesion in diaphysis (white star)
- Onion peel appearance of periosteum of diaphysis (white arrow)
- Permeated appearance
- Epiphysis and growth plate of distal femur are normal

Diagnosis. Ewing sarcoma of left side femur

Few salient features of Ewing's sarcoma

1. Common in diaphysis of long bones of kids aged between 5 and 10 years.
2. Differential diagnosis: Osteomyelitis until biopsy proven
3. Treatment: Neoadjuvant chemotherapy, wide excision of the tumor followed by adjuvant chemotherapy. *Chemo drugs* are *vincristine, ifosfamide, doxorubicin, etoposide.*
4. It is also a radiosensitive tumor.

Osteochondroma/Exostosis

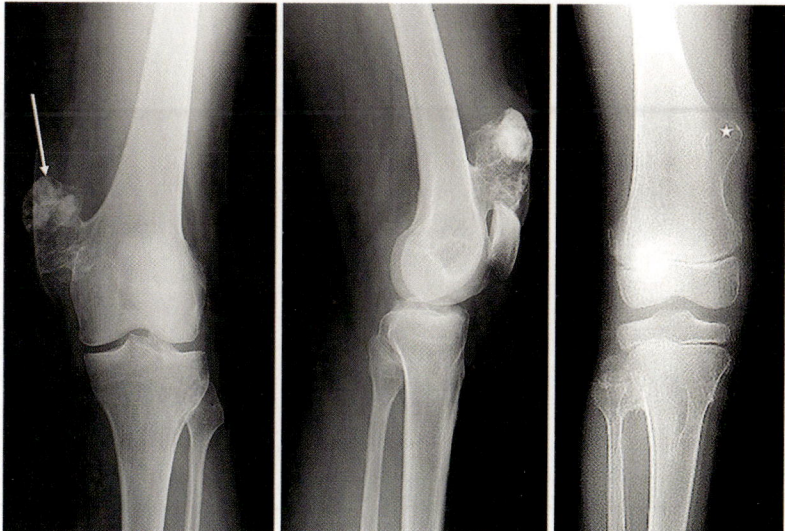

AP radiographs of both knee joint of skeletally immature patient show:
- Bony projection from metaphysis [pedunculated (white arrow) or sessile (white star)] of distal end of femur
- Growing away from joint
- Well-defined margin
- No periosteal reaction
- No soft tissue involvement

Diagnosis. Osteochondroma or exostosis

Few salient features of osteochondroma
1. Commonest benign tumor of bone.
2. Involves metaphysis of long bones, and grows away from joint
3. **Treatment:** If symptomatic.
4. **Complications:** Malignant transformation, fracture of peduncle, bursa over the cap, neurovascular compression and mechanical block of joint.
5. *Solitary exostosis has 1–5% chance of malignant transformation into chondrosarcoma.*
6. *Hereditary multiple exostosis or diaphyseal aclasis has higher incidence (up to 5–25%) of malignant transformation.*

Giant Cell Tumour/Osteoclastoma

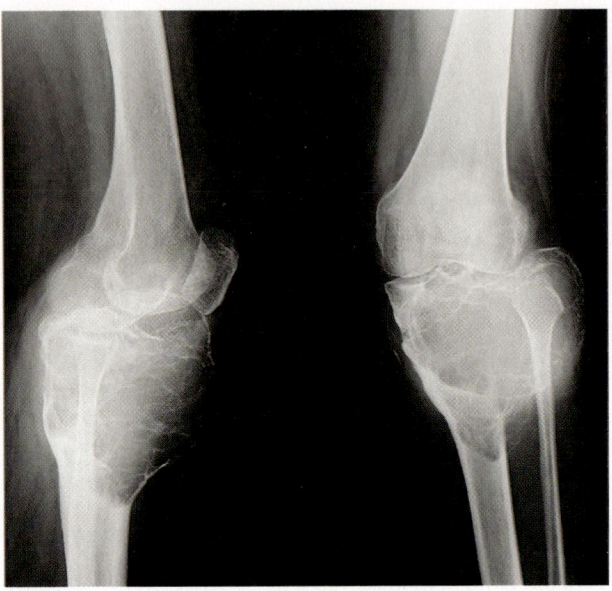

AP and lateral radiographs of knee joint of skeletal mature patient show:
- Osteolytic lesion in proximal "Epiphysis" of tibia
- **Expansile**
- **Eccentric**
- **Epiphyseal lesion**
- Soap bubble appearance
- No sclerosis of the margin

Diagnosis. Giant cell tumor of proximal tibia

Few salient features of giant cell tumor
1. Common in skeletally mature patients, epiphysis of long bones. *(Note: Another epiphyseal lesion is chondroblastoma which occurs in skeletally immature patient).*
2. Locally aggressive tumor and can very rarely metastasize.
3. Treatment: Curettage, treat lesion with phenol, liquid nitrogen and bone grafting/bone cement.

Simple Bone Cyst

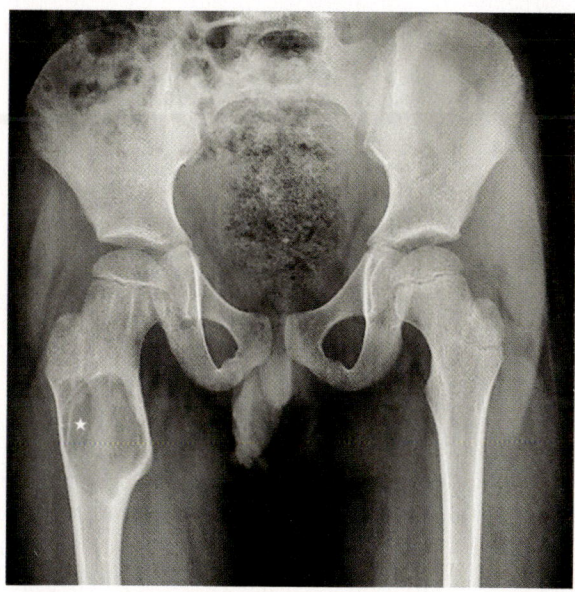

AP radiograph of pelvis with femur of skeletally immature child shows:
- **Well-defined, centred, non-expansile osteolytic lesion** in **metaphysis** of proximal end of femur
- Thinning of the cortex of proximal femur
- No periosteal reaction

Diagnosis. Unicameral bone cyst (simple bone cyst)

Few salient features of simple bone cyst

1. Common in second decade, metaphysis of long bones.
2. Benign in nature
3. Pathological fracture is the commonest complication
4. Treatment: Curettage and bone grafting

Aneurysmal Bone Cyst

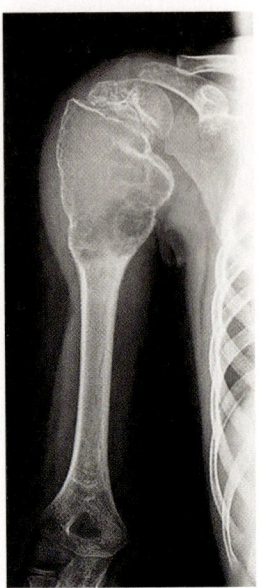

AP radiograph of right side humerus of skeletally immature child shows:
- Well defined radiolucent cyst in **metaphysis** of the proximal end of humerus
- Expansile
- Thinning of the cortex of proximal humerus
- No periosteal reaction

Diagnosis. Aneurysmal bone cyst

Few salient features of aneurysmal bone cyst
1. **Common sites:** Metaphysis of long bones, spine and pelvis.
2. **Treatment:** Sclerotherapy, curettage with bone grafting.

Multiple Myeloma

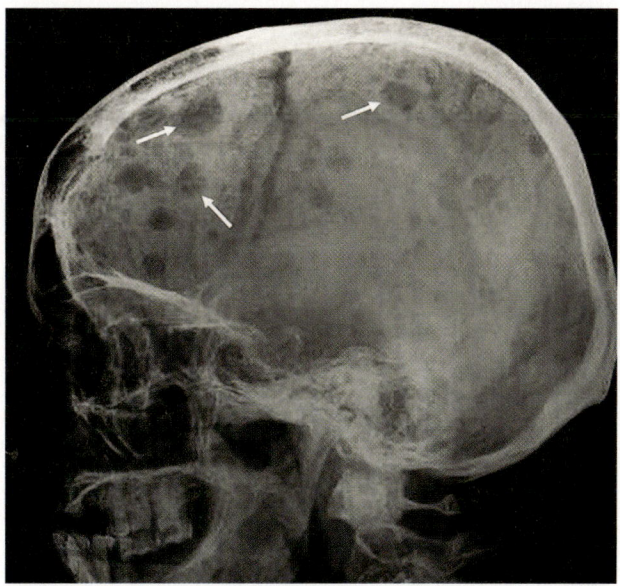

Lateral radiographs of skull of skeletally mature patient show:
- Multiple punched out osteolytic lesion (white arrows)
- Generalised osteopenia.

Diagnosis. Multiple myeloma

Few salient features of multiple myeloma
1. It is malignant tumor of **plasma cells**.
2. Diagnosis: Serum protein electrophoresis (**M band**), bone marrow biopsy
3. Common complications: Hypercalcemia, nephropathy, anemia, osteoporosis, pathological fracture.
4. Multi-drug chemotherapy is mainstay of treatment (melphalan, prednisolone, vincristine, adriamycin)
5. Bone marrow/stem cell transplant is results in remission.

4. DEGENERATIVE
Osteoarthritis of the Knee

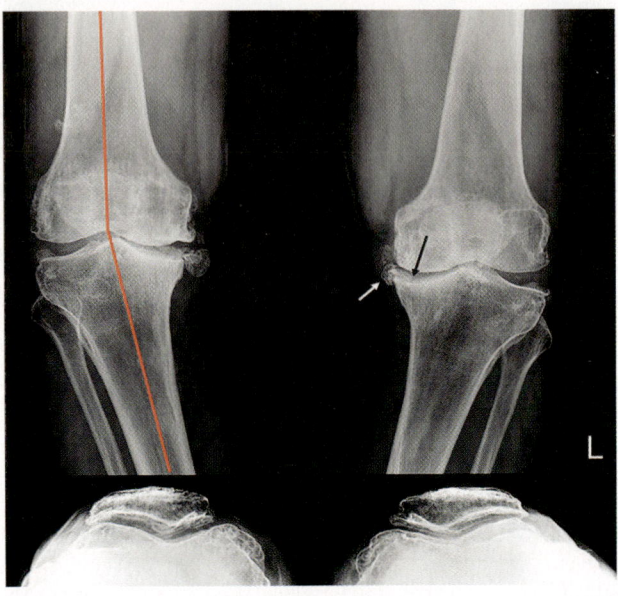

Bilateral AP and skyline radiograph (lower X-ray) of knee joints of skeletally mature patients shows:
- Medial joint space reduction (black arrow)
- Osteophyte formation (femur, tibia, patella: White arrow)
- Subchondral sclerosis
- Subchondral cyst
- Varus deformity (angled red line towards midline)
- Patellofemoral arthritis

Diagnosis. Osteoarthritis of the knee

Few salient features of osteoarthritis of knee

1. Common in older, obese patient.
2. **Clinical features:** Mechanical pain in knees.
3. **Medical treatment:** Weight reduction, physiotherapy, activity modification, analgesics, glucosamine.
4. **Surgical treatment:** Arthroscopic debridement, high tibial osteotomy, total knee replacement.

5. INFLAMMATORY DISEASE

Rheumatoid Arthritis

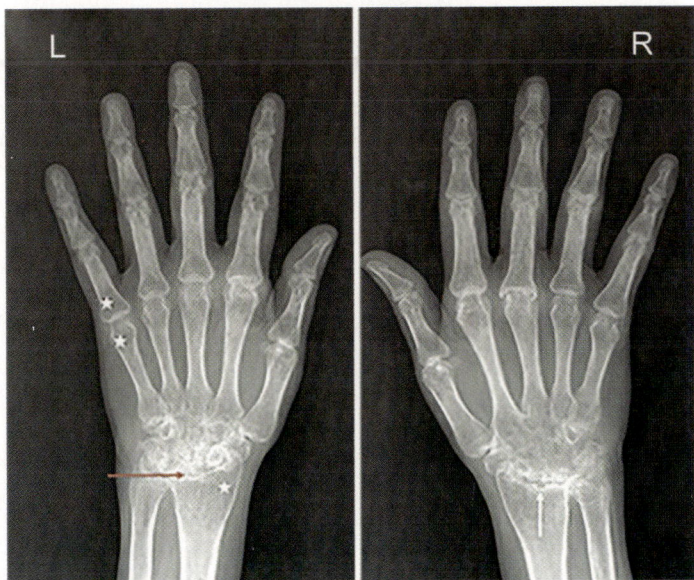

AP radiographs of both hands show:
- Symmetrical joint space reduction of wrist (red arrow) and joints of MCP and PIP joints
- Erosion of articular margin (white arrow)
- Subchondral cyst
- Juxta-articular osteopenia (starred areas)

Diagnosis. Rheumatoid arthritis

Other radiological features
Soft tissue shadow, deformity

Few salient features of the rheumatoid arthritis
1. Common in young female. HLA DR4, DR1+
2. **Clinical features:** Wrist, small joints of hand (MCP, PIP) involved, symmetrical involvement with morning stiffness are commonest symptoms.
3. Non-**operative treatment:** NSAIDs, DMARD, physiotherapy
4. **Surgical treatment:** Synovectomy, total joint replacement, arthrodesis, interpositional arthroplasty.

Ankylosing Spondylitis

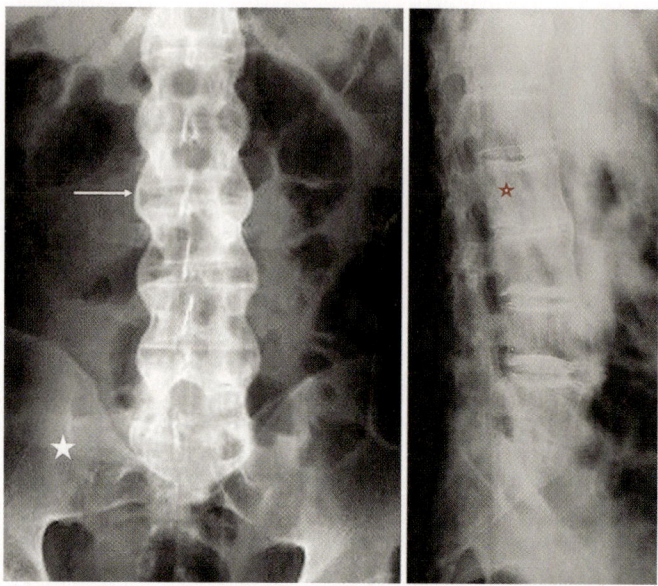

AP and lateral radiographs of lumbar spine of skeletally mature patient show:
- Loss of lumbar lordosis (lateral view)
- Squaring of vertebrae (red star)
- Bamboo spine appearance (white arrow)
- Bridging osteophytes (syndesmophytes)
- Fused sacroiliac joint (white star)

Diagnosis. Ankylosing spondylitis

Few salient features of ankylosing spondylitis
1. Common in young, male patient. **HLA-B27 + in 90% cases**
2. **Common sites of involvement:** Sacroiliac joint and spine
3. **Clinical features:** Low back pain with morning stiffness, reduced chest expansion, positive modified Schober's and positive wall test.
4. **Treatment:** Maintain spine mobility and prevent deformity, chest physiotherapy. Sulphasalazine and now TNF blockers (Infliximab, Etanercept) are tried with variable success.

6. METABOLIC DISEASE

Rickets

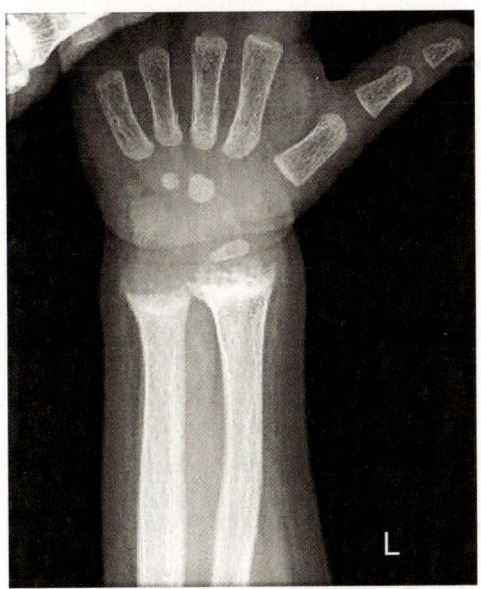

AP radiograph of wrist joint of skeletally immature child shows:

- Epiphysis: Thinned
- Physis: Widened
- Metaphysis of radius and ulna: Widened, cupping, splaying and frayed edges.
- Diaphysis: Generalized osteopenia, thinned cortex.

Diagnosis. Rickets

Few salient features of rickets
1. **Definition:** Inadequate mineralisation of bone matrix in growing skeleton.
2. **Etiology:** Hypocalcemic, hypophosphatemic.
3. **Clinical features:** Various deformities in limb.
4. **Treatment:** Healthy diet, adequate sunlight, vitamin D, splintage, deformity correction.

Scurvy

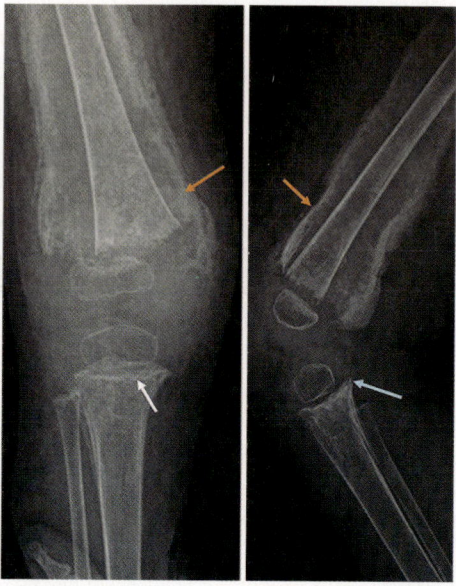

AP and lateral radiographs of right knee joint of skeletal immature child show:
- Periosteal reaction of diaphysis and metaphysis (subperiosteal hemorrhage) of distal femur (orange arrow)
- Severely osteopenic metaphyses
- Marginal spurs (Pelken sign) (light green arrow)
- "White line of Frankel" which is dense calcification at metaphysis (white arrow)
- The epiphyseal nucleus is markedly radiolucent with relatively sclerotic margins, producing an appearance of ringed epiphyses (i.e. Wimberger sign).

Diagnosis. Scurvy

Few salient features of scurvy

1. Common in children (developing world) due to deficiency of vitamin C
2. Commonest presentation—pseudoparalysis of the limb
3. Treatment—vitamin C supplementation, plaster/bracing

Osteomalacia

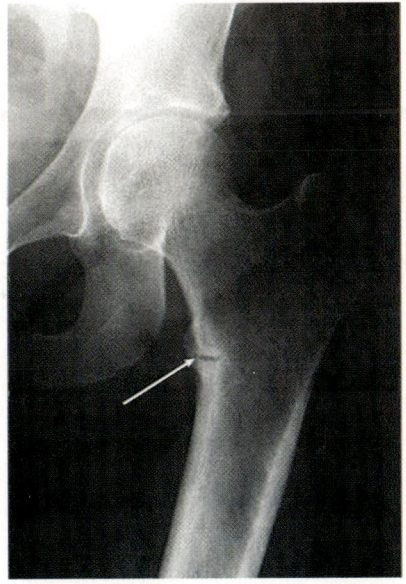

AP radiograph of hip of skeletally mature patient shows:
- Osteopenia
- Pseudofracture (i.e. looser zone) at medial cortex of the neck of the femur (white arrow)

Diagnosis. Osteomalacia

Other radiological features (not present in this radiograph)—other sites of looser zone—scapula, ribs, pubic rami
Occasionally triradiate pelvis and protrusion acetabula.

Few salient features of osteomalacia
1. Common in adult due to deficiency of vitamin D
2. Clinical presentation—bone pain, fracture
3. Treatment—rule out the secondary cause of osteomalacia, vitamin D supplementation, treatment of complication.

Osteoporosis

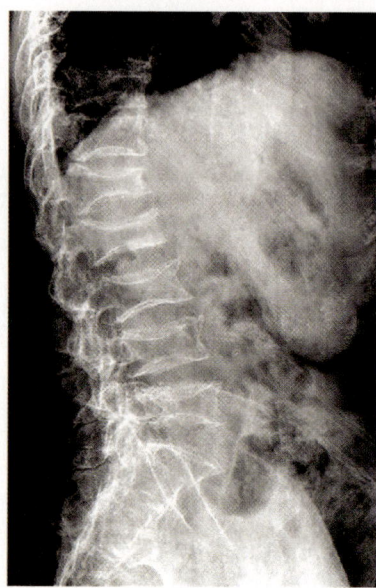

Lateral radiographs of lumbar spine of skeletally mature patient show:
- Gross osteopenia, loss of bony trabaculae
- Biconcave lumbar vertebral bodies
- Biconvex intervertebral spaces (codfish mouth sign)
- Wedging of lumbar vertebra (L1–L5) indicating pathological fracture.

Diagnosis. Osteoporosis

Few salient features of osteoporosis
1. **Etiology:** *Primary* (Type 1—postmenopausal; Type 2—senile), secondary
2. **Clinical presentation:** Deformity of spine, backache, fracture
3. **Investigation:** X-ray, dual-energy X-ray absorptiometry (DEXA) **(gold standard)**.
4. **Treatment:** Bisphosphonate therapy, teriparatide (parathormone), raloxifene, denosumab, calcium, vitamin D.

7. OTHERS

Avascular Necrosis of Hip

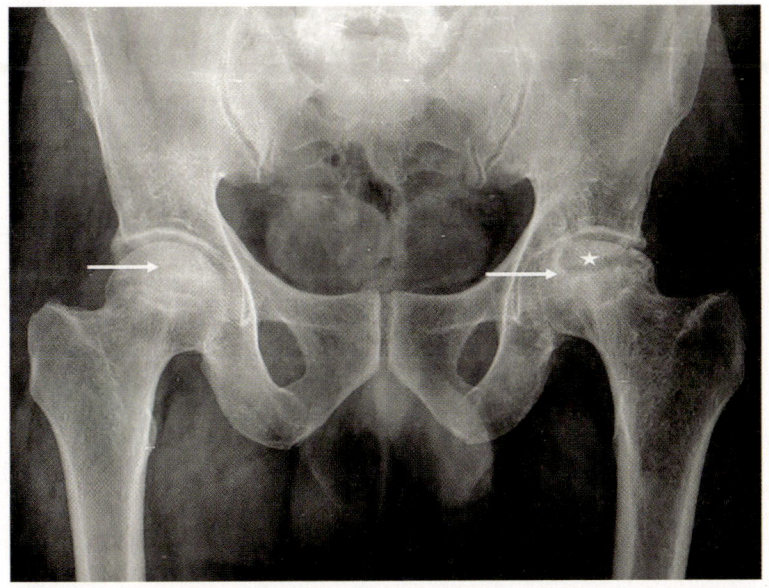

AP radiograph of pelvis with both hips of skeletally mature patient shows:
- Sclerosis of the superolateral part of femoral head both side (white arrow)
- Subchondral cyst left side (star)
- Collapse of the subchondral bone left side
- Reduction in joint space (left hip joint space)

Diagnosis. Avascular necrosis of the femoral head

Few salient features of avascular necrosis of the hip

1. **Common etiologies:** Steroid intake, post-traumatic (fracture neck femur, hip dislocation), decompression sickness, sickle cell anemia
2. **Clinical presentation:** Pain and stiffness of the hip joint, limited abduction and external rotation
3. **Diagnosis:** MRI
4. **Treatment:** Alendronate, core decompression, fibula strut grafting, total joint replacement.

Section

III

Orthopedic Implants

17. **Implants**

Implants

HIP HEMI REPLACEMENT PROSTHESIS

Austin Moore's prosthesis (AMP)

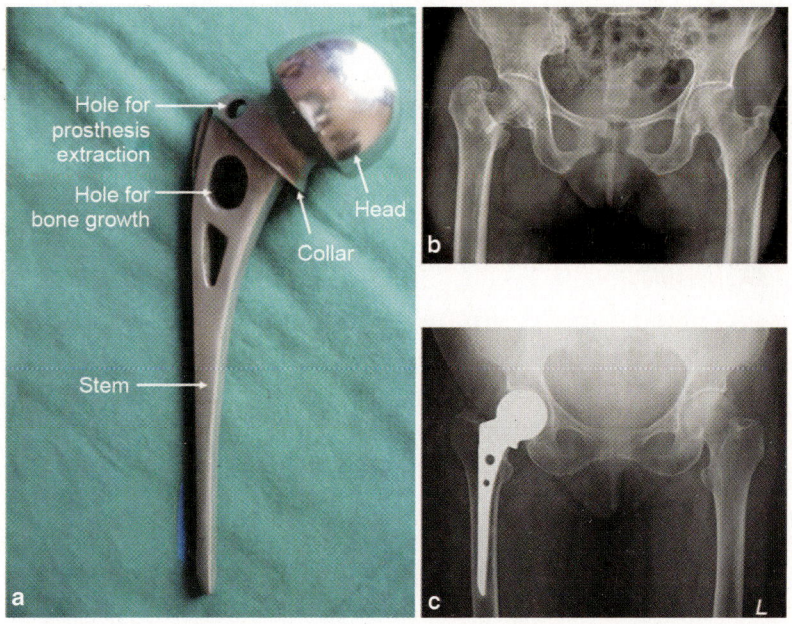

Figure: (a) Austin Moore's prosthesis; (b) Right fracture neck femur; (c) AMP *in situ* (right side)

Points to identify AMP

1. Head
2. Neck and collar
3. Curved stem with fenestrations (fenestrations for future bone in growth which imparts stability to the stem)
4. Small hole on top for prosthesis removal

Description. After the removal of femoral head and neck, the AMP stem sits into the femoral canal and head of prosthesis goes into the acetabulum. The collar rests onto the calcar or neck of femur (Fig. 1a).

Indications

1. Hemi replacement arthroplasty in fracture neck of femur in patients **aged more than 60 years**.
2. Used in patients with **good calcar and non-osteoporotic** bone.
3. The stem fixation in femoral canal is designed to hold on by virtue of thick cortices, and, therefore, it should be used without bone cement. **It is not recommended to be used in a very osteoporotic bone.** If bone cement is used for AMP stem fixation in femoral canal, presence of cement in the fenestration would render its removal very difficult.

Certain important tips

1. Plan of management of fracture neck femur according to patient's age
   a. *Age <60 years:* Closed reduction/open reduction and internal fixation by DHS/ 6.5 mm cannulated cancellous screws.
   b. *Age >60 years:* Hemi/total hip replacement depending upon arthritis status of acetabulum.
      i. Non-arthritic acetabulum-hemi replacement (uni- or bipolar prosthesis)
      ii. Arthritic acetabulum: Total hip replacement
2. There are two types of hemireplacement prosthesis: Uni- and bipolar
   Unipolar: AMP/Thompson prosthesis is also known as unipolar prosthesis as there is a single head in the prosthesis.
   Bipolar: It has a head within a head. It was designed to reduce the wear of the acetabulum.
3. Hemi replacement prosthesis which can be used with bone cement: Thompson unipolar and bipolar prosthesis (as there no holes in the stem).
4. Bone cement is used to fix implant stem firmly into the femoral canal which could be quite wide due to osteoporosis.
   Loose prosthesis stem into wide femoral canal would render the prosthesis unstable.

Prosthesis used for arthritic hip is total hip replacement. Austin Moore/Thompson/bipolar is NOT used in an arthritic hip as these prosthesis do not replace the acetabulum.

THOMPSON PROSTHESIS

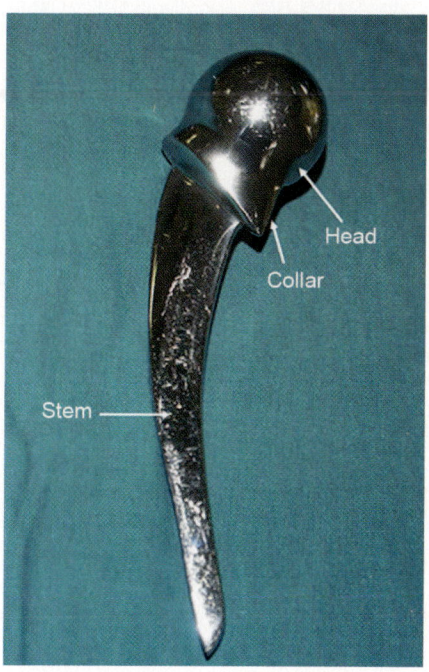

Points to identify

1. Head
2. Neck and long, oblique collar. The long collar is designed to compensate for the shorter/absent neck of the femur.

Note: The collar of Austin Moore is more horizontal as compared to Thompson as former is designed to sit over a normal length of the neck of femur.

3. Curved stem with NO fenestrations

Indications

1. Unipolar hemireplacement arthroplasty in fracture neck of femur in patients whose older than 60 years.
2. Used in patients with **poor** or **no calcar** and **osteoporotic** bone.
3. It is used with **bone cement**.

BIPOLAR PROSTHESIS

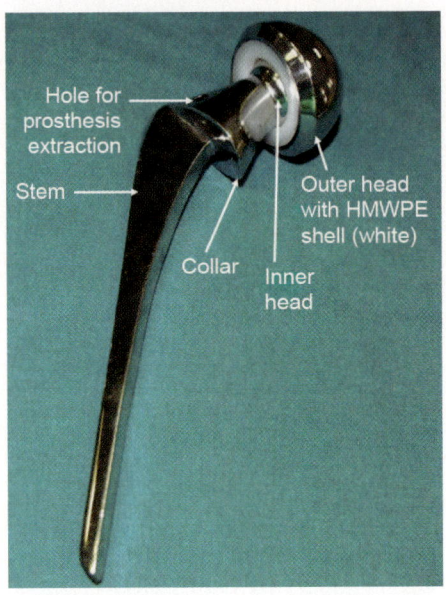

Points to identify
1. Mobile larger outer head over static smaller inner head.
2. Neck and collar
3. Curved stem with NO fenestrations

Indications
1. Bipolar hemireplacement arthroplasty in fracture neck of femur in patients older than 60 years.
2. Used in patients with **normal** or **osteoporotic** bone.
3. It can be used **with or without bone cement.**

Advantage and disadvantage of bipolar prosthesis

Advantage: Since both larger outer head over smaller inner head are mobile over each other, it therefore, helps in distribution of shear and stress forces between the 'femoral head and acetabulum' over larger areas and two different surfaces. Thus, theoretically less stress is transferred over acetabulum and prevents its degeneration.

However in due course of time, the two mobile bearing surfaces become less mobile and later tend to act as unipolar prosthesis (like Austin Moore and Thompson).

Disadvantage: Expensive as compared to unipolar prosthesis.

COMPARATIVE PICS OF THREE PROSTHESIS

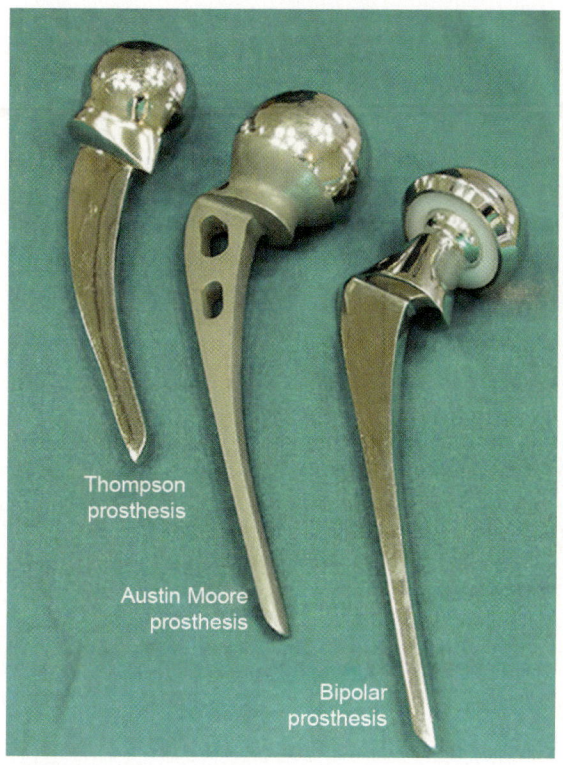

Important tip to differentiate AMP with others.

AMP has fenestration in the stem whereas other prosthesis do not have it.

DYNAMIC HIP SCREW (DHS)

The combined picture shows parts of DHS (left image), X-ray of right side intertrochanteric femur (top right image) and DHS *in situ* (below right image)

Points to identify
1. **Cannulated barrel along with side plate with holes for screw.** The angle between barrel and side plate is 135°.
2. **Richard's lag screw** (thread diameter 12.5 mm, shaft diameter 8 mm) which slides inside the barrel.
3. **Compression screw:** It is applied over Richard's screw to achieve compression at the fracture site.

Description
1. Richard's screw goes into the head and neck of femur through the barrel.
2. Side plate is fixed onto the shaft with cortical screws
3. Later compression screw is applied over Richard's screw to achieve on-table or intraoperative compression at the fracture site.

Indications
1. Fracture intertrochanteric femur
2. Fracture neck femur <60 years
3. Fracture subtrochanteric femur

Certain important tips

It is known as DHS because 'dynamic' compression at the fracture site can be achieved twice, i.e.
1. Immediately after the fracture fixation when compression screw is tightened over the Richard's screw, and
2. Secondly while weight bearing when Richard's screw telescopes inside barrel leading to compression at # site.

Since there is dynamic movement happening at the fracture site, hence the name, dynamic hip screw.

PEDIATRIC FRACTURE NECK FIXATION
"AUSTIN MOORE PIN"

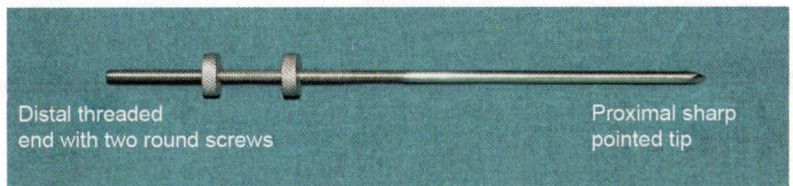

Distal threaded
end with two round screws

Proximal sharp
pointed tip

Points to identify
1. Proximal smooth end with sharp pointed tip
2. Circular cross section
3. Distal end threaded with two circular screws to slide over threads.

Indications
Internal fixation of fracture neck femur in pediatric population (<8–10 years)

Description
1. Proximal smooth end with sharp tip crosses the fracture followed by growth plate and engages the femoral head. The smooth proximal femoral end ensures minimal damage to the physis while crossing it.
2. Distal threaded portion lies on the greater trochanter.
3. Two round screws lock over each other to prevent migration of the pin.

PEDIATRIC FRACTURE NECK FIXATION KNOWLES PIN

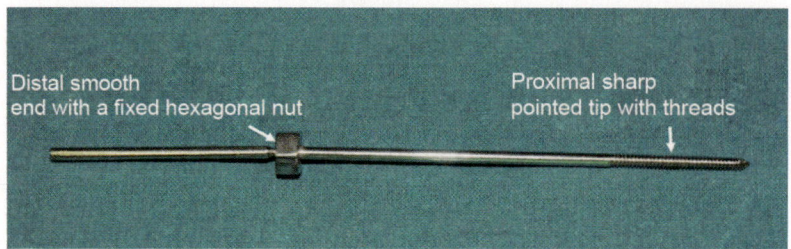

Distal smooth end with a fixed hexagonal nut

Proximal sharp pointed tip with threads

Points to identify
1. Proximal threaded shaft with sharp pointed tip
2. Circular cross section
3. Distal end is smooth and has fixed hexagonal nut

Indications
Internal fixation of fracture neck femur in pediatric population (<8–10 years)

Description
1. The threaded proximal end with sharp tip crosses fracture site followed by physis and engages in the femoral head.
2. Although it has better hold in the femoral head as compared to Austin Moore pin due to the threaded shaft, the **threaded shaft** has theoretically more potential to damage the physis of the femoral head.
3. After the insertion of Knowles pin, the shaft distal to the hexagonal nut is broken. Later, the nut is engaged with a driver to remove the Knowles pin, if required.

DYNAMIC CONDYLAR SCREW

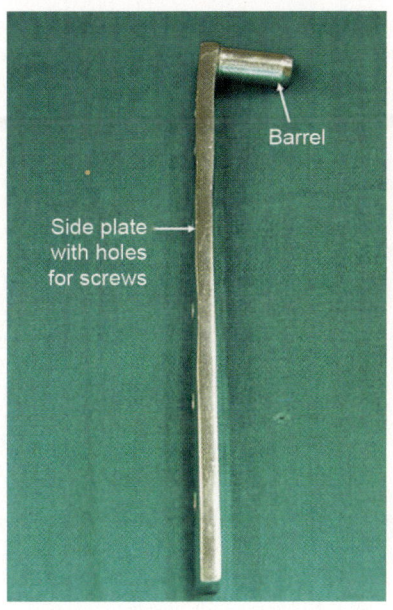

Points to identify

1. Cannulated barrel (similar to DHS)
2. Side plate with holes for screws (similar to DHS)
3. *Angle between the barrel and side plate is 95°* with second curve to accommodate the shaft (difference with DHS).
4. Richard's screw which slides inside the barrel (similar to DHS).
5. Compression screw applied over Richard's screw (similar to DHS)

Description

1. Richard's screw goes into the femoral condyles or head and neck of femur through the barrel
2. Side plate is fixed onto the shaft with cortical screws

Indications

1. Supracondylar fracture femur
2. Fracture intertrochanteric femur
3. Fracture subtrochanteric femur

Note: It is known as dynamic condylar screw (DCS) because it was designed to be used for supracondylar femur fractures where Richard's screw goes in femoral condyles. However, unlike in intertrochanteric fracture, compression at the fracture site is only while fixation. Later, there is no compression while weight bearing.

TOTAL KNEE REPLACEMENT PROSTHESIS

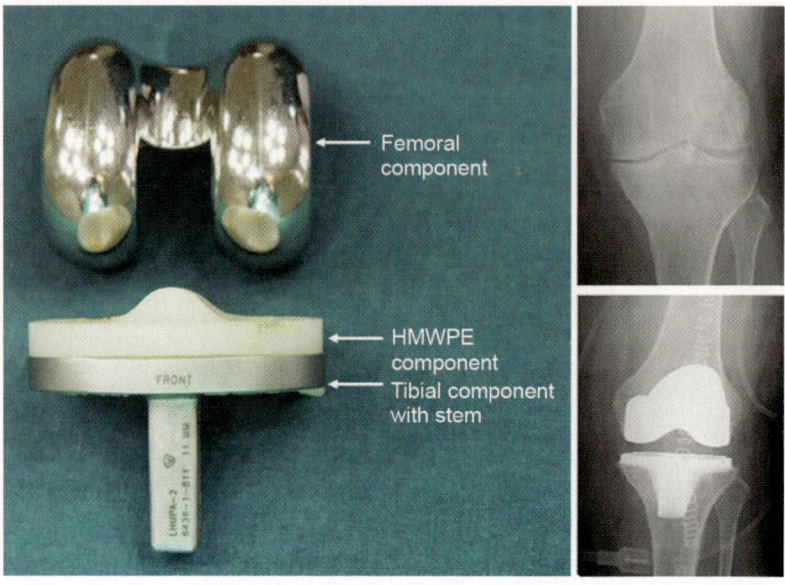

Figure shows various components of total knee prosthesis; femoral component, HMWPE (high molecular weight polyethylene) insert and tibial component. Top right X-ray reveals osteoarthritis of left knee. Below right X-ray shows postoperative radiograph of total knee replacement with prosthesis *in situ*

Indication

Total knee replacement in case of severe osteoarthritis (primary or secondary)

KÜNTSCHER'S INTRAMEDULLARY NAIL

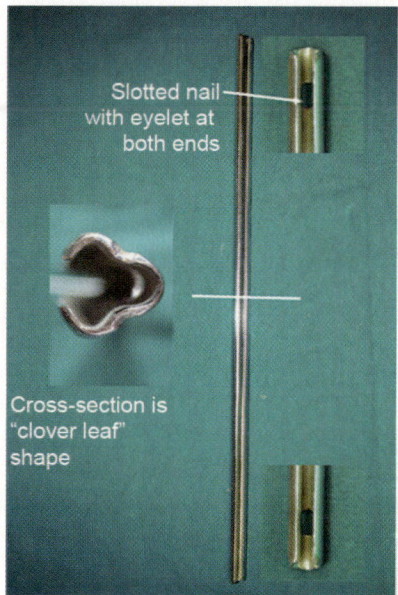

Slotted nail with eyelet at both ends

Cross-section is "clover leaf" shape

Points to identify
1. Unlocked, slotted, straight long nail
2. Clover leaf cross-section
3. Eyelet on both ends

Note: There is no side or superior-inferior end of the nail. Therefore, it could be used for any side of the femur and it can be used upside down too.

Description
1. K-nail is inserted into the femoral intramedullary canal with *slot anterolaterally and eyelet facing posteromedially.*
2. It provides *stability by three point fixation* in femoral canal;
   - Proximally: In the greater trochanter,
   - Middle: In the isthmus, and
   - Distally: In lower end of femur where nail is burried into cancellous end
3. The *Cloverleaf cross-section* of nail also helps in securing the purchase in the canal.
4. Eyelet is for removal.
5. Nail can be inserted *antegrade* (from pyriformis fossa to the fracture site and then distally) or *retrograde* (fracture site is opened, then nail is first inserted retrograde up to pyriformis fossa and hammered back distally).

Indications
Transverse fracture shaft of femur at the level of **isthmus** in **young adults.**

Demerits of nail
1. Since it is a non-interlocked nail, it **cannot prevent rotational stability** at the fracture site.

2. It provides best fixation in transverse fractures at the level of isthmus, and not recommended in comminuted, oblique or spiral fractures.

   It is used in isthmus level # as femoral canal is narrowest at the level of isthmus, and hence stability is better. It should not be used for levels above and below the isthmus as femoral canal is wide.

3. Since the fracture fixation is not as stable as by the fixation with interlocking nails, mobilization of the knee and weight bearing are delayed. This leads to slower rehabilitation and can cause stiffness at the knee joint.

FEMORAL INTERLOCKING INTRAMEDULLARY NAIL

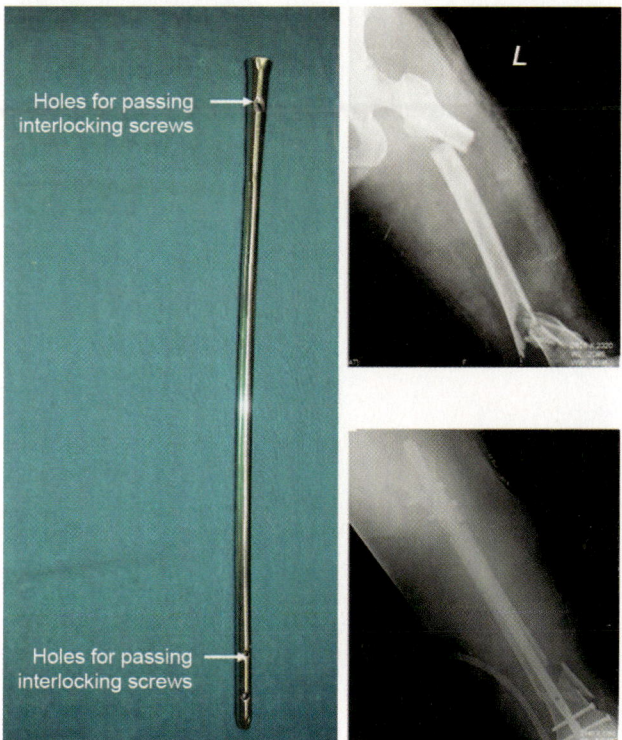

Holes for passing interlocking screws

Holes for passing interlocking screws

Points to identify
1. **Curved** long nail
2. **Round** cross-section
3. **Locking holes on proximal and distal** ends

Description
1. Nail is inserted into the intramedullary canal through the pyriformis fossa or tip of the greater trochanter.
2. Nail is fixed into the shaft in the femoral canal at proximal and distal ends by interlocking bolts which are inserted through the interlocking holes (*see* pre- and postoperative X-rays).

Indications
Fracture shaft of femur at any level and any type (transverse/comminuted/oblique/segmental).

Advantages of nail
1. Being an **interlocked nail, it prevents rotational deforming forces** at the fracture site, and therefore provides additional rotational stability at the fracture site along with torsional and bending stability.
   Therefore, it can be used for any type of femoral shaft fracture unlike unlocked nails which can be used only for midshaft fractures.
2. Early mobilization and weight bearing is permitted due to stable fracture fixation.

TIBIAL INTERLOCKING INTRAMEDULLARY NAIL

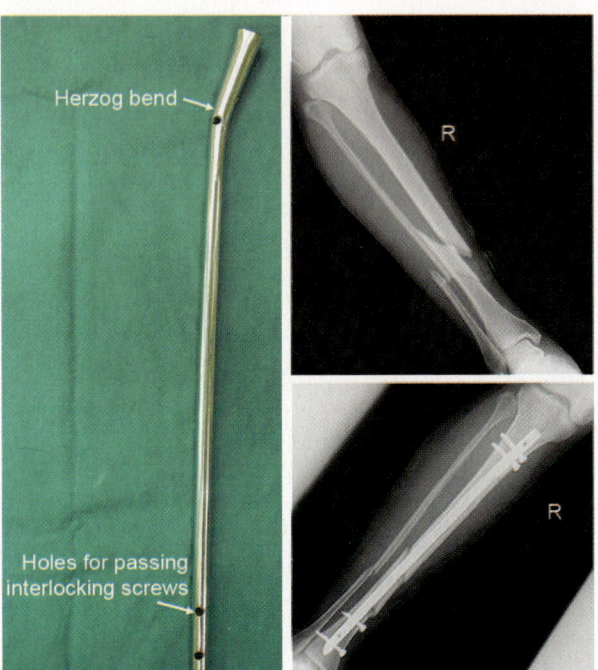

Points to identify
1. **Curved** long nail with acute bend in proximal third known as **Herzog's bend**
2. **Round** cross-section
3. **Locking holes on proximal and distal** ends

Description
1. Nail is inserted into the tibial intramedullary canal medial to the tibial tuberosity.
2. Nail is fixed onto the shaft in canal by proximal and distal ends by interlocking bolts through the holes (pre- and postoperative X-rays).

Indication
Fracture shaft of tibia of any radiological type.

Advantages of nail
1. Since it is an **interlocked nail,** it **prevents rotational deforming forces** at the fracture site providing more stability at the fracture site. Therefore, early mobilization and weight bearing can be initiated.
2. It can be used in any radiological type (transverse/oblique/spiral/comminuted). The stability at the fractures site is better due to interlocking of nail into the shaft.

Remember
There is no side of tibial interlocking nails, can be used for both left and right.

RUSH INTRAMEDULLARY NAIL

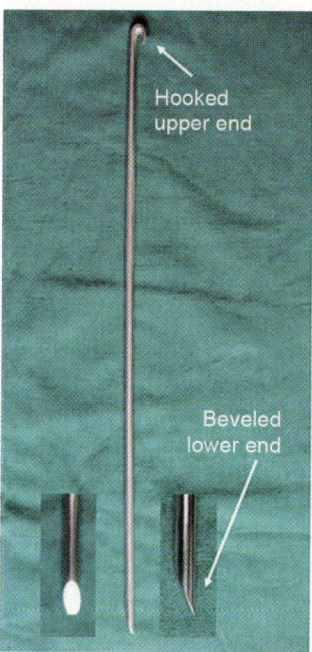

Hooked
upper end

Beveled
lower end

Points to identify
1. **Straight** nail
2. Round cross-section
3. Upper end is like a hook
4. Lower end is beveled

Note: Whole nail looks like a walking stick!

Description
Nail is inserted into the intramedullary canal with hook end superiorly.

Indications
Transverse fracture shaft of long bones like humerus, ulna, tibia **'in children'** (who have narrow canal diameter).

Demerits of nail
1. Since it is a non-interlocked nail, it cannot prevent rotational forces at the fracture site. Hence, additional support to the limb in form of brace or plaster of Paris cast might be required for few weeks.

Remember. There is no side of the nail, can be used for both right and left sides.

TALWALKAR'S SQUARE INTRAMEDULLARY NAIL FOR RADIUS AND ULNA

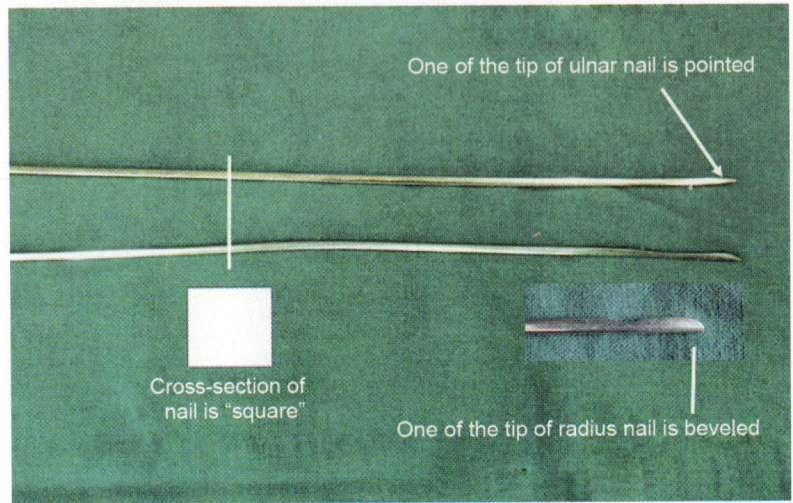

One of the tip of ulnar nail is pointed

Cross-section of
nail is "square"

One of the tip of radius nail is beveled

Points to identify
1. **Straight** long nail
2. **The end of nail which enters into bone has pointed tip for ulnar nail and beveled tip for radius**
3. **Square** cross-section
4. **Other end** is threaded (required for removal)

Description
1. Ulnar square nail is inserted into the ulnar intramedullary canal from tip of the olecranon process.
2. Radial square nail is inserted into the intramedullary canal from the tip of radial styloid process/adjacent to Lister's tubercle.

Indication
Fracture shaft of radius and ulna, in mid shaft level

Disadvantages of nail
Since it is a **non-interlocked nail,** it cannot **prevent rotational deforming forces** at the fracture site. Hence, additional support to the limb in form of brace or plaster of Paris cast might be required for few weeks.

Also, poor stability could lead to malunion or nonunion of #.

Further, early mobilization of elbow and wrist is delayed due to inferior stability of the fixation.

Remember
1. The name is **TAL-WAL-KAR** and not TAL-WAR-KAR.
2. Preferred implant for fracture forearm fixation is plate and not square nail because former provides absolute stability at the # site.
3. **Forearm # malunion** leads to **loss of pronation-supination.**

DYNAMIC COMPRESSION PLATE (DCP)

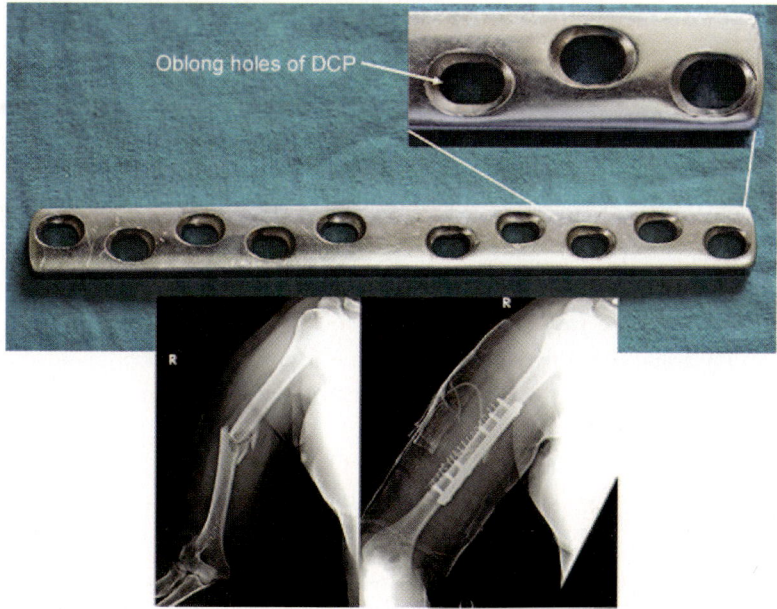

Oblong holes of DCP

Top image shows DCP. Lower left image shows a comminuted fracture midshaft humerus fracture while lower right image shows ORIF with DCP.

Points to identify
1. Plate with oblong holes
2. Plate has hole which is **smooth** (unlike locked compression plate which has smooth and threaded portion)
3. Undersurface is flat/concave.

Description
1. Plate is applied over the bone
2. Screws are passed through the hole of plate onto the bone via a predrilled and tapped pilot hole.
3. After the first screw close to # site is inserted and tightened, the second screw on other side of the # is tightened. While second screw is tightened over plate in the oblong slanted hole of DCP, it leads to movement of two ends of fracture towards each other causing compression at the fracture site. Hence the name, dynamic compression plate (DCP).

Indication
Open reduction and internal fixation of **fracture of long bones** like humerus, radius, ulna, femur and tibia.

Important tips
The strength of DCP fixation depends upon quality of bone. So, when used in osteoporotic bone, it may lead to loosening of implant (screws) during cyclic loading.

LOCKING COMPRESSION PLATE (LCP)

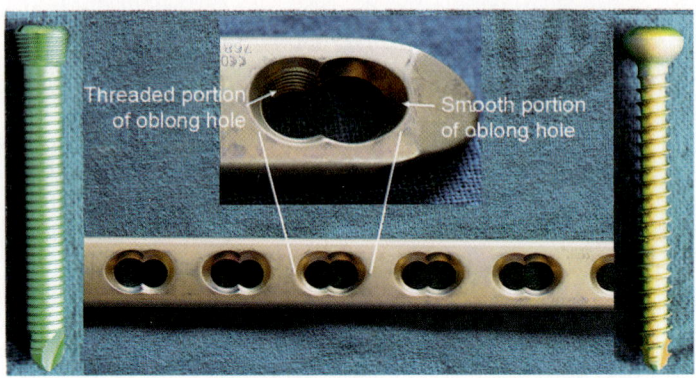

The combined figure shows LCP with oblong combi hole (smooth, threaded) along with locking screw (green) and conventional screw (yellow).

Points to identify
1. Plate with oblong holes
2. It is characterized by **combination holes** through which screws are passed into the bone. Combi-hole has **smooth** and a **threaded portion oriented like "8"**.
3. Undersurface is notched.

Description
1. Plate is applied over the bone.
2. Screws are passed through the predrilled holes into the bone.
3. Green color locking screws pass through the threaded portion of holes (locking hole) are locked onto the plate, whereas yellow color screws pass through the smooth portion (compression hole), and are not locked.

Indication
Internal fixation of fractures of long bones like humerus, radius, ulna, femur and tibia especially in **periarticular fractures and osteoporotic bones**.

Certain important tips
LCP with its **combi-hole** gives an option to surgeon to achieve **compression like DCP at the fracture site** through the smooth portion of hole exactly like DCP. Locking screws onto the bone through the **threaded portion of screw hole are also locked** onto the plate. Use of locking screws converts the entire construct into a quite rigid and stable fixation, and therefore screw pull out/implant loosening is minimised/prevented during cyclic loading. Rigid fixation is quite important for:
a. **Fractures involving osteoporotic bones** which carry a high chance of implant loosening and
b. **Periarticular #** (fracture) which require rigid/absolute fixation.

ONE-THIRD TUBULAR PLATE

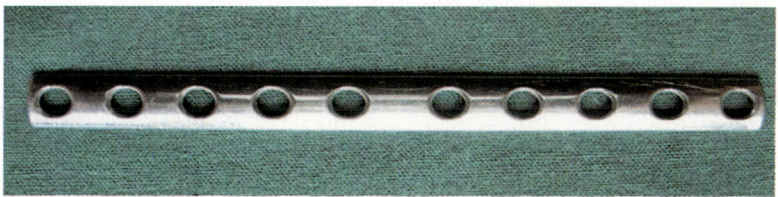

Points to identify
1. Plate with round holes
2. Cross-section of plate is 1/3rd of a circle or a tube (that is why name is 1/3rd tubular plate)
3. Holes for screw

Description
1. Plate is applied over the bone
2. Screws are passed through the predrilled and tapped hole onto the bone

Indications
Internal fixation of fractures of long and thin bones like ulna and fibula.

Remember. There is another implant which looks like 1/3rd tubular plate k/a **semi-tubular plate**.
It is k/a semitubular because it is half of a circle (1/3rd plate is 1/3 of a circle).

KIRSCHNER'S WIRE

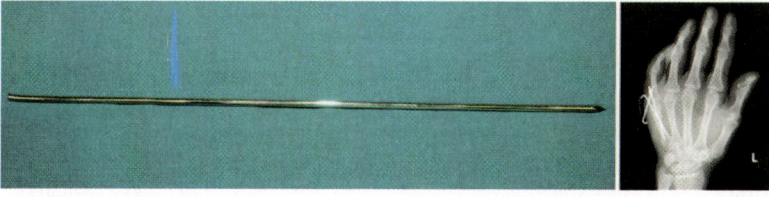

Points to identify
Thin wire pointed on both ends

Indications
1. Internal fixation of **small fragments** such as malleolus, patella, greater tuberosity of humerus "directly" or by "tension band wiring".
2. Internal fixation of fracture of **small bones** like carpals, metacarpals, phalanx, tarsals or metatarsals.
3. Upper limb skeletal traction.

STEINMANN PIN

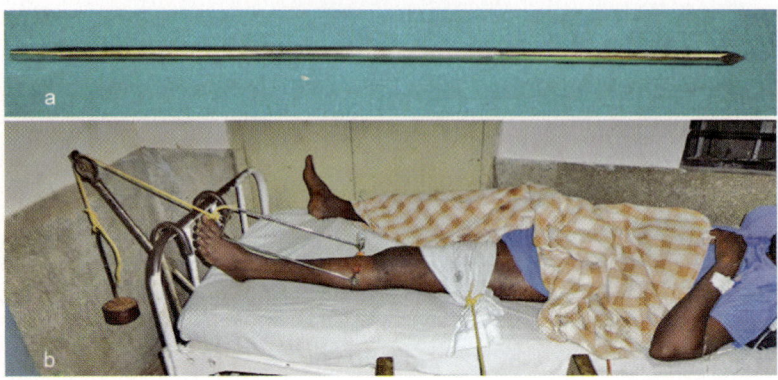

Points to identify
1. Thick pin with pointed tip on one end whereas other end is blunt (c.f. K wire whose both ends are pointed)
2. Smooth shaft with round cross-section

Indications
1. Skeletal traction
2. Used in external fixation

Points to remember
1. One can get confused between K wire and Steinmann pin. Steinmann pin is thick, pointed at one end and the other end is blunt, whereas K wire is pointed at both ends and is thin.
2. Most common complication of skeletal traction is pin tract infection and sometimes neurovascular injury while applying the pin.

Sites for lower limb skeletal traction
1. Calcaneum
2. Lower end tibia
3. Upper end tibia
4. Lower end femur
5. Greater trochanter

Sites for upper limb skeletal traction
1. Through 2/3rd metacarpal
2. Through distal end radius
3. Through olecranon

After inserting the Steinmann pin in a bone for skeletal traction, the other end of the Steinmann pin is covered by an empty vial which could be an antibiotic vial. When asked from students on why there is an antibiotic vial covering the end, the most frequent answer is that antibiotic diffuses into the pin via capillary action and prevents pin tract infection!!!

In fact, the antibiotic vial has nothing to do with prevention of infection. It is merely used to cap the pointed end of the pin to prevent injury to the other limb. Anything can be applied over the pointed end to cap including xylocaine vial/mere plastic cap!! Then one must NOT answer that xylocaine will diffuse through pin to reduce pain!! Steinmann pin does not have nano-pores for capillary action!!

SCREWS

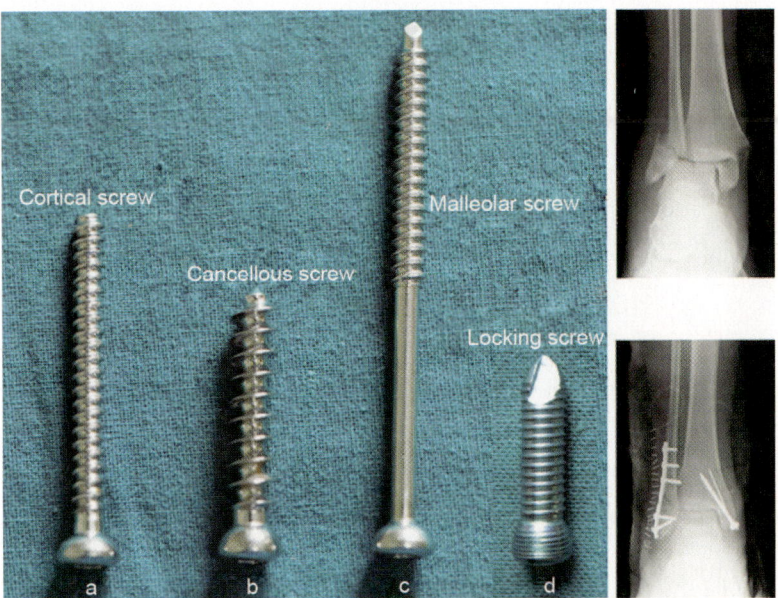

Left image shows four type of screws. Top right image shows bimalleolar fracture. Lower right image shows medial malleolus fixation by a cancellous screw and K-wire

Points to identify
1. Screws with thread on the shaft
2. Head with slot for screw driver
3. Locking screw is identified with threads on head

Type of screws
1. Cortical screw (A) (used in cortical bone)
2. Cancellous screw (B) (used in cancellous bone)
3. Malleolar screw (C) (used in fixation of medial malleolus)
4. Locking screw (D) (used in locking hole of locking compression plate)

Indications
1. Internal fixation of **small fragment** like malleolus, patella, tuberosity of humerus.
2. Internal fixation of fracture of **small bones** like carpals, metacarpals, phalanx, tarsals or metatarsals.

EXTERNAL FIXATOR SET: SCHANZ PIN, TUBULAR ROD AND CLAMPS

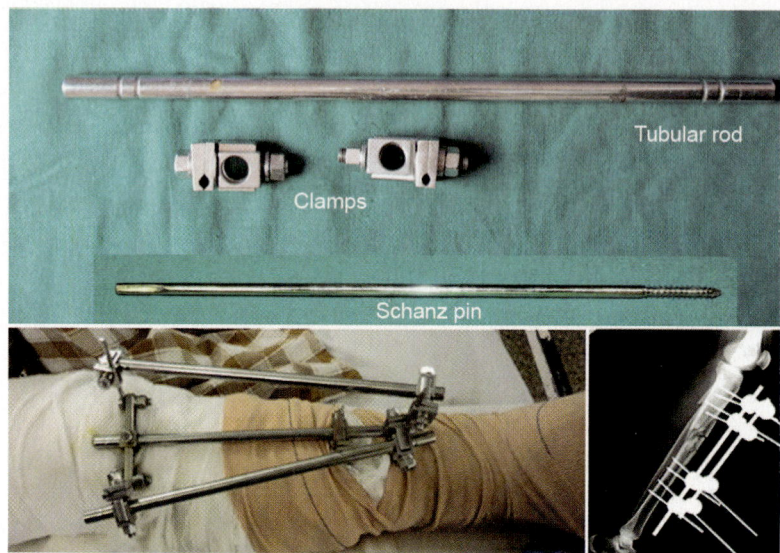

Top image shows parts of an external fixator. Lower left image shows external fixator on right tibia and lower right image shows X-ray of the tibia with external fixator *in situ*

Points to identify
Schanz pin
1. Pin with pointed tip on one end which is threaded
2. Mid-shaft of pin is smooth
3. Other end is blunt

Tubular rod and clamps
Clamps and rods are used to connect pins to each other and give a stable frame.

Indication
Used in external fixation

External fixator use
Open fracture.

IV

Orthopedic Instruments

Instruments

BONE LEVERS (HOHMANN, TRETHOWAN AND LANE)

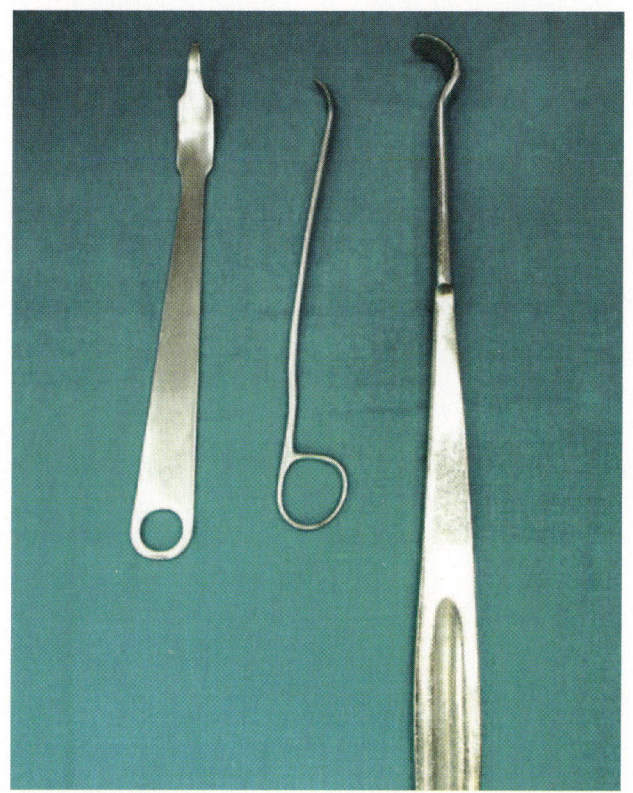

Use: To retract muscle and soft tissue from the bone

PERIOSTEUM ELEVATOR

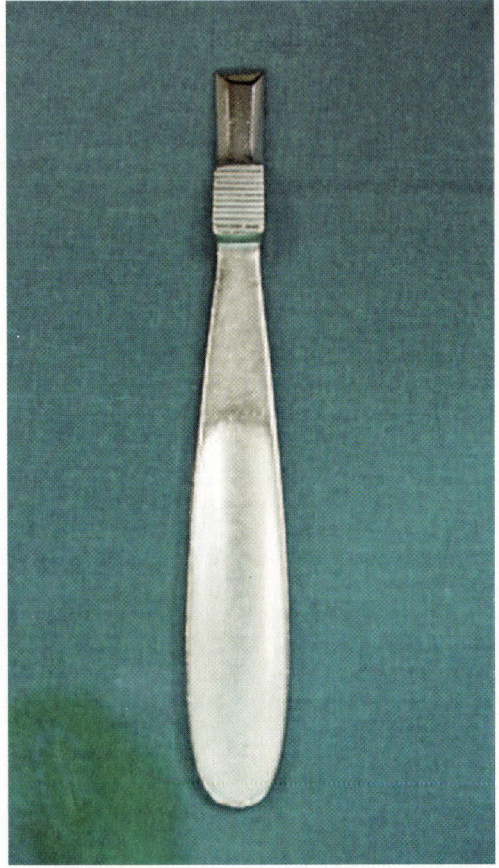

Use: To elevate periosteum from bone to expose the bone for procedures such as fracture fixation, tumor excision or infection.

CHISEL

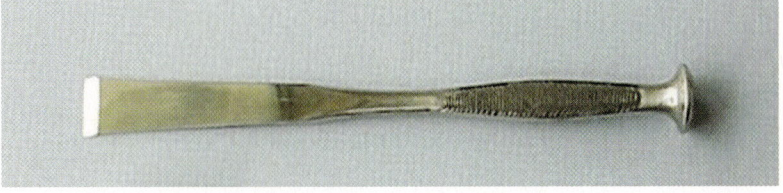

Use: It has a sharp and a bevelled edge. Used to cut/taper the bone

OSTEOTOME

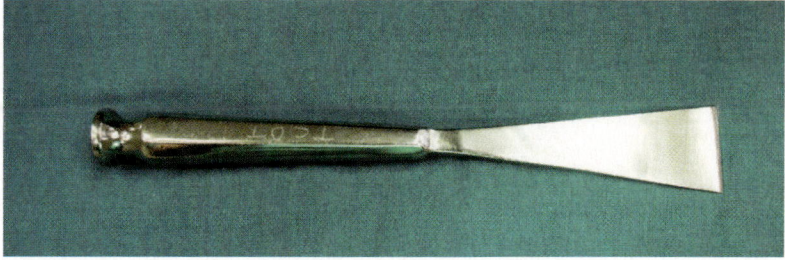

Use: Both edges are bevelled, and is used to cut a bone.

MALLET

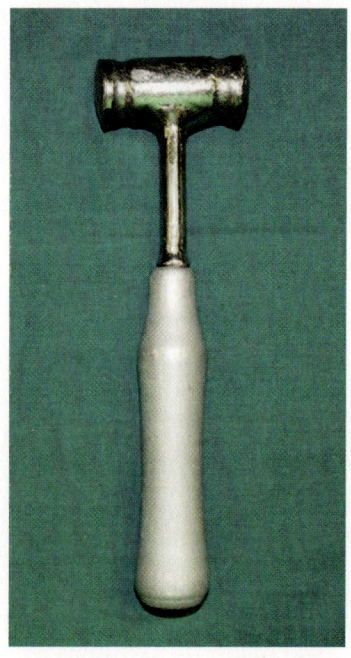

Use: To hit upon the chisel, osteotome, bone gouge, etc.

BONE NIBBLER

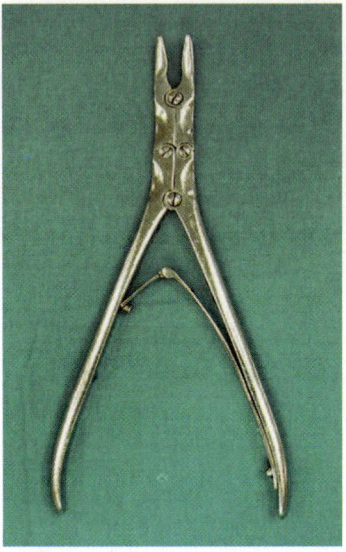

Use: To nibble the infected/dead tissue or bone

CURETTE

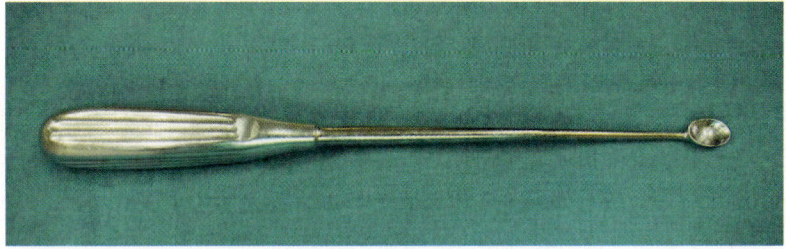

Use: To remove or curette infected granulation tissue/hematoma

BONE GOUGE

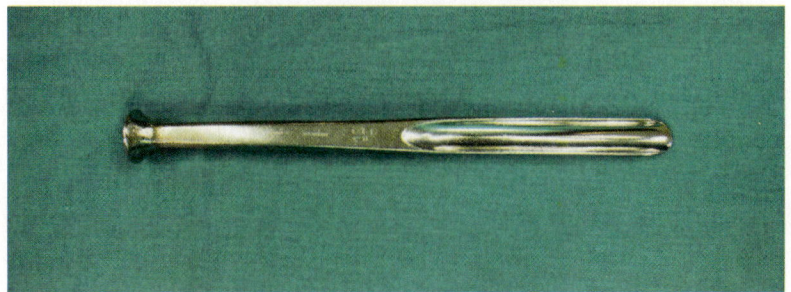

Use: To extract the bone graft from iliac crest

Prosthesis and Orthosis

Prosthesis

PATELLAR TENDON BEARING PROSTHESIS

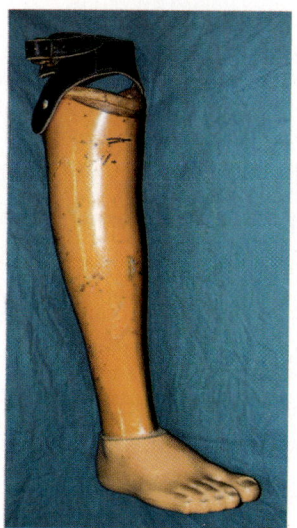

Indication
Patients with below knee amputation

Parts
- Suspension
- Socket
- Shank/shin piece
- Ankle-foot assembly

ABOVE KNEE PROSTHESIS

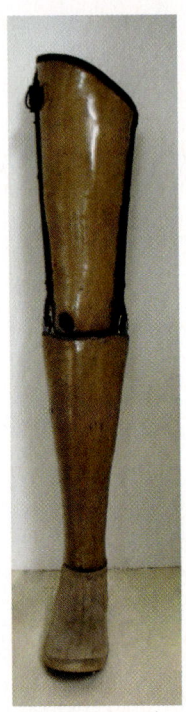

Indication

Above knee amputation

Parts

- Suspension
- Socket
- Knee joint
- Shank/shin piece
- Ankle-foot assembly

SOLID ANKLE CUSHION HEEL (SACH) FOOT

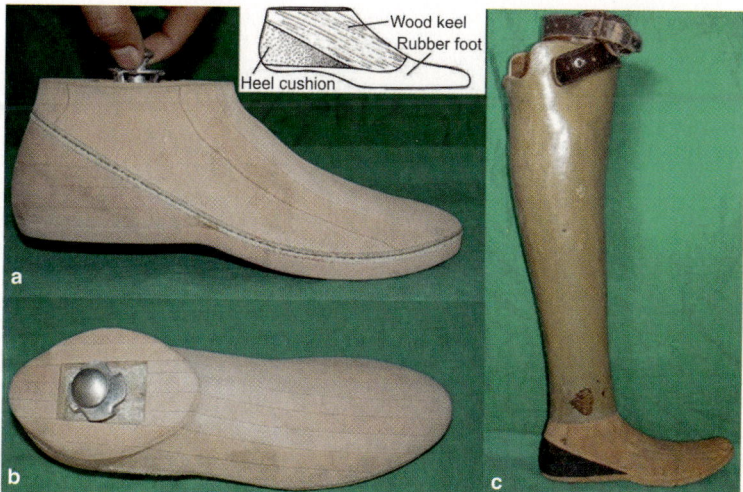

Figure (a) SACH foot with neel held by finger (cross-section in inset); (b) SACH foot from above; (c) SACH foot fitted over a below knee PTB prosthesis

It is a non-articulated foot wherein there is no separation between foot and ankle.

It is quite frequently used in our country. It provides slight inversion–eversion and plantar–dorsiflexion by heel compression.

- Structure
  - Ankle joint is solid with wooden keel,
  - Heel has alternating layers of hard and soft rubber (MCR) which helps in simulating movement at heel (plantar and dorsiflexion)
- Walking
  - Suitable only for walking on a even ground.

Indication

Used as a part of lower limb prosthesis.

Parts

- Central wooden keel
- Alternate layers of hard and soft rubber
- Rubber body

Advantages

Available in various sizes and fitted in most shoes.

Disadvantages

- Does not look like normal foot, needs footwear
- Not waterproof
- Squatting and sitting cross leg not possible
- Costlier than Jaipur foot

JAIPUR FOOT

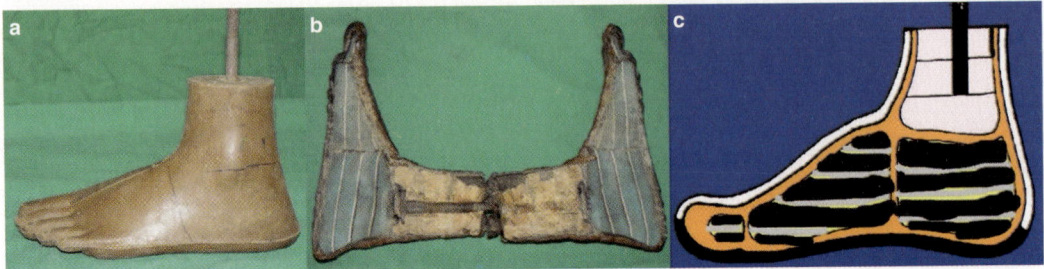

Figure (a) Jaipur foot; **(b)** Cut section of Jaipur foot showing MCR blocks; **(c)** Diagrammatic representation of the same

- Developed by PK Sethi (Jaipur)
- Structure
  - Solid wooden block at ankle
  - 3 MCR blocks (forefoot, hindfoot and toes)
  - MCR blocks enclosed in vulcanised rubber (outer covering)

Indication
Used as a part of lower limb prosthesis

Parts
- Rubber core
- Wooden block
- Vulcanised rubber coating

Advantages
- Economical, cosmetically acceptable
- It can be used with or without footwear (barefoot walking is possible)
- Squatting is possible as it allows enough dorsiflexion
- Easy to walk on uneven ground and sit cross leg due to possible inversion–eversion and forefoot movement.

Disadvantages
- Height is about 7 inch
- Cannot fit into Syme's prosthesis

MADRAS FOOT

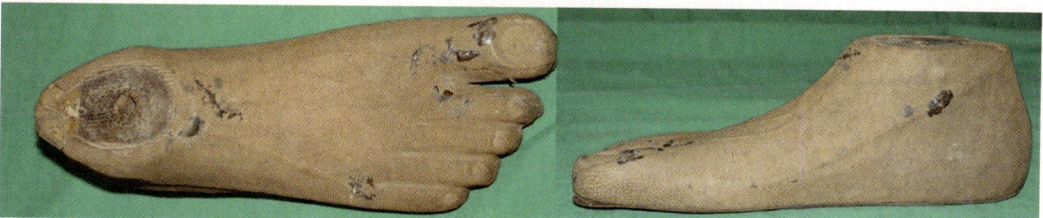

- Modified SACH foot
- Made of wooden kneel, hard and soft rubber, canvas rubber and swade leather
- Bare foot walking is possible

ABOVE ELBOW PROSTHESIS

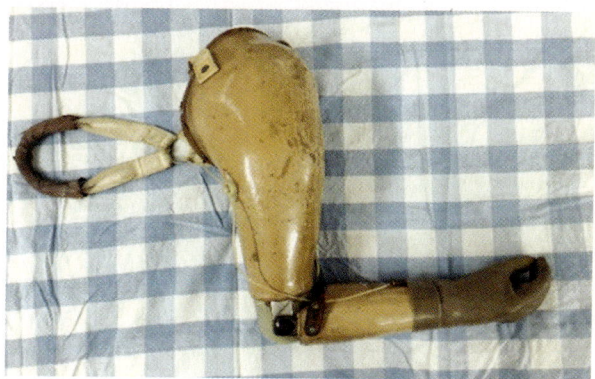

Indication: Above elbow amputee.

Orthosis

CLAVICLE BRACE

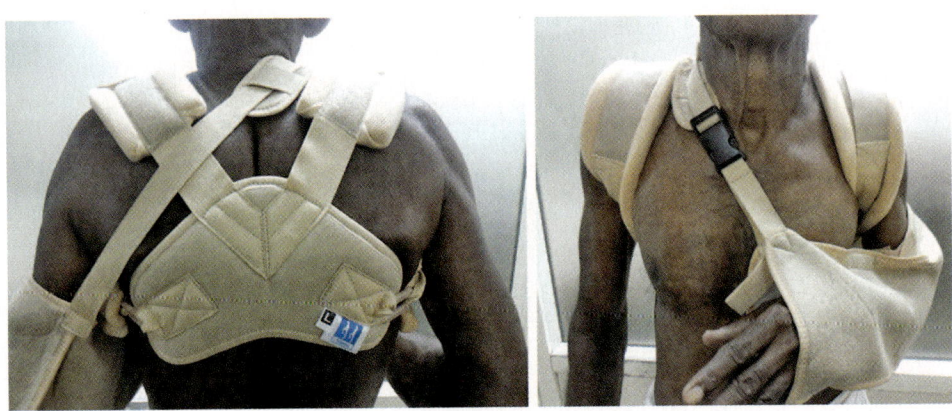

Indication

Mid-shaft fracture clavicle.

Description

1. Brace is applied for conservative treatment of mid-shaft fracture clavicle.
2. It is always **applied along with arm sling.**
3. Brace is given for 6–8 weeks.

ARM SLING

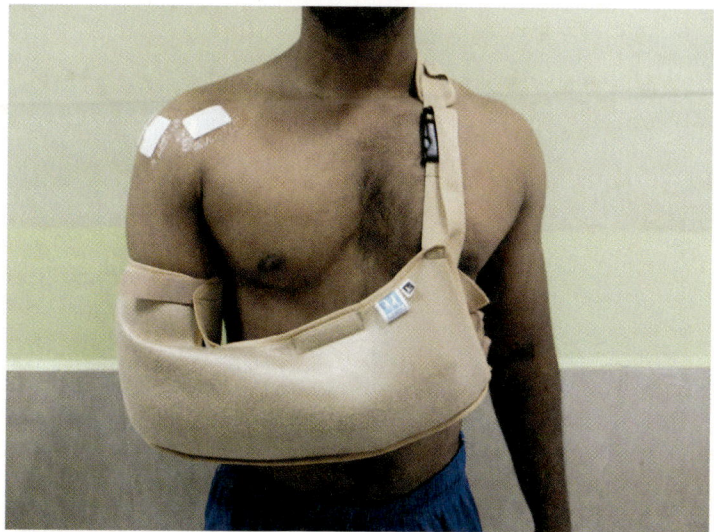

Use. To give rest to upper limb.

Indication

Soft tissue and bony injuries of upper limb.

SOFT CERVICAL COLLAR

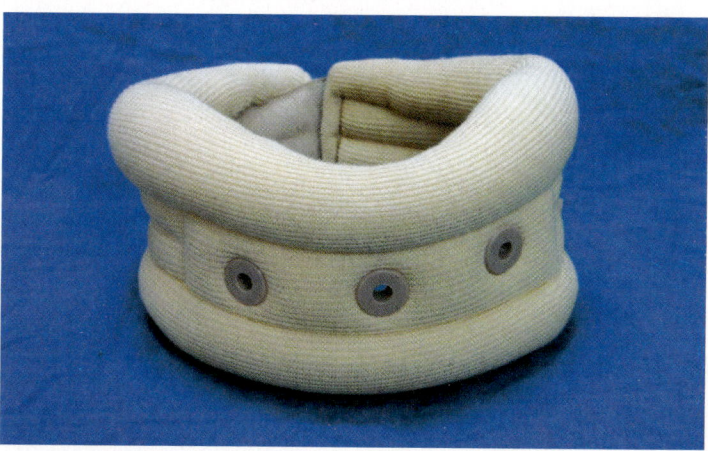

Indications

1. Cervical spondylitis
2. Cervical intervertebral disc prolapse
3. Neck sprain

Contraindication. It is **never prescribed** for **cervical fractures and/or dislocation** as it cannot provide adequate immobilization.

HARD CERVICAL COLLAR

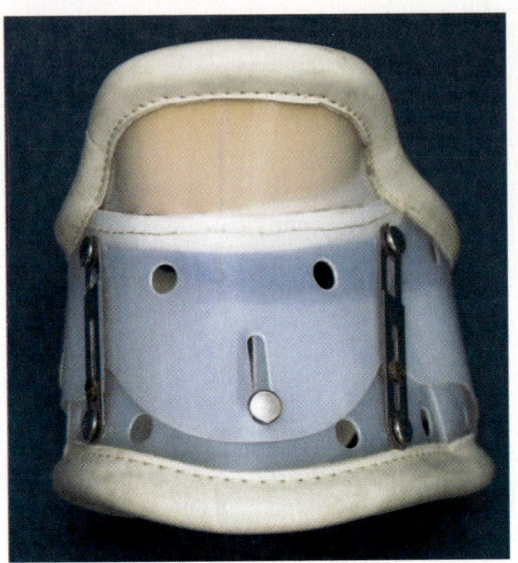

Indication
Fracture of cervical spine

Description
1. Hard cervical collar is given in fractures and/dislocation of cervical spine.
2. Unlike soft cervical collar, it provides **"relatively rigid immobilization"** to cervical spine which is desired in cases of fracture to avoid or exacerbate any spinal cord injury.

Soft cervical collar should not be given in cervical spine injury as it cannot prevent side-side/rotation/flexion-extension movement at neck. It will jeopardize the spine stability and can lead to/exacerbate spinal cord injury in case of cervical spine #

PHILADELPHIA COLLAR

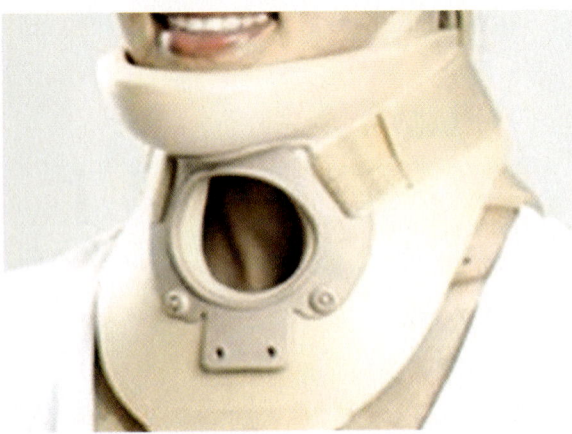

- Semirigid cervical orthosis made of Plastazote foam
- Anterior opening for tracheostomy
- Upper part supports mandible and occiput, lower part extending till sternal notch anteriorly and T3 posteriorly
- Limits 50 to 60% of cervical motion(both flexion and rotations)
- *Indication:* Cervical spine injuries

KNEE ANKLE FOOT ORTHOSIS (KAFO)

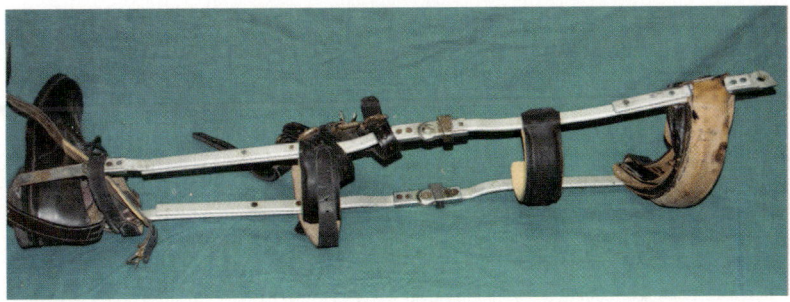

Parts
- Shoe attachment, stirrup, ankle joint
- Metal upright, calf bands
- Knee joint
- Thigh bands

Indication
Applied in patients with poliomyelitis, muscular dystrophy or spinal cord injury who have paralytic weakness at knee and ankle foot.

DDH SPLINT

Use: It is a flexion abduction orthosis used for DDH of hip before 6 months of age (before child starts crawling). It maintains femoral head in acetabulum.

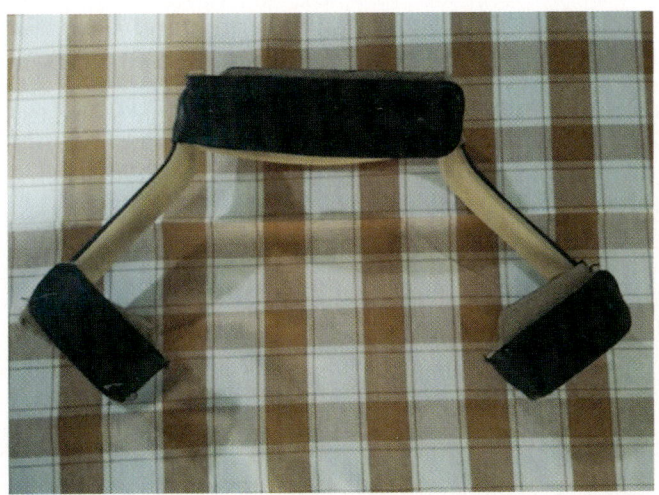

AXILLARY CRUTCH

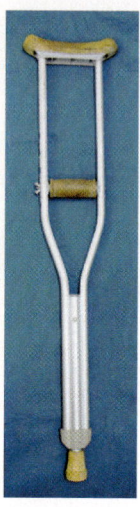

Indication

Lower limb injuries (fractures of pelvis, femur, tibia, knee, ankle foot, etc.) where patient has been advised partial or non-weight bearing walking.

Parts

- Axillary pad
- Handpiece
- Two uprights
- Adjustable rod
- Rubber ferrule

Length measurement of the crutch

Patient standing: 5 cm below the anterior axillary fold to 6" front and 6" laterally to 5th toe.

Patient supine: Anterior axillary fold to bottom edge of the heel of the shoe.

Once, axillary crutch are applied, shoulders are depressed and palm rests on the hand grip of the crutch with elbows in 30° flexion.

Note: Axillary crutch is **never held in axilla**. It is held against chest wall, **2" below the anterior axillary fold**. If it goes high up in axilla, it can lead to pressure upon posterior cord leading to radial nerve palsy k/a "**crutch palsy**".

DROP SPLINT DYNAMIC (COCK-UP SPLINT)

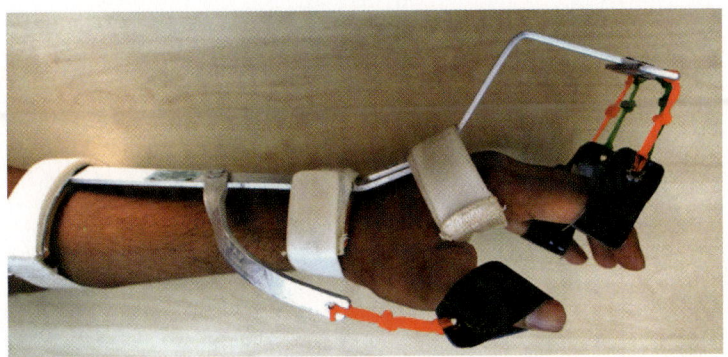

Indications

1. Wrist drop due to radial nerve palsy.
2. Finger drop due to posterior interosseous nerve palsy.

Description

1. This is a **dynamic wrist drop splint.** In resting position, it keeps wrist and fingers in **functional position also k/a "glass holding position"**, wherein wrist remains in 15–20° dorsiflexion; metacarpophalangeal (MCP) and interphalangeal (IP) joints in flexion. **The forearm, wrist and hand is supported by** velcro **straps, whereas fingers are supported by elastic straps** suspended from aluminium bar by rubber band.

2. In patients with radial nerve palsy, wrist and fingers are "dropped position" as patients cannot dorsiflex his wrist and fingers. With dynamic cock-up splint, wrist and hand is held in functional position at rest. However, patient can flex his MCP and IP joints and then it goes back to glass-holding position due to elastic bands. This leads to active mobilization of uninvolved hand muscles.

3. This splint is better than static cock up splint as active mobilization of MCP and IP joints can be continued avoiding stiffness.

Note: Static wrist drop splint is meant to keep wrist and hand in functional position but does not allow any active mobilization of MCP and IP joints. Static splint need to be removed to flex MCP and IP joints.

KNUCKLE BENDER SPLINT

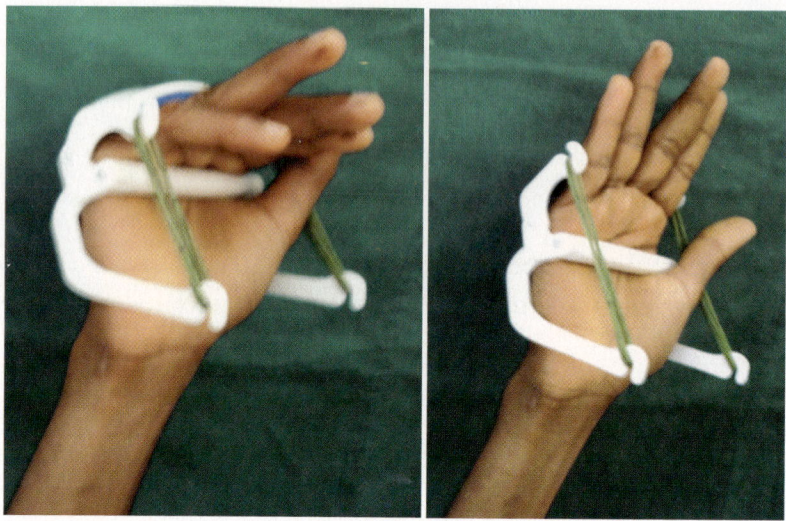

Indication

Applied in isolated ulnar nerve injury or combined median and ulnar nerve injuries with clawhand to prevent contracture.

Description

Knuckle bender splint keeps the MCP joint in flexed position and IP joints in extension (intrinsic plus position).

Functional position of wrist and hand is **"glass-holding position"**.

Splint for Isolated Median Nerve Injury

- After median nerve injury, the thumb stays in adduction due to abductor pollicis brevis palsy. This would result in adduction contracture.
- Thumb abduction splint is kept between thumb and index finger to maintain thumb in abducted position.

FOOTDROP SPLINT/ANKLE FOOT ORTHOSIS (AFO)

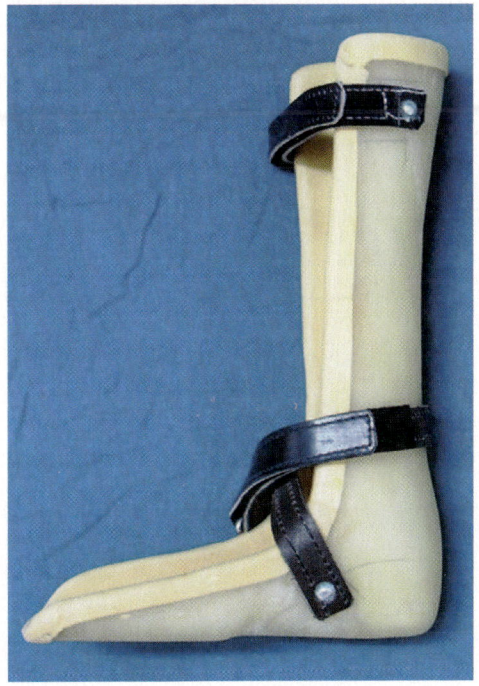

Indication
- Applied in footdrop due to common peroneal nerve injury/sciatic nerve injury/ extensor tendon injury.
- Maintains ankle stability in neuropathic foot, post polio residual deformity.

Description
1. After the footdrop, the ankle stays in gravity assisted plantarflexed position which could result in equinus deformity. Ankle foot orthosis (AFO) is meant to keep ankle and foot in functional position (neutral) after the footdrop to prevent equinus contracture.
2. It is a static splint needs to be removed to perform actively plantar flexion and passively dorsiflexion to maintain flexibility of the foot and ankle.

Functional position of ankle and foot is neutral position where ankle is at neutral of dorsiflexion or plantar flexion.

DENIS BROWNE (DB) SPLINT

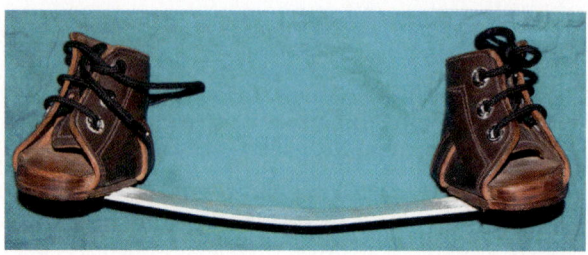

It is named after Australian surgeon Dr John Dennis Wolko Browne (1934).

Indication

Congenital talipes equinus varus (CTEV) foot to maintain corrected position (achieved by manipulation or surgically) of foot.

Parts

- *Curved bar:* Equal to width of shoulder and it maintains dorsiflexion at ankle.
- Pair of CTEV shoes.
- Winged nuts to allow abduction of each foot.

Description

1. It is applied **after CTEV correction** is achieved either by sequential manipulations and cast application or surgery, **to maintain the correction** for full time in **children <1 year**. Children >1 year of age are given DB splint in night and CTEV shoes in the daytime.
2. It is a **dynamic splint** and not a static splint. When the child kicks one side of foot, other foot goes in eversion, abduction and dorsiflexion due to the interconnecting bar between two sides of shoe.

CTEV SHOE

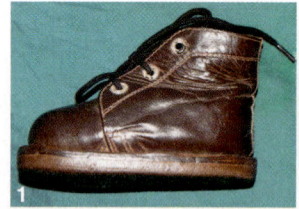 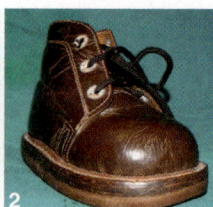 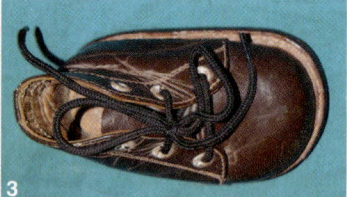

Indications

Congenital talipes equinus varus to maintain corrected position of foot in children >1 year of age while walking.

Description

1. It is applied **after CTEV correction** is achieved either by sequential manipulations and cast application or surgery **to maintain the correction in children >1 year**. It is given during the daytime.
2. CTEV shoe has three characteristics
    a. **No heel**: To prevent equinus recurrence (Fig. 1)
    b. **Lateral border shoe raise**: To prevent inversion recurrence (Fig. 2)
    c. **Straight and stiff medial border**: To prevent forefoot adduction (Fig. 3)
3. Shoe is worn till 7–8 years of age while walking.

THOMAS KNEE SPLINT

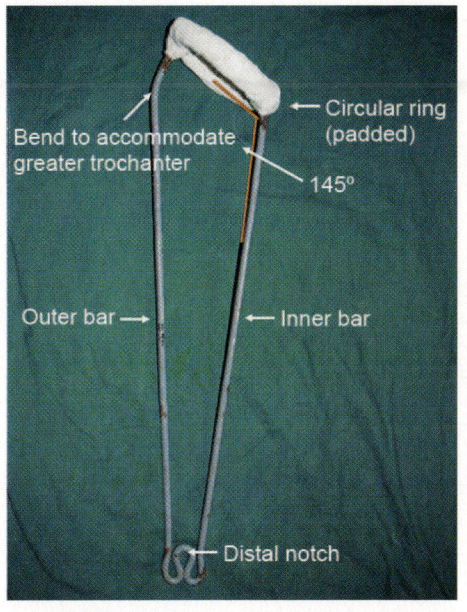

Bend to accommodate greater trochanter
Circular ring (padded)
145°
Outer bar
Inner bar
Distal notch

Thomas knee splint was designed by Hugh Owen Thomas (1876) **to provide rest to tuberculosis of the knee**. Later, it was extensively used in 1st world war to immobilise fracture femur and thereby considerably reducing the morbidity and mortality due to fracture femur from 80% in 1916 to 8% in 1918.

Parts
1. Padded circular ring on the top: To rest below ASIS, over the ischial tuberosity and around the groin.
2. Two bars; outer and inner. Inner bar is straight, whereas outer bar makes angulation to accommodate the greater trochanter. The angle between ring and inner bar is 145°.
3. The two bars join as W shape joint where traction cord from limb can be tied.

Measurement of the TK Splint
1. **Ring size measurement:** Measure the diameter of the unaffected thigh and add 2" to the measurement. This 2" is to accommodate the swelling of the affected side.
2. **Length of the Thomas knee splint:** It is calculated by measuring the distance from crotch to the tip of the heel and add 6–9" to the length. This distance equals the length of the inner bar.
3. The Thomas knee splint can be used for both sides. It means that it does not has any side.

Indications
1. Fracture shaft femur
2. Fracture intertrochanteric femur
3. Fracture subtrochanteric femur

Complications
1. Ring sore around groin, under ASIS and over ischial tuberosity
2. Footdrop if the outer bar is too close to the head of fibula and, if it is NOT well padded.

BOHLER BRAUN FRAME/SPLINT

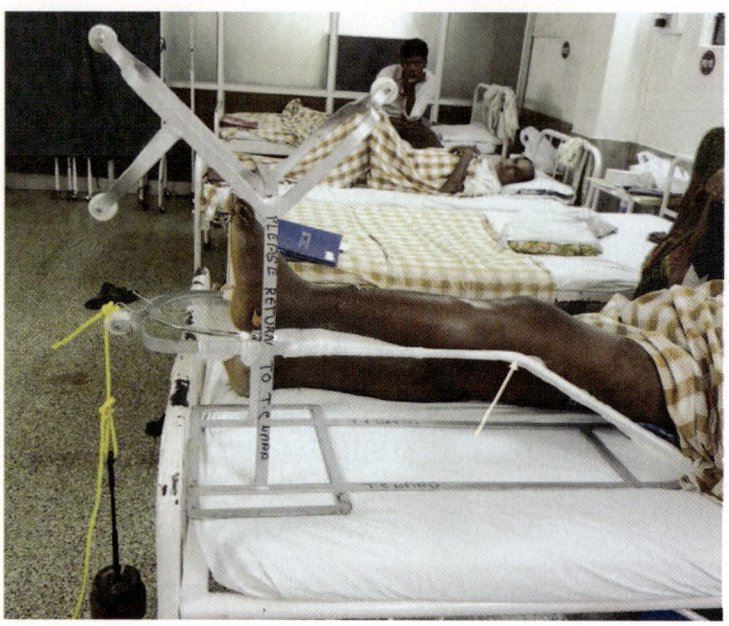

Indications

Bohler Braun frame is recommended for fractures of **lower end of femur and upper end of tibia** to be managed with skeletal traction. Various pulleys are for traction.

- The distal most pulley for: Calcaneal fracture/distal tibia fracture
- *2nd pulley:* Supracondylar fracture (distal tibia traction)/distal femur traction for femoral shaft.

Disadvantages of Bohler frame:

1. Bohler frame rests on patient's bed, and cannot move with patient. Hence, it hampers ease of transportation or patient's nursing care (unlike Thomas knee splint).
2. As the frame has no control over the proximal fragment of the fracture, the latter can move along with patient's movement causing displacement of fracture which could result in deformity, non-union of the fracture.

#Note: The bend (yellow arrow) in the BB splint is meant to keep the knee flexed which relaxes hamstring and gastrocnemius muscle. In case of supracondylar # femur and # upper end of tibia, the distal and proximal fragments tend to angulate posteriorly due to pull from hamstring and gastrocnemius respectively. This posterior angulation of fragment can endanger the integrity of the posterior neurovascular bundle crossing the popliteal fossa.

Therefore, bend in the Bohler Braun frame keeps the knee bent and this relaxes the above said muscles. Avoiding overangulation of fragments preventing neurovascular injury.

Various pulleys over Bohler frame is used to pass traction cord over it according to various fracture site.

VI

Ward Round

21

Common Plasters, Traction (skin, skeletal) and External Fixator

PLASTER OF PARIS (POP)

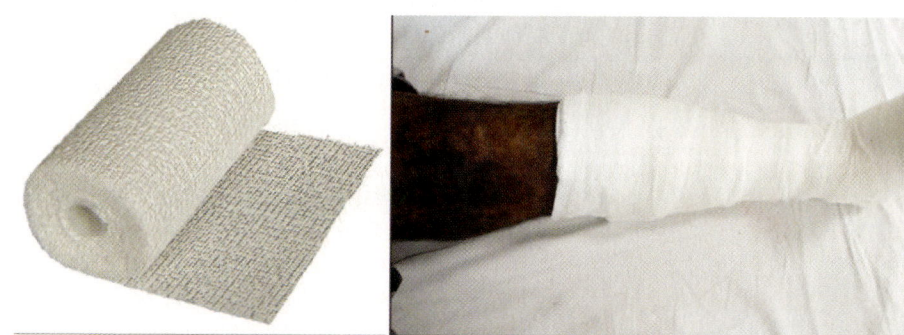

POP is made from gypsum, a naturally occurring material. The name POP is said to stem from an accident involving a house in Paris which was built over deposit of gypsum. Accidentally, the house got burnt down. A lot of people walked over the charred remains of house and floor having gypsum powder. When rain felled over the floor, footprint in the floor mud set rock-hard. This lead to discovery of gypsum hardening properties. POP is prepared by heating gypsum ($CaSO_4 \cdot 2H_2O$).

$$CaSO_4 \cdot 2H_2O + heat \rightarrow CaSO_4 \cdot 1/2H_2O + 3/2H_2O \text{ (released as steam)}$$

Chemically, **POP is calcium sulphate hemihydrate ($CaSO_4 \cdot \frac{1}{2} H_2O$).**

When water is added to it, the original material (gypsum: $CaSO_4 \cdot 2H_2O$) is re-formed and heat is released. Since, first introduction by Mathijesen in 1852, it has been used as orthopaedic cast.

Orthopedic use of cast

1. To support reduced fracture and dislocation
2. To stabilize and rest joints in case of soft tissue injury (ankle sprain, ligament injury, etc.)
3. To correct a deformity (CTEV)
4. For postoperative immobilization to rest tissues

Advantages of POP	Disadvantages of POP
• Cheap • Easily available • Accurate casting possible • Easy to cut in case of tight POP	• Heavy • Can be broken easily • Loosen and disintegrate if come in contact with water

Instructions after cast application

1. Limb elevation
2. Active mobilization of finger/toes and other free joints
3. Watch for any bluish discoloration of finger/toes
4. Excessive tightness to be reported immediately

Complications of cast application

1. *Compartment syndrome:* A disastrous complication especially if tight cast is applied. If compartment syndrome is suspected, cast should be immediately released till the skin and should be removed.
2. Nerve compression at tight points
3. Skin ulceration
4. Thermal injury: Due to the heat release at the time of casting.

SYNTHETIC CAST

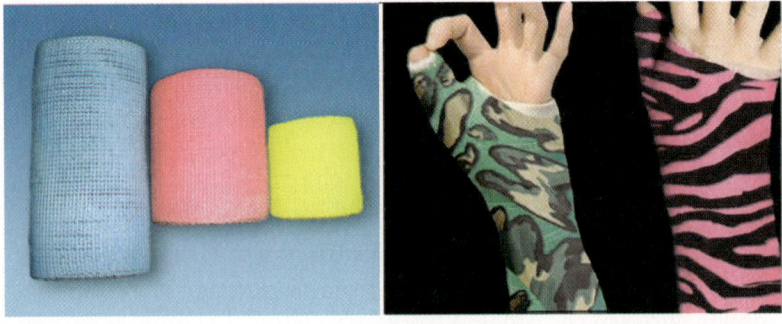

It is made up of fibreglass impregnated with polyurethane polymer which undergoes polymerization after addition of water/chemical solvent, and become very rigid.

Advantages of synthetic cast	Disadvantages of synthetic cast
• Light weight (63% lighter than conventional POP) • Very hard, so more durable • Water resistant/repellant • Minimal heat release while application	• Costly • Difficult to accurately cast • Very hard to cut

ABOVE ELBOW CAST

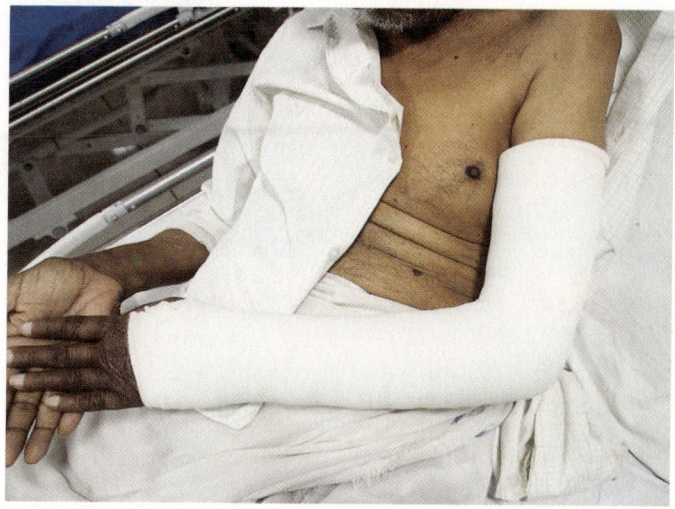

Proximal and distal extent of AE cast/slab

Proximal: Upper 1/3rd of arm

Distal: Just proximal to metacarpophalangeal joint or just proximal to proximal palmar crease.

Indications: After closed reduction in:
1. Both bone forearm fracture
2. Colles' fracture
3. Elbow dislocation

BELOW ELBOW CAST

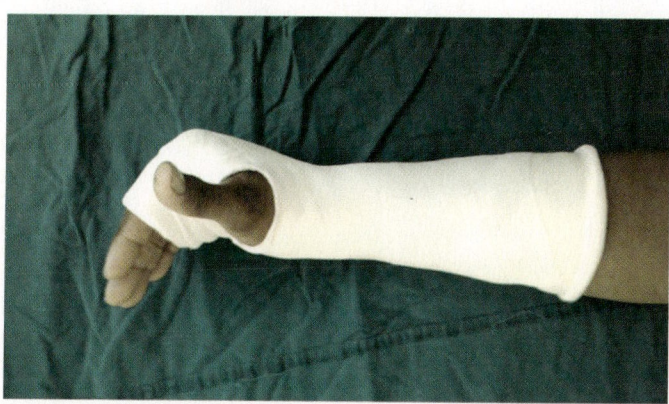

Proximal and distal extent of BE cast/slab

Proximal: Upper 1/3rd of forearm

Distal: Just proximal to metacarpophalangeal joint

Indication: Closed reduction in Colles' fracture.

ABOVE KNEE CAST

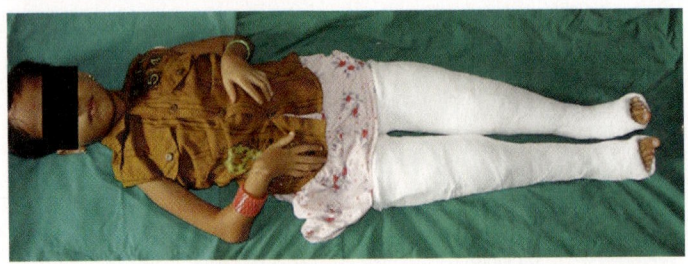

Proximal and distal extent of the AK cast/slab

Proximal: Upper 1/3rd thigh

Distal: Just proximal to metatarsophalangeal (MTP) joint. IN some cases, the POP is extended till the tip of all toes on plantar aspect but dorsum is spared till MTP joint.

Indications

After closed reduction in:

1. Both bone leg fracture
2. Undisplaced patella fracture

Note: In patella fracture, the distal extent of the AK cast can be just kept above the two malleolus which is also known as **above knee cylindrical cast**.

BELOW KNEE CAST

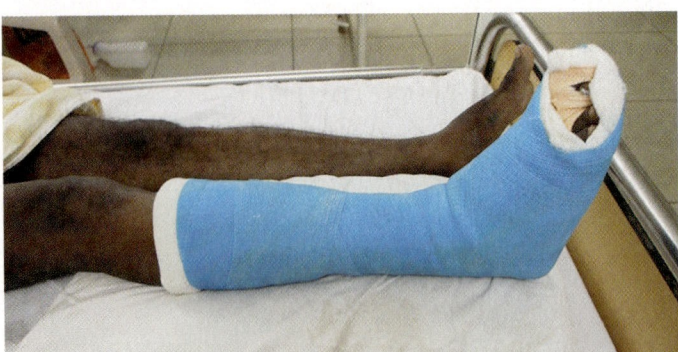

Proximal and distal extent of the BK cast/slab

Proximal: Upper 1/3rd of the leg, four fingers below the tip of the fibula.

Distal: Just proximal to metatarsophalangeal joint of dorsal aspect whereas the POP can extend up to the tip of toes on plantar aspect.

Indications: After closed reduction in:

1. Ankle dislocation
2. Undisplaced malleolar fracture
3. Ankle sprain
4. Soft tissue injuries of foot and ankle

ONE AND HALF HIP SPICA

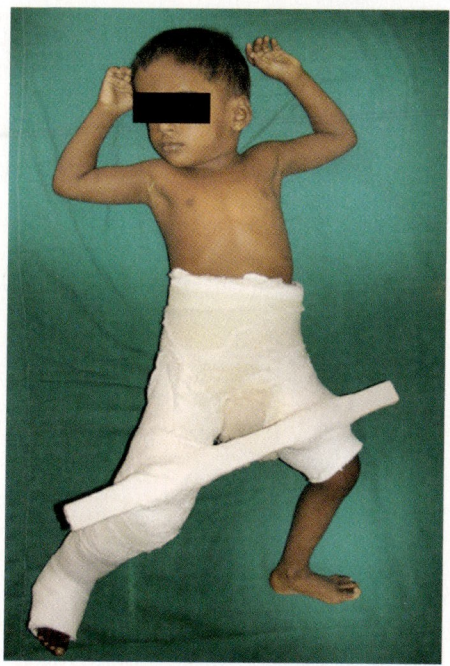

Proximal and distal extent of plaster

Proximal: Up to navel/rarely up to axilla on affected side.

Distal: Up to the metatarsophalangeal joint on affected side, and just above the knee on unaffected side.

The two thighs could be connected with a wooden bar to reinforce the strength of the plaster.

Indications

After closed reduction in:
1. Pediatric femur shaft fracture
2. Pediatric undisplaced fracture neck femur

ABOVE KNEE SKIN TRACTION

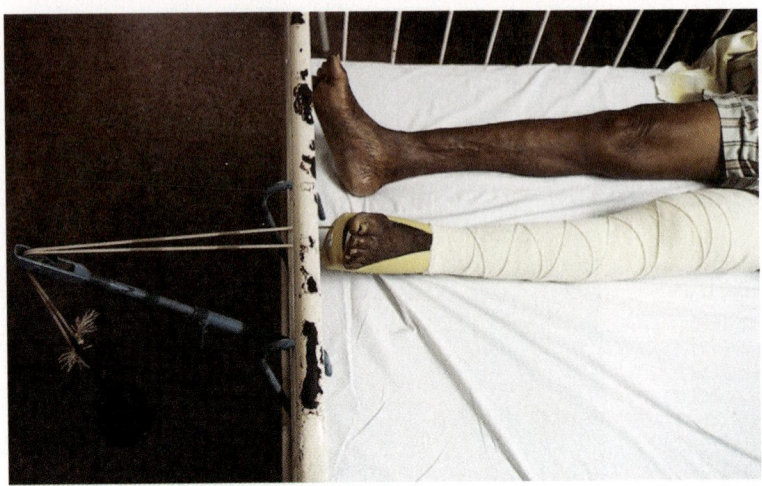

- The above knee skin traction is applied from mid thigh up to the ankle using a commercial above knee traction kit/custom made materials.
- Maximum skin traction which can be applied is 6.7 kg (approx. 8–10% of body weight).

Indication
- To relieve pain and spasm due to hip pain arising out of synovitis, arthritis of hip or fracture neck femur/intertrochanteric femur.
- To prevent or correct hip deformity (tuberculosis).

Advantages of skin traction	Disadvantages of skin traction
• Easy to apply	• Cannot apply more weight, hence heavy traction cannot be applied
• Cheap	• Skin reaction, blister formation
• Can be applied by paramedics too	• Cannot apply for long
• Non-invasive procedure	• Slippage of traction can lead to loss of reduction in case of fractures
• No chance of bone/joint infection	• Tight traction can lead to neurological injury, if close to nerve (below knee skin traction can compress common peroneal nerve over fibular neck)

CERVICAL TRACTION (GLISSON'S TRACTION)

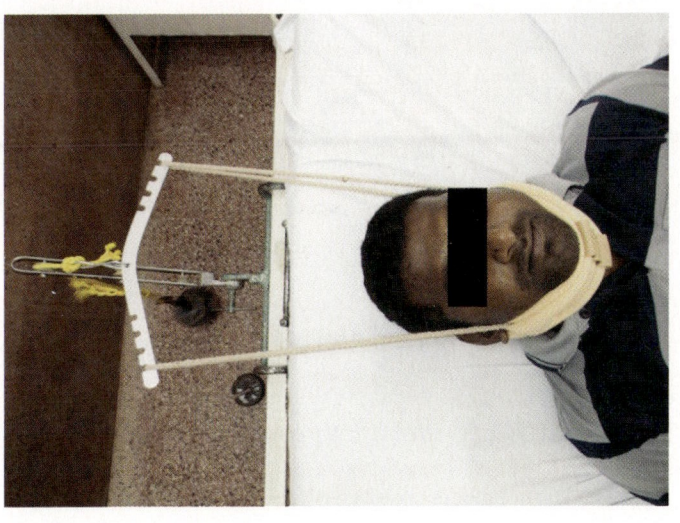

It is a **'skin traction'** applied around the neck.
Indication: Cervical spondylitis, cervical intervertebral disc prolapse.

LUMBAR TRACTION

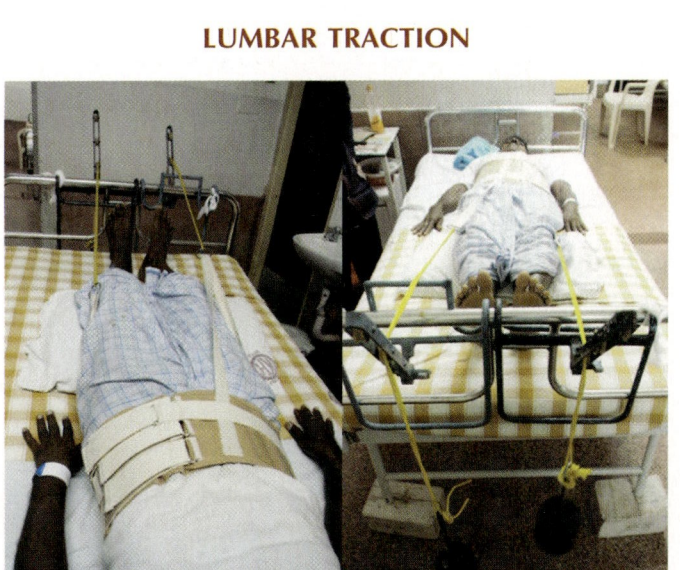

It is a **'skin traction'** applied around the waist.
Indication: Lumbar spondylitis, lumbar intervertebral disc prolapse.

UPPER TIBIAL SKELETAL TRACTION

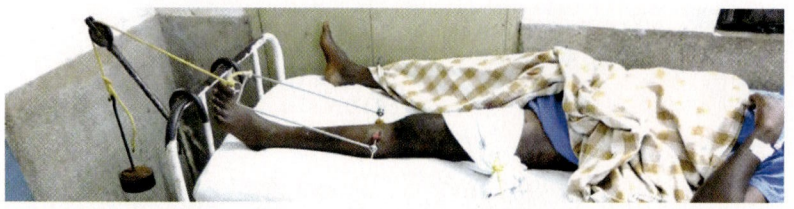

Indications: Femur fractures, reduced hip dislocation for maintenance of reduction.

Implant used for upper tibial traction
Steinmann pin, Denham pin (if bone is too osteoporotic).

Site for upper tibial traction
- The pin is inserted 2 cm below and 2 cm posterior to the highest point of the tibial tuberosity.
- The pin is inserted from lateral cortex of tibia to medial side.

Risk of upper tibial traction
Injury to common peroneal nerve.

Site of skeletal traction
Lower limb:
1. Proximal femur (in trochanter)
2. Distal femur
3. Proximal tibia
4. Calcaneum

Upper limb
5. 2nd, 3rd metacarpal
6. Olecranon

Advantages of skeletal traction	Disadvantages of skeletal traction
• Can apply more weight (up to 11–18 kg; hence heavy traction can be applied)	• Invasive procedure
• No chance of slippage of traction	• Neurovascular injury while pin insertion, e.g. common peroneal injury while upper tibial traction application.
• Can apply for long duration	• Specialized procedure has to be performed by surgeon only
• Can apply in skin lesion/ wounded skin/open fracture	• Pin tract infection; rarely leading to osteomyelitis
	• Large traction force can distract fracture

CALCANEAL SKELETAL TRACTION

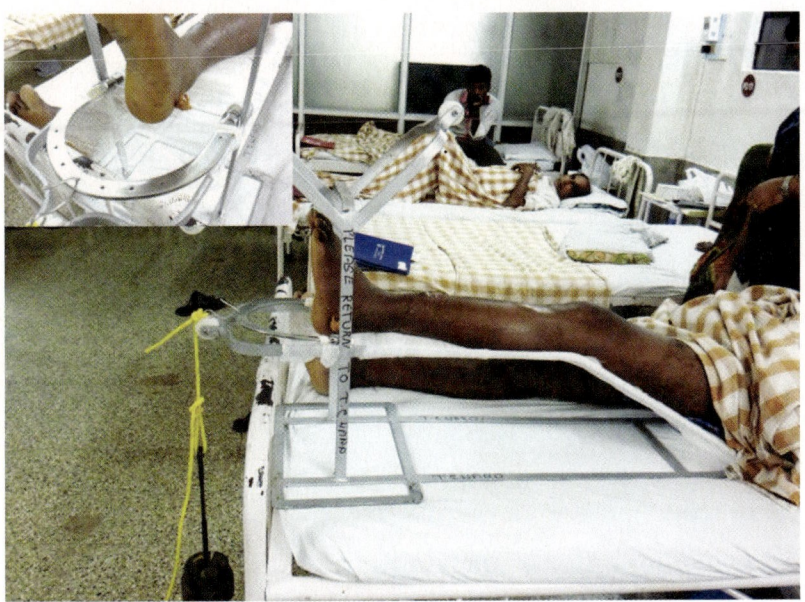

Indications: Tibia fracture

Implant used for calcaneal traction
- Denham pin (like a Steinmann pin but has thread in center to have better purchase in cancellous calcaneum)
- K-wire tensioned traction

Site for calcaneum traction
- The pin is inserted 1 cm below and 1 cm posterior to the medial malleolus
- The pin is inserted from medial side of calcaneum.

Risk of calcaneum traction
Injury to medial neurovascular bundle (tibial nerve, posterior tibial artery).

SKULL TRACTION (GARDENER-WELLS TONGS)

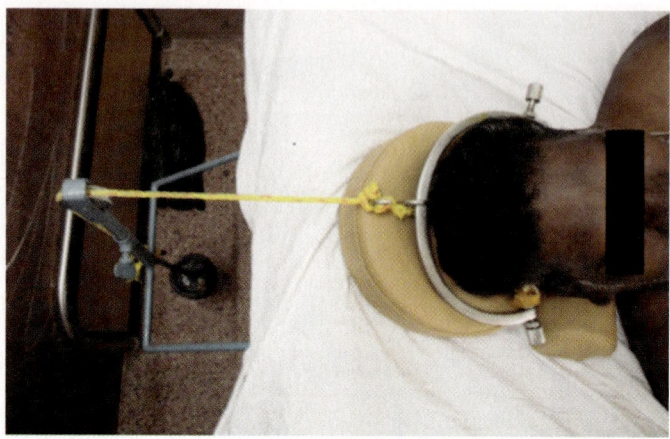

Indication: Cervical spine fracture/reduced dislocation of cervical spine for maintenance of reduction.

Other device to apply skull traction: Crutchfield tongs.

EXTERNAL FIXATOR

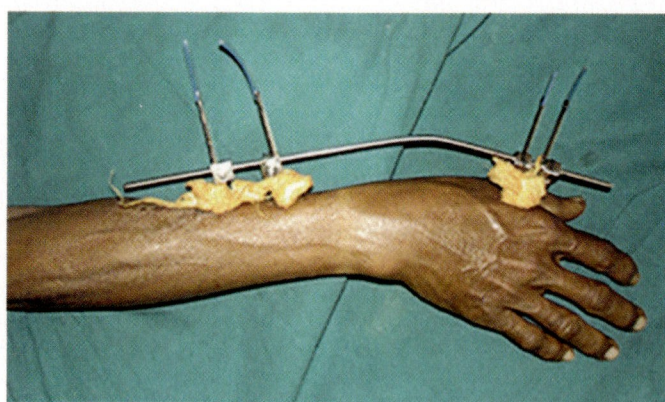

Indication
Maintenance of fracture reduction especially open fractures.

Advantage of external fixator
* The chance of deep bone infection is less as there is no internal implant.
* Daily dressing of the open wound/surgical wound could be done easily.
* Future plastic surgical procedure (skin grafting, flap surgery) can be easily performed while the fracture reduction is retained.

Disadvantage of external fixator
* Chance of pin tract infection/osteomyelitis
* Daily dressing of pin tract is required

Index